Exploring the History of Neuropsychology

EXPLORING THE HISTORY OF NEUROPSYCHOLOGY

Selected Papers

ARTHUR BENTON
Emeritus Professor of Neurology and Psychology
University of Iowa

With an Introduction by
KENNETH M. ADAMS

OXFORD
UNIVERSITY PRESS
2000

OXFORD
UNIVERSITY PRESS

Oxford New York
Athens Auckland Bangkok Bogotá Buenos Aires Calcutta
Cape Town Chennai Dar es Salaam Delhi Florence Hong Kong Istanbul
Karachi Kuala Lumpur Madrid Melbourne Mexico City Mumbai
Nairobi Paris São Paulo Singapore Taipei Tokyo Toronto Warsaw

and associated companies in
Berlin Ibadan

Published by Oxford University Press, Inc.
198 Madison Avenue, New York, New York, 10016
http://www.oup-usa.org
1-800-334-4249

Library of Congress Cataloging-in-Publication Data
Benton, Arthur Lester, 1909–
Exploring the history of neuropsychology : selected papers /
Arthur Benton ; with an introduction by Kenneth M. Adams.
p. cm. Includes bibliographical references and index.
ISBN 0-19-513808-2
1. Neuropsychology—History.
2. Clinical neuropsychology—History.
3. Aphasia—History. I. Title.
QP360 .B487 2000 616.8—dc21 99-088047 Rev.

2 4 6 8 9 7 5 3 1

Printed in the United States of America
on acid-free paper

To
Robert James Joynt

Preface

The impetus that led eventually to the writing of historical and quasihistorical papers, some of which form the collection in this book, arose several decades ago. At the time I was struck by the extreme divergence in the acceptance and usage of concepts and terms such as "agnosia," "amnesic aphasia," "apraxia," and the like by the leading figures in the then very young field of neuropsychology/behavioral neurology. It seemed to me that this state of affairs could not be the product of objective observation. More likely it represented a heritage of the past. I therefore explored the relevant literature of nineteenth-century neurology to trace the evolution of thought and practice with respect to these concepts and terms. The exploration was rewarding. I began to see how current concepts and practice were more often than not the outgrowth of diverse earlier formulations. I also began to appreciate the place that my own research efforts occupied in the continuum from the past to the present (including the realization that some insights on my part, which I thought were original, had been expressed in vaguer form by earlier writers). This outcome whetted my appetite to continue to explore the past, and in due course I became a part-time amateur historian.

There is no unifying theme in this collection of essays. They are explorations of diverse aspects of the field, the choices reflecting my own special interests. They were written at different times and in different contexts. Consequently, there is much repetition in making points and in citing the literature. Some essays are systematic accounts of developments in thinking in a particular area (e.g., the prefrontal region, spatial thinking), some consider the contributions of a single individual (e.g., J. A. P. Gesner, Albert Pitres), and others deal with methodological issues. Many other aspects of the history of clinical neuropsychology/behavioral neurology remain to be explored. I am convinced that the effort would pay rich dividends in the form of increased sophistication and enhanced judgment by clinicians and researchers.

I am too close to these papers to have a fair idea of what significance or value they may hold for neuropsychologists and behavioral neurologists. Hence

I was very pleased that so knowledgeable and astute a judge as Kenneth Adams accepted the invitation of the publisher to write a brief analysis of the collection and discuss its implications. I am grateful to him.

My heartfelt thanks go to Jeffrey House and Fiona Stevens of Oxford University Press for their constant encouragement and help during the course of the project.

It is a great pleasure to dedicate this book to my longtime friend and colleague, Robert Joynt, who is himself a distinguished historian of neurology.

Iowa City, Iowa A. B.
January 2000

Contents

Part III Methodology and Assessment

Part IV Hemispheric Cerebral Dominance

Part V Pediatric Neuropsychology

Introduction

KENNETH M. ADAMS

My great pleasure in being invited to write the introduction to this book will be matched by the lasting enjoyment and insight this book will give to its readers. Students, teachers, and researchers delving into this volume will find it to be very different from almost any other book on neuropsychology they might happen to have, save perhaps an earlier collection of some of Arthur Benton's papers edited by Louis Costa and Otfried Spreen.[1] The introduction of that book is well worth consulting because it provides a description of the evolution of Benton's own career as a scientist and clinical neuropsychologist.

The present volume is a collection of papers by Arthur Benton that have a distinctive historical emphasis. His treatment of certain key issues deepens one's understanding of the evolution of neuropsychology from the perspective of a scholar in the field whose own career has helped to define the modern context of neuropsychology.

I should point out that the ideas, descriptions, and interpretations presented in this volume could be produced only by an effort to examine scientific writings and their historical context that is of a kind not familiar to those who have grown up in the age of the automated literature search. This quest involves first the identification and procurement of literature that is often very difficult to obtain. In some instances it is obscure. Having obtained the source reference, it may often involve a translation from the predominant French, German, and Italian linguistic corpus of neurological literature of the time. Occasionally, it necessitates a translation from an unfamiliar language by colleagues. For Benton, the work also involved a continuous communication with a worldwide network of colleagues and friends developed over the course of 60 years as an academician. Finally, weighing the import of the work required a steady, wise, and sometimes forgiving human perspective.

This volume is organized into five topical sections, but readers should resist the temptation to limit their exploration to their areas of interest or expertise. It

1. Costa, L., & Spreen, O. (1985). *Studies in Neuropsychology: Selected Papers of Arthur Benton.* New York: Oxford University Press.

is in reading Benton's exploration in areas *less* familiar to one that readers may appreciate his engaging, informed, and insightful style even more. The first section of the book, called "Evolution of the Discipline," contains six papers ranging over the years 1982–1994. Chapter 1, written for the Elsevier *Handbook of Neuropsychology*, paints the history of neuropsychology on a grand historical canvas. Here at the outset Benton defines neuropsychology implicitly in his selection of topics and literature ranging over psychology, neurology, and psychiatry. Look deliberately at the weaving of the story across disciplines, cultures, periods, and contexts. The appraisal of the status of the concepts of localization, hemispheric dominance, memory and perception, and the aphasic disorders written in 1988 would be not off the mark if it were applied today.

Chapter 2 is an appreciative portrait of four outstanding contributors to neuropsychology that was given to the International Neuropsychological Society (INS) when it was presented as a 1987 invited master lecture on the occasion of a celebration of the 15th anniversary of the reorganized INS (an organization Benton helped to create and bring back to life in 1972 after a faltering organizational start in 1967). His personal relationships with these colleagues make their contributions come to life in this paper. Even those (myself included) who had the opportunity to meet, or to be taught in their professional youth by one or more of these four eminent scholars, will find Benton's appraisal of them over the years to be heartwarming and most informative.

Chapter 3, a briefer piece on the fate of three neuropsychological concepts, is enormously instructive today. Those who feel that they have done good but unheralded work will certainly want to examine and relish these three parables. Benton points out that the three discoveries in the areas of astereognosis (by Puchelt), vision and the occipital lobes (by Panizza), and prosopagnosia (by Quaglino and Borelli) were initially unappreciated, though they were later seen as important advances. The reasons for this initial lack of appreciation may have varied, but Benton's injunction that all of us are "more or less prisoners of the *Zeitgeist*" could not be more apt today. The measured response he recommends to results that don't "fit" is well taken.

The fourth chapter on the history of our understanding of the prefrontal region is a must, particularly for those who may think that the issues confronting us in gaining a full understanding of this most anterior of brain regions dropped unexpectedly out of the sky in the 1940's. Contributors back then and even at the start of the twentieth century may be seen to have been the beneficiaries of a large corpus of existing work on animals and humans. I invite the reader's attention to the way in which Benton pans for scientific gold—reporting, selecting, considering, and judging temperately. Much reinvention of long-identified qualities and problems related to the prefrontal area could be moderated by a careful reading of this paper. Current neuropsychologists, in researching this brain region, have discovered some things that are new. For reasons that will become clear after study of this chapter, their research could be even more cogent with this context in mind.

In a similar way, but more briefly, Chapter 5 on cerebrovascular disease provides examples of how certain dilemmas in understanding the effects of cerebrovascular disease have informed—and at times misinformed—us about localization.

The final chapter in this section, a 1982 essay on the evolution of spatial thought in clinical problems and practice, may be the most salutary for those neuropsychologists who feel a bit too comfortable in their understanding of the independent and complementary functions of the right cerebral hemisphere. Those contemplating the creation of new tests sensitive to right hemisphere disease and dysfunction will do well to study this history. I especially liked the way in which Benton builds the story of how modern appreciation for the manifold features of right hemisphere function developed. In at least one sense, the reader might be able to see why some clinicians and researchers still have found it reasonable to think of the right hemisphere as the "minor" hemisphere even as recently as a decade ago (see also Chapter 17).

Part II contains six papers on aphasia that were published in the years 1960–1988. Each sheds a different light on this area of neuropsychology. Together, they indicate why aphasiological studies were in the forefront of behavioral neurology for so long. The first is a 1960 *Archives of Neurology* paper that has no peer. The descriptive examples from literature and history going as far back as ancient Greece inform us of the essential origins of the terms we take for granted today. The paper takes us through historical observations and lays the foundation for the explosion of knowledge about brain–behavior relationships in language in the second half of the nineteenth century. To teach a course in any aspect of the clinical neuropsychology of language and send a student away without having absorbed the scholarship in this paper would be a loss.

The second chapter of this section looks in more detail at the development of knowledge regarding aphasia from 1800 to the "fateful" case report of Broca in 1860. Presented first at the inaugural meeting of the Academy of Aphasia in 1963, this is material not covered in the previous chapter, and is a further scrutiny of French thinking in this period and a setting of the stage on which Broca's findings would come to stand.

The third offering here is a 1964 neurology paper about the memoir of Marc Dax. This is a more fateful lesson from the history of aphasia about scientific discovery and reporting than Broca's case report. It is of considerable interest to anyone seeking to master the history of language disorders; any neuropsychologist might profit from this cautionary tale regarding the fate of Dax's initially obscure conference paper. One can only imagine the legal wrangles over the intellectual property case that might be the final chapter to such a story today.

The next chapter, a comparative essay about the observations of Sigmund Freud and Henri Bergson on aphasia, is a treat. Both made important contributions to an understanding of the disorder that contradicted the dogma of the time. This paper reminds one that, as Benton puts it, "what a clinician sees, or at least deems worthy of note, in his assessment of aphasic patients is determined in large part by his own preconceptions." It would be a great lesson to use in a supervisory context for students.

The final two chapters in this section define and highlight the contributions of Gesner and Pitres in the realms of jargon and amnestic phenomena in aphasia. They give readers an excellent grasp of some of the nuances that characterize studies of language behavior when done well. Aphasiologists will enjoy the way in which Benton appraises the impact of these nineteenth century workers on thought in aphasia.

Part III, devoted to methodology and assessment is unique. Benton obviously means something rather different than many clinical neuropsychologists today would think from this section's moniker. The first chapter is a 1978 account of how animal studies, clinical observation, and experimentation can blend into a relatively seamless tapestry of knowledge. The departure point of the narrative is the work of several European animal researchers, and in particular the Berlin physiologist Hermann Munk. The road that follows will be fascinating to the reader.

The second chapter in this section sets forth some *desiderata* for neuropsychological assessment worth heeding. Chapter 15 calls attention to some useful procedures for the assessment of the amusias, including protocols that could be implemented in the clinic today despite the effects of vanishing music education budgets, dysphasic rappers and chanteuses, music videos, and other *impedimenta* to the expression and appreciation of music.

The fourth and final selection in this section is an excellent summing up of clinical neuropsychology in the 30 years between 1960 and 1990, given first as the twentieth Herbert Birch lecture at the 1992 INS meeting. It appraises the field during what has been unquestionably its major thrust toward recognition as an independent psychological specialty and as a critical nexus for continued interdisciplinary inquiry and progress.

Part IV is a trio of contributions on hemispheric dominance. The first one, a 1972 contribution to a medical history journal, has long been a favorite of mine. It offers a very informed historical perspective on the term "minor hemisphere."

The second of these chapters provides a scholarly framework for the commonplace question that occurs in science when we look back at the time before a discovery and wonder why nobody could see what seems obvious or elementary now. This tale of tantalization appeared first in a 1984 *Neuropsychologia* number. The foreshadowing evidence that led to Broca's initial clinical case and its subsequent elaboration is fascinating.

Finally, a 1991 *Neuropsychology Review* paper exploring the legacy of Henry Hécaen and Oliver Zangwill informs us about the value and limits of hemispheric dominance as a rubric for the exploration of brain–behavior relationships. In my view, this is the most complete and balanced assessment one will find of a topical paradigm that was one of the major foci of neuropsychology in the last half of the twentieth century.

The last two chapters comprise Part V, devoted to pediatric neuropsychology, an abiding interest of Benton. The first, an appraisal of the evolution of dyslexia as a concept, was first presented at the Orton Society in 1980. This is a rendering of a topic central to the provenance of the child neuropsychologist's claim to be numbered as essential in schools, clinics, and homes. It also presages the mapping of subtypes so critical in the advancement of a mature learning disorder taxonomy. The closing chapter is a complementary piece looking more broadly at the status of developmental neurospsychology. It draws together various currents extending beyond dyslexia to point the way ahead at the start of the 1990s.

I cannot imagine that this collection will be matched at any point. The scholarship in these papers is remarkable. In my view, the book is particularly important for students given that modern information science can sometimes foster an uncoupling between information and knowledge. Reading and thinking about Benton's integrative work as seen here is an antidote to that.

Will scholarship of this kind endure in the next century? If not, we will rediscover the same ideas and experiences in successively shorter cycles. If we do not conduct our scholarly inquiry with at least a modicum of Benton's scope and vision, how will we come to understand the development of our concepts about brain and behavior?

This book offers a perspective on modern neuropsychology and behavioral neurology one could not hope to secure in any other way. It also points the way for future inquiry in more ways than are immediately obvious. The reader should attend carefully to those many places in these pages where Benton points to ideas not completed, controversies unresolved, and questions not yet well-formulated.

This book reflects a lifetime of understanding of the field. Read it with a sense of the inspiration and dedication with which it was prepared.

Part I

EVOLUTION OF THE DISCIPLINE

1

Neuropsychology: Past, Present, and Future

Introduction

Human neuropsychology is the discipline that investigates on an empirico-scientific level the interrelations of the brain with mentation and behavior. It is a compound discipline in that it represents the confluence of several fields of study—neurology and psychology, neuroanatomy and neurophysiology, neurochemistry and neuropharmacology. Addressing one of the oldest of philosophic themes, the mind–body problem, neuropsychology has a long past. However, the term itself is relatively new (Bruce, 1985), having gained currency only in the 1950s when it displaced older terms, e.g., psychoneurology (Bekhterev), brain pathology (Kleist).

Since it is an amalgam of a number of fields of study, the status of neuropsychology through the ages has been dependent upon the status of its contributory disciplines. For example, on the psychological level, when mentation was classified into a few broad categories such as "perception," "cognition" and "memory" (as was the case up to 1800) or personality dissected into complex traits such as "benevolence," "acquisitiveness" and "reverence" (as Gall did), there was little hope of identifying specific cerebral correlates in them. On the anatomic level, it was scarcely possible to relate cortical variables to behavior when, as was generally the case up to the 1820s, the gyri of the cerebral cortex were regarded as "enteroid processes" that were not even deemed worthy of being given a name (cf. Schiller, 1965). Nor could much understanding of the neural mechanisms mediating normal and disturbed speech be gained when, despite excellent clinical descriptions of aphasic disorders, eighteenth-century

---

Reprinted with permission from F. Boller and J. Grafman (Eds), *Handbook of Neuropsychology, Vol. 1*,

physiology proposed that sluggishness in brain function caused by dryness and rigidity caused these disabilities (cf. Benton and Joynt, 1960). Thus the history of neuropsychology has been one of irregular progress as advances in one or another of its contributory disciplines were achieved and made an impact on thinking and practice in the field.

The period of 1861–1875 stands out as one of very rapid progress when concurrent advances in clinical neurology, anatomy, physiology and psychology combined to effect a transformation of the field and give it a new structure. Broca's (1863, 1865) correlation of nonfluent aphasic disorder with anterior left hemisphere disease initiated a new era of lesional localization and gave rise to the concept of hemispheric dominance. Meynert's (1867) research identifying projection, association and commissural pathways, as well as regional differences in the cellular architecture of the cerebral cortex, provided an anatomic basis for the postulation of neural mechanisms underlying cognitive functions, the most important of which were Wernicke's (1874) models of the neurological basis of diverse language performances (cf. Geschwind, 1967). The psychological counterpart of Wernicke's neural connectionism was the associationist psychology of Wundt, presented in his published lectures in the 1860s and his book on "physiological psychology," the first edition of which appeared in 1874 (cf. Boring, 1950). Wernicke's correlation of fluent aphasic disorder with left posterior temporal lobe disease complemented Broca's earlier localization of nonfluent speech disorder and was of major clinical and theoretical significance. The demonstration of the excitable motor cortex by Fritsch and Hitzig (1870) provided a powerful impetus for animal experimentation by physiologists and directed the attention of clinicians to the possibilities of cortical localization of function. Indeed, the Fritsch-Hitzig stimulation experiment was repeated on a human subject by Bartholow (1874).

The contemporary period is also one of very rapid change. The advent of the newer neurodiagnostic techniques of computed tomography (CT), magnetic resonance imaging, positron emission tomography, cerebral blood flow determination and evoked potential recording has ushered in a new era of lesional localization in which structural and functional abnormality of the brain can be demonstrated with greater clarity and precision than ever before. At the same time, advances in neurophysiology and neuropharmacology (won largely through the development and applications of single and multiple cell recording) and in anatomy (where hitherto unknown pathways have been identified) are providing valuable indications of the neural mechanisms underlying cognitive processes and leading to a revision of conceptions about the functional organization of the brain. On the behavioral side of the equation, application of standardized quantitative methods of assessment has disclosed performance deficits that had escaped attention and has served to correct biased observation.

Some topics have played a dominant role in the history of neuropsychology. The oldest are the perennial questions of localization of function in the brain and the nature of the cerebral mechanisms underlying thought and action. After Broca's revolutionary discovery in the 1860s, hemispheric cerebral dominance (itself a form of localization) became an issue of major importance. Certain types of behavioral disability were subjects of special interest, perhaps because of their striking character as well as their debilitating consequences. The earliest were disorders of memory and of speech. In the latter half of the nineteenth century, disturbances in perception, recognition and orientation (chiefly visual but also auditory and somesthetic) became prominent topics of study. General intellectual impairment, i.e., dementia, was recognized very early but did not become a major topic for research until well into the twentieth century. On the other hand, the cognitive and personality changes associated with frontal lobe disease attracted special interest as early as the 1880s.

This chapter presents a brief and, of necessity, highly selective account of some aspects of the evolution of knowledge and thinking in the field of human neuropsychology. Current trends predictive of the likely directions of future development will then be considered.

Concepts of Cerebral Localization

Early Conceptions

The earliest attempts to relate discrete mental functions or faculties to the brain (dating back to about A.D. 100) took the form of a localization of functions along its anterior-posterior axis, either in the brain substance or in the ventricles. Of the two possibilities, ventricular localization was favored for a number of reasons. It accorded well with the doctrine of the circulation of animal spirits and, in addition, the hollow spaces within the brain seemed to be the more appropriate place for the noncorporeal soul to exert an influence on the body (cf. Pagel, 1958). In the scheme of Nemesius (ca. A.D. 400), sensation and perception were located in the anterior ventricles, thinking and reasoning in the third ventricle and memory in the fourth ventricle. The concept provided a structural framework for a dynamic process wherein sensory impressions were received and integrated into perceptions in the anterior ventricles, moved to the third ventricle to be reflected upon, and deposited as memories in the fourth ventricle. In the absence of a more convincing model, ventricular theory survived for a remarkably long time and derangement of the humors was often invoked to account for the occurrence of isolated defects in mentation. For example, the fifteenth-century physician, Antonio Guanerio, explained anomia and paraphasic speech by postulating an excessive accumulation of phlegm in the posterior ventricle (the "organ of memory") in the affected patients (cf. Benton and Joynt, 1960).

Localization of function in the substance of the brain largely displaced ventricular localization as a dominant approach in the seventeenth and eighteenth centuries. Thomas Willis conceived of sensation taking place in the corpus striatum, proceeding to perceptual integration in the corpus callosum and surrounding territory and progressing to memory in the cerebral cortex (cf. Clarke and Dewhurst, 1972). The eighteenth-century French surgeon, La Peyronie, having observed that most parts of the cerebral hemispheres could be injured without producing obvious mental impairment, concluded "from the facts and by way of exclusion" that the corpus callosum was the seat of intellect (cf. Soury, 1899). Transmission of animal spirits along distinct pathways was the physical basis of mentation and blockage in transmission produced disturbance in one or another mental function (cf. Clarke and O'Malley, 1968).

Gall

While relatively broad concepts of localization of function were the rule before 1800, a quantum leap to another mode of thinking was introduced by Franz Joseph Gall in the first decades of the nineteenth century. Placing mental functions in the cerebral hemispheres and insisting that the brain was in reality an assemblage of organs, each of which subserved a specific intellectual faculty or character trait, Gall made cerebral localization a central issue in neuropsychology. Although, with a few exceptions, his placement of these faculties and traits and his absurd phrenology provoked ridicule, his basic premise that the cerebral hemispheres formed a highly differentiated structure permitting precise localization of function, was taken quite seriously and engendered a decades-long controversy between "localizationists" and "antilocalizationists." During this period (1820–1860), the systematic detailed descriptions of the cerebral hemispheres, the basal ganglia and the thalamus by Rolando, Burdach, Leuret, Gratiolet and other anatomists showed that the brain was indeed a highly differentiated organ, the parts of which were interconnected (cf. Meyer, 1971). For example in 1854, Gratiolet presented the first description of the optic radiations arising from the lateral geniculate nucleus and fanning out to the occipital and parietal cortex, thus providing an anatomic basis for the subsequent dethronement of the "optic thalamus" as the cerebral center of vision and the placement of that center in the occipital lobes (cf. Polyak, 1955).

The specific aspect of Gall's scheme that aroused the greatest scientific interest was his placement of two centers of language, one for speech articulation and the other for the "memory of words," in the orbital region of both frontal lobes. Conflicting clinicopathologic findings fueled an acrimonious debate that was not resolved until the 1860s (cf. Benton, 1964).

The "Golden Age"

Broca's discovery ushered in the "golden age" of cerebral localization, extending roughly from 1870 to 1890. This period of intense activity, involving both animal experimentation and clinicopathologic correlations in patients, resulted in the localization of a variety of functions and capacities: e.g., visuosensory and visuoperceptive capacities in loci in the occipital lobes (Munk, 1878; Wilbrand, 1887), somatosensory and somatoperceptual capacities in the parietal lobe (Wernicke, 1895), learning capacity and memory in the frontal lobes (Bianchi, 1895). From a scientific standpoint, it seemed clear to most students that specific regions of the cerebral hemispheres subserved specific functions and that systematic study of these regions and their interconnections would provide an adequate model of the neural basis of mentation. As has been noted, the anatomic researches of Meynert in the 1860s fitted in well with these expectations.

The Critics

A long-standing tradition, preeminently represented by Flourens, who maintained (from ablation studies on the pigeon!) that all parts of the cerebral hemispheres were functionally equipotential and later by Goltz who subsequently took a less extreme position, denied that focal lesions had the specific effects attributed to them and hence that the assumption of the existence of circumscribed cortical centers was false (Clarke and O'Malley, 1968). But this holistic view of a more or less functionally homogeneous brain could not survive the massive accumulation of observations on animals and patients indicating that, in fact, lesions in different regions did produce radically different behavioral consequences.

However, another line of thought had greater weight. It was concerned primarily with the neural mechanisms underlying normal and disordered behavioral function. The dominant concept, held explicitly or implicitly, was that the cortical centers somehow contained the information reaching them in the form of images or representations and that the integration of these representations via pathways connecting the cortical centers constituted a person's immediate perceptual knowledge of his environment. If these images or representations were retained over time, they became memory-images. For example, Wernicke (1895), having described two patients with tactile object agnosia, ascribed the defect to "a loss of memory-images of the tactile sensations of concrete objects which are located in the middle third of the postcentral gyrus."

Some clinicians and experimentalists could not accept this relatively simple formulation of the control of mentation by circumscribed cortical areas and their connections, whether through the arrangement of a storage of "memory-images" or not. They were not antilocalizationists in the Flourens sense nor did they deny that lesions in a specific region could produce specific behavioral defects. However, they did emphasize that these facts did not mean that specific mental capacities were subserved by specific parts of the brain.

Jackson's (1878) oft-quoted dictum that "to locate the lesion which destroys speech and to locate speech are two different things" expressed this view concisely. Essentially the same position was taken by the physiologist Jacques Loeb (1886), when he insisted that it was simply not possible to locate mental functions in the brain and that efforts to do so were, in principle, not different from the earlier attempts of theologians to identify the seat of the soul. Pointing out that the concept of "function" is only a shorthand term for a whole series of events, he defined "cerebral localization" as a description of how the course of events is changed by defined changes in the nervous system. Decades later, Hebb (1949) introduced his concept of interacting, overlapping cell assemblies and Lashley (1950) described his fruitless "search for the engram." The implication of these views was that the neural mechanisms underlying mentation and behavior were far more complicated and extensive than those envisaged by the localizers with their assignment of specific functional properties to demarcated cortical areas and the connections between them.

These opposing conceptions of the nature of the neural mechanisms underlying mental performances applied with particular force to the analysis of the aphasic and agnostic disorders. Aspects of the debate will be considered in the sections on aphasia and perceptual disorders.

Hemispheric Cerebral Dominance

The concept of hemispheric cerebral dominance was born when Broca (1865; Berker et al., 1986) was led to conclude from his observations that "we speak with the left hemisphere." Over the ensuing decades the concept of left hemisphere dominance acquired a larger significance, encompassing intellectual capacities beyond the realm of speech. The cognitive or "noetic" school of aphasiology, as represented by Jackson, Finkelnburg (who introduced the concept of "asymbolia") and Marie, held that aphasia was essentially an intellectual disorder and not merely an affection of speech as an instrument of communication. The aphasic patient was "lamed" in thinking (Jackson), he was not able to grasp the import of nonverbal symbolic actions such as gestures (Finkelnburg), he was particularly deficient in the capacity for abstract thought (Goldstein, 1924). Later

Liepmann (1900) and Kleist (1923; Strauss, 1924) described diverse forms of apraxia as a consequence of focal left-hemisphere disease and Gerstmann (1930) associated certain disorders of the body schema with a lesion in the territory of the left angular gyrus. The cumulative effect of these observations and correlations was to establish the idea that the left hemisphere was the "major" hemisphere in that it subserved not only speech functions but also certain distinctive aspects of human mentation and activity.

Somewhat paradoxically, during this period when the left hemisphere was being assigned ever greater importance for intellectual processes, there were scattered attempts to show that the right hemisphere also possessed distinctive functional properties with respect to the mediation of cognitive behavior (cf. Benton, 1972). But these proposals had no significant influence on neuropsychological thought until after World War II when the researches of Hécaen (Hécaen and Ajuriaguerra, 1945; Hécaen et al., 1951) and Zangwill (Paterson and Zangwill, 1944; McFie et al., 1950) showed that impairment in visuoperceptual and visuoconstructional performance was closely associated with lesions of the right hemisphere. These pioneer studies were followed by demonstrations of the association of right hemisphere disease with defects in nonverbal auditory discrimination (Milner, 1958, 1962) and tactile-spatial performance (Carmon and Benton, 1969). The concept of "dominance" thus gave way to the concept of "asymmetry of hemisphere function," which assigned special behavior-mediating roles to each hemisphere.

Hemispheric Dominance and Language

The issue of the role of lateral hand preference as a determinant of hemispheric dominance for speech arose very early, indeed immediately after Broca made his correlation between speech and the left hemisphere. As observations of cases which did not follow the rule accumulated, both he and other clinicians added the qualification that left hemisphere dominance for speech held only for right-handers. In left-handers the right hemisphere was dominant for speech. This symmetrical or "mirror-image" formulation of the association between handedness and hemispheric specialization for speech was accepted for three-quarters of a century until observations after World War II showed that it was untenable. Studies by Conrad (1949), Humphrey and Zangwill (1952) and Goodglass and Quadfasel (1954) of aphasic patients with unilateral lesions disclosed that aphasic disorder in the left-hander was in fact more frequently produced by a left-hemisphere lesion than one in the right hemisphere. Obviously the contralateral relationship between hand preference and the hemisphere dominant for speech held only for right-handers. The additional observation by Conrad that aphasia was likely to be less severe and longlasting in left-handers suggested that speech was bihemispherically "represented" in some left-handers, a concept which was subsequently confirmed by the Wada test studies of Milner and co-workers (1966; Milner, 1973).

In addition, a sinistral familial background had been invoked occasionally to explain unusual and unexpected clinical findings. The uncommon occurrence of crossed aphasia in right-handed patients has been ascribed to the circumstances that they belong to families in which left-handedness is prominent (cf. Kennedy, 1916; Ettlinger et al., 1956), although it is acknowledged that crossed aphasia is also seen in right-handed patients with a completely dextral familial background (cf. Clarke and Zangwill, 1965). Familial sinistrality has also been advanced as a possible explanation for the finding that some right-handed patients show only a partial syndrome of fluent aphasia (i.e., conduction aphasia) from a lesion in Wernicke's area instead of an expected full syndrome (cf. Benson et al., 1973; Mendez and Benson, 1985).

The question of whether the right hemisphere (in right-handers) possesses any language capabilities also arose fairly soon after Broca's discovery. Clinicians were inclined to think that it did. Jackson believed that automatic, interjectional and emotional speech in aphasic patients was produced by the undamaged right hemisphere while impairment in propositional speech was the consequence of left-hemisphere damage. Recovery from aphasic disorder was attributed to the assumption of speech functions by the undamaged right hemisphere.

Subsequent observation has provided some support for these ideas. Patients who have undergone left hemispherectomy for removal of a malignant neoplasm are, of course, severely aphasic but nevertheless are still capable of emotional and very simple propositional speech as well as a limited degree of understanding of oral speech (cf. Smith, 1966; Burkland and Smith, 1977). Another type of evidence pointing to the participation of the right hemisphere in expressive speech has been the observation that pharmacologic inactivation of the right hemisphere in some aphasic patients through injection of amobarbital renders them completely mute, suggesting that their disordered speech was mediated by the right hemisphere (cf. Kinsbourne, 1971; Czopf, 1972). Studies of "split-brain" patients after section of the corpus callosum for relief of epilepsy showed clearly that the right hemisphere does have a limited capacity for understanding oral and written language (cf. Gazzaniga, 1970; Zaidel, 1977; Bogen, 1985). Finally, an indication that the right hemisphere plays a role in recovery from aphasic disorder comes from cerebral blood flow findings that reduced reactivity in both frontal areas is seen in patients with persisting Broca's aphasia, while recovered patients show normal reactivity in the right-frontal area (cf. Meyer et al., 1980).

However, limitations in this concept of right-hemisphere participation in language functions are also apparent. Occasional case reports have described patients who, having recovered from aphasia after a left-hemisphere stroke, once again became aphasic after a right-hemisphere stroke and this sequence of events has been interpreted as evidence that language functions had been transferred to the right hemisphere after the first stroke (cf. Nielsen, 1962). But the far more numerous instances of recurrence of an aphasic disorder after a second left-hemisphere stroke, as well as those of permanent and severe aphasic disability from a left-hemisphere lesion, indicate that post-stroke interhemispheric transfer, if it is real, is not a common occurrence. In addition, recent observations indicate that bilateral lesions of the third frontal gyrus do not produce a more severe or lasting motor speech disorder than do lesions confined to the left hemisphere (cf. Levine and Mohr, 1979).

Hemispheric Dominance and Nonverbal Performance

The early indications of a specialization of the right hemisphere for perceptuospatial performance in the several sense modalities led to a massive research effort focused on the question of the functional properties of the "minor" hemisphere. The field of inquiry expanded beyond perceptual capacities to encompass motor performances, attentional processes, emotional reactivity, musical functions, developmental trends and individual and class differences. The hundreds of relevant studies are summarized in many books and reviews (cf. Harnad, 1977; Hécaen and Albert, 1978; Walsh, 1978; McGlone, 1980; Bradshaw and Nettleton, 1981; Bryden, 1982; De Renzi, 1982; Kertesz, 1983; Lezak, 1983; Young, 1983; Springer and Deutsch, 1985). Some fundamental issues arising from this research will be considered.

One problem raised by the findings is that, although defective performance on these nonverbal tasks is generally more frequent and more severe in patients with right-hemisphere lesions, impairment is also shown by many patients with lesions of the left hemisphere. To cite a representative observation, visuoconstructional disability, which is presumably a consequence of right-hemisphere dysfunction, is also seen in 10–15% of patients with left-hemisphere disease, a figure which may be compared to the 1–2% incidence of aphasic disorder in patients with right-hemisphere disease (cf. Arrigoni and De Renzi, 1964; Benton, 1967). Obviously, the "dominance" of the right hemisphere for constructional praxis is not comparable to the dominance of the left hemisphere for speech. The task of discriminating unfamiliar faces provides another example of a preponderance of defective performances occurring among patients with right-hemisphere damage coupled with a smaller but notable frequency of failure in patients with left-hemisphere lesions (cf. Hamsher et al., 1979). These results are congruent with those of visual field studies of facial discrimination in normal right-handed subjects showing that, while a majority of them perform better on left-field presentations, a substantial minority (20–25%) manifest either no difference between the fields or an unexpected right-field superiority (cf. Hilliard, 1973; St. John, 1981).

These findings of a rather modest "dominance" of the right hemisphere for so many nonverbal task performances are sometimes explained by postulating that different hemispherically related mechanisms are involved in the mediation of these performances. The explanation raises a question of how the functional properties of each hemisphere are best described. The first distinction that was made is the obvious one of designating the left hemisphere as verbal and the right as nonverbal, i.e., defining the difference largely in terms of the type of information that was processed. According to this view, the left hemisphere processes verbal information directly while it processes nonverbal information by first encoding it in verbal terms; the right hemisphere processes information in pictorial terms. Hence, although it is adept in processing nonverbal information, it can process only very simple verbal information that can be apprehended pictorially, e.g., short monosyllabic words representing concrete objects.

For a number of reasons (no single one of which would seem to be compelling), the dichotomizing of hemispheric function into verbal and nonverbal categories has been viewed as inadequate and a variety of other formulations have been advanced. For example, the left hemisphere is specialized for serial (sequential) processing and the right for parallel (simultaneous) processing; the left hemisphere employs an analytic strategy, the right a holistic strategy; the left hemisphere focuses on details, the right on the total configuration; the left hemisphere apprehends the semantic aspects of a stimulus, the right hemisphere the physical features.

There is no agreement among theorists and researchers about which formulation is most valid, about how one formulation can be distinguished from another on empirical grounds, and indeed whether any single formulation can be shown to be congruent with the facts (cf. Bradshaw and Nettleton, 1981, and accompanying commentary). The traditional verbal/nonverbal dichotomy receives substantial support from clinical findings that the great majority of left-hemisphere-damaged patients who fail visuoperceptual and visuoconstructional tasks are aphasics with significant impairment in language comprehension (cf. Benton, 1973; Hamsher et al., 1979). The semantic–physical distinction is supported by results indicating that pre-experimental instructions to normal subjects to attend to the physical or social attributes of faces presented in the left or right visual fields has opposite effects on the pattern of performance, the "physical" instructions favoring a left-field superiority and the "social" instructions favoring a right-field superiority in recognition (cf. Galper and Costa, 1980).

Neuropsychology of Memory

Background

Accounts of loss of memory can be found in the earliest medical writings, where disabilities are described both within a setting of general mental impairment and as a more or less isolated disorder. As has been noted, ventricular theory provided a special cerebral localization for memory functions. Pure alexia was considered to be a restricted "loss of memory for letters" and anomia a "loss of memory for words" (cf. Meunier, 1924; Benton and Joynt, 1960). Case reports in the mid–nineteenth century described patients who exhibited various features of today's amnesic syndrome (cf. Levin et al., 1983).

The first systematic study of memory disorders was that of the French philosopher–psychologist Ribot (1882) who offered a classification and proposed theoretical formulations that had a decisive influence on subsequent thought in the field. His classification distinguished clearly between anterograde and retrograde amnesia and included the categories of modality-specific amnesia and loss of memory for symbols. But surely his most important contribution was his well-known "law of regression" stipulating that memory for recent events is more susceptible to disruption than older memories because it is less well-organized and less deeply consolidated. Moreover, he pointed out that the placement of events in a time frame was particularly vulnerable to disruption. A second major event of the 1880s was the publication of Ebbinghaus's (1885) pathbreaking study of learning and retention which introduced new methods of experimentation and recording that are in use today and which established "laws of learning" that still retain their validity.

Still another major event of the 1880s was the description by Korsakoff (1887; English translation by Victor and Yakovlev, 1955) of the distinctive syndrome of striking memory loss, confabulation, general mental impairment and polyneuritis that bears his name. Once explicitly described, the syndrome was readily observed by clinicians and its causative factor identified as a nutritional deficiency. The remarkable defect of memory was the subject of much study and was determined to be primarily a pervasive impairment in the capacity to learn and retain new experiences and knowledge (i.e., anterograde amnesia) coupled with a forgetting of experiences antedating the onset of the disorder (i.e., retrograde amnesia). The patient's tendency to confabulate (which, in any case, was not always present) was generally interpreted as an attempt to cover up the failure of memory.

It was first assumed that cortical-subcortical disease provided the neuropathological basis for the syndrome; Korsakoff himself postulated that destruction of subcortical association tracts produced the disorder (cf. Brierly, 1966). However, autopsy studies soon established that lesions in diencephalic structures, particularly the mammillary bodies, were a constant finding in the brains of Korsakoff patients (Gudden, 1896; Bonhoeffer, 1899, 1901; Gamper, 1928). This correlation between a well-defined disorder of memory and lesions in the mammillary bodies, hypothalamic and thalamic nuclei added a new chapter to the study of brain—behavior relationships in its demonstration of a crucial role of the diencephalon in the mediation of memory processes. Later it was discovered that specific impairment in learning and retention could be produced by lesions of the hippocampal formation in the mesial temporal lobes. Surgical experience demonstrated clearly that an amnesic syndrome followed bilateral excisions in this area (Scoville and Milner, 1957). The circumstances that the two crucial loci, diencephalic and mesial temporal, are connected via the fornix, gave rise to the concept of a hippocampal-mammillary neural system subserving new learning and recent memory (Ojemann, 1966).

Current Developments

At the present time no areas of human neuropsychology are being more actively investigated than disturbances of learning, retention and memory. No doubt the steadily increasing prevalence of dementing illness and of longtime survival from severe head injury, both of which conditions represent major public health problems, is one reason for this concern. A number of interrelated research questions have been addressed, among them: comparison of the features of memory impairment in specific disorders such as the Korsakoff syndrome and Alzheimer's disease; identification of the site of the neural mechanisms underlying memory performances (e.g., diencephalic, mesial temporal, frontal); analysis of memory defects in terms of its components (e.g., registration, consolidation, encoding, retrieval); study of the role of neurotransmitters in the mediation of memory functions (cf. Squire and Butters, 1984). A few highlights of this vast research effort will be briefly considered.

A development of major importance has been the incorporation of the theories, models and techniques of cognitive psychology into the study of memory disorders in patients (cf. Cermak, 1982; Squire and Butters, 1984). No less important is the growing rapprochement between animal experimentation and clinical observation, as exemplified by the demonstration (in contrast to the negative outcome of earlier studies) (cf. Douglas, 1967) that experimental lesions of the hippocampus and surrounding structures in animals can produce memory deficits that are comparable to analogous amnesic symptoms in the human subject (cf. Mishkin, 1982; Zola-Morgan, 1984).

Diencephalic and Temporal Amnesia

It has long been known that there are characteristic behavioral differences between Korsakoff patients and those with temporal lobe amnesia. The confabulation so frequently shown by the Korsakoff patient is rarely seen in the temporal lobe amnesic who acknowledges that he has a memory problem while the Korsakoff patient frequently denies it. On the other hand, it was assumed that the memory defect in the two classes of patients was essentially the same—a severe impairment in learning and retention of new information and a retrograde amnesia of variable length. However, recent investigative work has produced evidence suggesting that the patterns of impairment are in fact different. Lhermitte and Signoret (1972) found that while their Korsakoff patients showed a less severe anterograde amnesia than their patients with presumed hippocampal lesions, they were far more impaired on tests of sequential memory. Huppert and Piercy (1979) have reported that Korsakoff patients showed a normal rate of forgetting of recently learned material while the single hippocampal patient who was studied showed extremely rapid forgetting. Findings of other studies have been inconsistent with respect to this question of an intergroup difference in rate of forgetting. A conclusion drawn by some theorists from the ensemble of findings is that the memory deficit of the Korsakoff syndrome occurs at the early stage of registration and encoding, while the defect of the temporal lobe syndrome occurs at the later stage of identification and storage (cf. Winocur, 1984). These differential deficits in processing may represent the effects of lesions at different loci in a single hippocampal-diencephalic neural system. Alternatively it may imply that there are discrete neural mechanisms underlying different elements of memory, a concept which is supported by the finding that bilateral destruction of the fornix (a key component of the hippocampal-mammillary system) generally does not produce impairment of memory (cf. Squire, 1980).

The Temporal Pattern of Retrograde Amnesia

As has been noted, Ribot's "law of regression" predicted that remote memories were more likely to be retained following brain disease than were recent memories. The "law" was generally accepted by clinicians who observed that, in contrast to their manifest defect in recent memory, demented patients and senile subjects could recount numerous events from their remote past. The gradual shrinkage of retrograde amnesia after head injury was also supportive of the proposition (cf. Russell and Nathan, 1946; Benson and Geschwind, 1967). However, systematic study has generated inconsistent results that prevent ready acceptance of the concept. Thus, Warrington and Sanders (1971), utilizing a test of recall of public events in past decades, found that both normal subjects and Korsakoff patients showed essentially the same modest decline in memory for events over a 40-year period, with the overall performance level of the patients being lower than that of the controls. In contrast, Seltzer and Benson (1974), employing a similar technique, found a pronounced superiority in recall for remote events (25 or more years before testing) as compared to recall for recent events (1–10 years before testing) on the part of Korsakoff patients. The findings of Albert and coworkers (1979) confirm those of Seltzer and Benson. The findings of H. S. Levin and co-workers (1985) confirm those of Warrington and Sanders. It is evident that uncontrolled factors of an organismic, cultural or procedural nature that may be determining these conflicting results need to be identified.

Perceptuomotor vs. Factual Learning

Beginning with Milner's demonstration that H. M., a patient with a pervasive hippocampal amnesic syndrome, learned a mirror-tracing task at an essentially normal rate, there have been many reports documenting the capacity for motor and perceptual learning of patients with either hippocampal or diencephalic memory impairment. Among the tasks in which patients have been shown to perform successfully are rotary pursuit (cf. Brooks and Baddeley, 1976), mirror-reading (Cohen and Squire, 1980), judgments of familiarity (Huppert and Piercy, 1976) and complex nonverbal puzzles (Cohen, 1984). The striking disparity between the patients' capacity to learn these skills and their utter inability to recall the occasions, contexts, and circumstances associated with their successful learning, has led theorists to postulate the existence of two independent (but perhaps interacting) memory systems with different functional properties. Different sets of labels have been applied to the distinction, depending upon the theorist's judgment of what constitutes its basis, e.g., semantic-episodic (Tulving, 1972), attributional-contextual (Huppert and Piercy, 1976), procedural-declarative (Cohen, 1984).

Aphasic Disorders

Background

Even during the pre-Broca period the aphasic disorders were of interest to at least some physicians and a fairly substantial literature had accumulated before 1860. Almost all the specific aphasic defects (e.g., paraphasia, alexia, jargon speech) had been described and a clear differentiation between fluent and non-fluent forms of speech impairment had been made. Gall's placement of speech centers in the frontal lobes had stimulated at least one large-scale clinicopathologic study by Andral (1840) whose findings did not support the Gall-Bouillaud thesis (cf. Benton and Joynt, 1960; Benton, 1964, 1981).

As aphasia became a major area in neuropsychology after the Broca revolution, two schools of thought about its essential nature emerged. The "associationist" school conceived of the disorder as a disturbance in the instrument of speech that was produced by neural disconnections, which resulted in impairment of associative processes—between speech and thought, between speech and sensorimotor processes, and between components of the speech system itself. A sharp distinction was drawn between aphasic disorders and disturbances in speech that reflected defective ideation. In contrast, the cognitive or "noetic" school (already mentioned in relation to hemispheric cerebral dominance) conceived of aphasia as being primarily an intellectual disability that was reflected in nonverbal as well as verbal behavior and particularly in an incapacity to engage in abstract reasoning and symbolic behavior. The debate on the issue, extending over several decades, began to approach resolution only with the publication of the comprehensive study of Weisenburg and McBride (1935) comparing the performances of aphasic, nonaphasic and control patients on an extensive battery of verbal and nonverbal tests. One major finding of this study, which generated a good deal of new information about aphasia and at the same time provided a methodological model for subsequent investigation, was that there was extreme variability in nonverbal test performances among aphasic patients. While cognitive defects (not necessarily restricted to symbolic thinking) were more the rule than the exception, there were severely aphasic patients who performed on a normal level.

The debate between the associationist and cognitive schools extended beyond the issue of the relationship between aphasia and thought to encompass the interrelated questions of classification, localization and underlying neural mechanisms. The classification schemes developed by Wernicke (1874, 1886), Lichtheim (1885) and Bastian (1898), the leading members of the associationist school, postulated the existence of discrete types of aphasic disorder that were produced by lesions in either localizable cortical centers or the specific neural pathways connecting them. Despite certain shortcomings, the scheme was found to be sufficiently useful that it was generally adopted and, in its essence, is still the dominant classification utilized in clinical neurology. The cognitive school, the leading members of which were Jackson (1878), Marie (1906) and Head (1926), viewed aphasia as a unitary disorder affecting all modes of verbal communication—oral expression, oral understanding, writing and reading—and hence regarded classifications based on specific defects as necessarily superficial. Nor could they accept the associationists' restrictive, relatively simple descriptions of the nature of the neural mechanisms underlying normal and disordered speech. Instead they thought in terms of far more widespread and complicated arrangements always involving a large part of the brain. As Head (1926, p. 474) put it, "the processes which underlie an act of speech run through the nervous system like a prairie fire from bush to bush."

The cognitive school made more extensive use of tests in investigating aphasic patients. Marie (Moutier, 1908) and Head (1926) constructed elaborate batteries which they used primarily to support their convictions about intellectual impairment in aphasia rather than as impartial assessment procedures. The tests were not standardized, ranged widely in difficulty level and were not always well designed. Indeed, when resident physicians in neurology and psychiatry were given the Head battery, they found some tests to be quite perplexing (Pearson et al., 1928). The first aphasia test battery to be constructed in accordance with modern standards was that of Weisenburg and McBride (1935), which was utilized in the study mentioned above.

The last decade of the nineteenth century saw a considerable expansion of knowledge about specific aspects of aphasia. The most important contribution was that of Déjerine (1892) who elucidated the neuroanatomic substrate of pure alexia on the basis of autopsy study of a patient with the disorder. Brissaud (1894) called attention to the phenomenon of dysprosodic speech which he called *aphasie d'intonation* and which he contrasted with *aphasie d'articulation*. However, no great attention was paid to these disturbances in the "melody of speech" until after Monrad-Krohn published his widely cited paper on the topic in 1947. Pitres (1898) described the syndrome of amnesic aphasia, the cardinal feature of which was a pronounced difficulty in naming and retrieving words in conversation within a setting of at least relative preservation of verbal understanding and expressive speech. Pitres (1895) also studied aphasia in polyglots and wrote an influential paper on the subject.

The conflict between the "noetic" and "connectionist" schools on the issues of the nature of aphasic disorder and its underlying neural substrate continued through the early decades of the twentieth century. It was a period in which many clinical contributions enriched knowledge of the varied symptomatology of aphasia without, however, any radical change in the approaches to the disorder. Head's (1926) conceptualization of aphasia as a unitary defect in symbolic formulation and expression and his derogation of the efforts of the connectionist "diagram makers" were a potent determinant of diagnostic approaches in Britain and the United States, where there was a definite waning of interest in the anatomical basis of the disorder. Marie's (1906) "iconoclastic" views had a considerable following in France but were countered by the localizationist position of Déjerine (1914) who emphasized specific anatomoclinical correlations. Goldstein's (1924) efforts to relate amnesic aphasia (and to some degree conduction aphasia) to impairment of the "abstract attitude" encountered strong opposition in the German-speaking countries (cf. Von Kuenburg, 1930; Isserlin, 1932; Lotmar, 1933) where, despite the attacks on it, the model of Wernicke was maintained.

The Modern Period

The decades since World War II have witnessed a tremendous surge of interest in the aphasic disorders, in part because stroke-produced aphasia is such an important cause of socioeconomic disability. At the same time neurodiagnostic procedures, such as CT and magnetic resonance imaging, permit investigators to collect a substantial amount of clinicopathologic data fairly quickly and new discoveries have modified concepts about classification and lesional localization.

Classification

Thanks to the development and application of objective assessment procedures that can subject the validity of different systems of classification to empirical test, this controversial issue is on the way (although not yet near) to resolution. One advance has been the demonstration that in fact there are fluent-paraphasic and nonfluent-articulatory *types* of aphasic disorder and not a normal distribution of cases along the dimension of fluency. The expressive speech of about 80% of aphasic patients can be classified with confidence as fluent or nonfluent (cf. Goodglass et al., 1964; Benson, 1967; Kerchensteiner et al., 1972; Wagenaar et al., 1975). Indeed it may be possible to augment this figure through a judicious selection of criteria of classification.

On the other hand, the cogency of classification of aphasic syndromes within the two broad categories such as those of Geschwind (1965; Benson and Geschwind, 1985) and Luria (1970), which necessarily involve assessment of the status of auditory comprehension, reading and writing as well as expressive speech, is less certain. Objective behavioral assessment criteria, such as have been utilized in establishing the fluency/nonfluency dichotomy, have rarely been applied to define these syndromes. In all probability, many cases now placed in a specific category would not survive an objective quantitative analysis. Anomic aphasia, classically described as impaired naming within the context of intact repetition and understanding, is one example. Conduction aphasia, classically described as impaired repetition and phonemic paraphasic speech within the context of intact understanding, is another. According to one estimate, only about 20% of cases in an unselected sample of aphasic patients could be classified with confidence as representative of one or another aphasic syndrome (cf. Prins et al., 1978). It is obvious that this problem deserves intensive study.

Another problem is posed by the observed instability of assigned diagnostic categories over time. It is well known that in the course of recovery a "Wernicke's aphasia" may become a "conduction aphasia" or an "anomic aphasia" and that a "global aphasia" may become a "Broca's aphasia." Shifts from nonfluent to a fluent expressive disorder, although uncommon, also may occur (cf. Prins et al., 1978; Knopman et al., 1983). This instability does not necessarily mean that the diagnostic syndromes are invalid but the changes must surely be taken into account when clinicopathologic relationships are investigated.

Lesional Factors

Important insights into the neuropathologic basis of specific aphasic syndromes have been gained even though some formulations may require revision because of looseness in behavioral classification. A few highlights will be mentioned.

Before the advent of CT scanning, relatively little attention was paid to the factor of size of lesion for the reason that this variable could be assessed with some degree of accuracy only in patients who had undergone surgery or had come to autopsy fairly soon after examination. It has now been established that size of lesion interacts with locus to determine both the severity and pattern of speech impairment as well as outcome. Taking the nonfluent aphasic disorders as an example, one finds several implications from recent studies: a lesion confined to Broca's area is more likely to produce an apraxia of speech than a classic Broca's aphasia; the latter is produced by a larger and deeper lesion involving not only Broca's area but also the surrounding posterior frontal and anterior parietal territory; moreover global aphasia is typically produced by even larger lesions involving the temporal lobe as well as frontal and parietal areas (cf. Hécaen and Consoli, 1973; Mohr et al., 1978; Naeser and Hayward, 1978; Kertesz et al., 1979; Mazzocchi and Vignolo, 1979; Tonkonogy and Goodglass, 1981). A tenable inference from the findings is that these nonfluent aphasic disorders represent a single syndrome, the breadth of which varies along a continuum of severity that is determined in large part by the size of the causative lesion.

Broadly speaking, the traditional localization of the causative lesion of Wernicke's aphasia in the posterior part of the first temporal gyrus (i.e., Wernicke's area) has stood the test of time. Nevertheless, recent study has indicated that the typical lesion is likely to involve other areas, such as the posterior parietal territory, the second temporal gyrus and primary auditory cortex, in varying degrees (cf. Hier and Mohr, 1977; Naeser and Hayward, 1978; Kertesz et al., 1979; Mazzocchi and Vignolo, 1979; Naeser, 1983). Indeed it appears that a lesion in Wernicke's area is not an absolutely necessary precondition for the appearance of a Wernicke aphasia. It has been suggested that variations in the symptom-picture of Wernicke's aphasia are related to variation in lesional locus within the broad temporoparietal territory, i.e., that the posterior parietal area is spared in patients who show better reading than oral comprehension and is importantly involved when the reverse performance pattern is manifested (cf. Hier and Mohr, 1977; Heilman et al., 1979).

Patients classified in the category of conduction aphasia have been found to have lesions in Wernicke's area and the posterior parietal territory as well in the insular region (cf. Naeser and Hayward, 1978; Kertesz et al., 1979; Damasio and Damasio, 1980). The size of the lesions is generally smaller than those seen in patients with Wernicke aphasia. Their locus indicates disruption of posterior–

anterior pathways (arcuate fasciculus and/or insula) and hence is in accord with the formulation that conduction aphasia is a specific disconnection syndrome (cf. Geschwind, 1965).

Study of the aphasic syndromes resulting from lesions outside of the traditional "zone of language," i.e., the transcortical, basal ganglia and thalamic aphasias, is a development of major importance. Until about 25 years ago, considerable skepticism about the reality of these disorders was expressed, but since then there has been a steady accumulation of irrefutable evidence (thanks to the utilization of CT scan) that they exist and in fact are not particularly rare (cf. Cappa and Vignolo, 1979; Damasio et al., 1982b; Mohr, 1983; Naeser, 1983; Graff-Radford et al., 1984). Although the clinicopathologic data are still sparse, a number of distinctive symptom-complexes have been described and tentatively related to lesions in specific loci within subcortical structures. In similar fashion, the symptomatology of the transcortical aphasic disorders and their lesional basis have been elucidated (cf. Rubens, 1976; Rubens and Kertesz, 1983).

Aphasia and Thought

Although the age-old controversy about the relationship of aphasia to cognitive status persists, it has lost much of its heat as an empirical approach to the question has supplanted the ex cathedra pronouncements of the protagonists of opposing schools. Studies of the intellectual status of aphasic patients have investigated a variety of cognitive performances, e.g., visuoperceptual and visuoconstructive performances, short-term memory, in addition to symbolic thinking and concept formation (cf. Zangwill, 1964, 1969; Archibald et al., 1967; Newcombe, 1969; Benton, 1973; Lebrun and Hoops, 1974; Hamsher, 1981).

A capsule summary of the findings and their implications might read as follows. A majority of aphasic patients do show impairment on one or another measure of cognitive function and their defects are by no means restricted to tests of abstract reasoning or symbolic thinking. They are generally more impaired than are nonaphasic patients with left-hemisphere disease but differences in size and locus of lesions prevent a straightforward interpretation of this observation. Among aphasic patients, those with significant defects in oral verbal comprehension are most likely to show defective nonverbal test performance. Moreover, certain nonverbal tasks, such as the identification of environmental sounds and pantomime recognition, are failed only by aphasics (and perhaps severely demented patients) but not by nonaphasics with brain disease (cf. Vignolo, 1969; Duffy et al., 1975; Varney, 1978; Varney and Benton, 1982). However, the overriding finding (often overlooked in intergroup comparisons) is one of extreme interindividual variability among aphasic patients, even among those with severe disturbances in comprehension. This variability indicates that in virtually every sample of aphasics some will perform normally, a fact which has been convincingly documented in case reports (cf. Alajouanine and Lhermitte, 1964; Zangwill, 1964). In addition, there is no evidence for a significant relationship between the degree of deficit in nonverbal task performance and the severity of aphasic disorder (cf. Basso et al., 1973).

Overview

The thrust of modern investigation has been to demonstrate that it is possible to describe the neural mechanisms underlying normal and disturbed speech in terms of the connectionist model formulated by Geschwind (1965). To be sure, these mechanisms are proving to be far more complex, involving progressions, parallel processing and interactions in information processing, than was originally specified. To this extent, current conceptions are compatible with the views of Head (1926) who insisted that the phenomena of aphasia could not be explained by the simplistic formulations of the nineteenth-century diagram makers, but who was unable to offer a more satisfactory model. Another development (more in line with the thinking of Head than with the static Wernicke-Lichtheim models) is the realization that aphasic disorders represent a dynamic changing state of affairs on both the anatomic–physiological level and the behavioral level. Finally, the concept of precisely localized centers has given way to that of broader "zones" representing critical junctures in more complex systems mediating speech and language performances.

Agnosic Disorders

"Higher-level" impairment of perception and recognition (i.e., not directly attributable to basic sensory defects) first engaged scientific attention in the late 1870s when Munk (1878, 1890), having identified "cortical blindness" following total occipital lobe excisions, went on to describe "mindblindness" as a consequence of less extensive occipital removals. His "mindblind" dogs, who evidently could see since they ambulated freely and avoided obstacles, would stare uncomprehendingly at objects and persons and failed to respond appropriately to stimuli such as pieces of meat or threatening gestures, but reacted normally to auditory and olfactory stimulation. Munk's formulation that the dogs "could see but not understand" was accepted by some clinicians who had observed a similar condition in patients with bilateral occipitoparietal disease (e.g., Wilbrand, 1887, 1892). Astereognosis, the somesthetic analog of mindblindness, was described by Hoffman in 1885 and related by Wernicke (1895) to the presence of lesions in the postcentral gyrus.

Visual agnosia, a term coined by Freud (1891), gradually displaced mindblindness as the preferred name for that condition. The most important early contribution to its understanding was made by Lissauer (1890), who proposed that the complete act of recognition involved two interacting processes—perceptual integration ("apperception"), which organized sensory data into a unity, and association, which linked the perceived entity with past experience. Failure in recognition could result from a primary defect in either process, which, however, was likely to involve a secondary defect in the other process. Thus all cases of visual agnosia reflect some degree of impairment in both processes, although one process might be more severely affected than the other. He considered his own patient, a mildly demented elderly man, with marked impairment in object recognition, to be an instance of a primarily "associative" agnosia since the patient could copy figures and showed adequate visuodiscriminative capacity.

From the very beginning the classical concept of agnosia encountered strong resistance and over the ensuing decades it has remained a controversial issue. Broadly speaking, three points of view regarding the nature of agnosic disorders emerged. First, without denying that there may be a number of levels of impairment of recognition, clinical investigators have published case reports supporting the real existence of the Munk-Wilbrand type of a relatively pure associative visual agnosia which could not easily be explained by sensory or perceptual defects (cf. Rubens and Benson, 1971; Taylor and Warrington, 1971; Hécaen et al., 1974; Albert et al., 1975; Mack and Boller, 1977).

On the other hand, a "reductionist" school attributed all disorders of recognition to the presence of elementary sensory defects and questioned the validity of the basic concept of agnosia (cf. Bay, 1953; Critchley, 1964; Bender and Feldman, 1965). To counter the argument that many non-agnosic patients show the same sensory defects to an equal or even more severe degree, Bender and Feldman (1965) defined "agnosia" as an expression of sensory defect complicated by dementia or general mental impairment. Finally, impairment in the perceptual-integrative component of visual recognition was considered to be primary by some investigators (cf. Gelb and Goldstein, 1920; Poppelreuter, 1923; Brain, 1941).

During its evolution the concept of agnosia was broadened to encompass disabilities that were not necessarily restricted to a single sensory modality such as autotopagnosia (Pick, 1908), anosognosia (Babinski, 1914, 1918), finger agnosia (Gerstmann, 1924,) and even "agnosia of utilization" (Morlaas, 1928) and "thumb–mouth agnosia" (Angyal, 1941). Inevitably this expanded application of the term led to a loss of precision in the definition of the concept. But at the same time, clinical observation fostered a trend in the opposite direction toward differentiating between subtypes of modality-specific agnosia. As early as the 1880s a dissociation between disability in recognizing things and disability in apprehending spatial relationships was noted and a distinction drawn between object agnosia and "spatial agnosia" (cf. Benton, 1969; De Renzi, 1982). Confirmed by subsequent clinical and experimental findings, the distinction led to the present formulation of two cortical visual systems, one (inferior occipitotemporal) subserving object recognition and the other (occipitoparietal) subserving the appreciation of spatial relationships (cf. Ungerleider and Mishkin, 1982; Levine et al., 1985). Continuing clinical observation led to further analyses of disturbances in visual recognition. Defective color identification and color-form association not attributable to acquired color blindness (achromatopsia) were described by Lewandowsky (1908) and Sittig (1921). Kleist (1934) distinguished between impairment in the discrimination of meaningless forms and impaired recognition of concrete objects. Loss of the capacity to identify familiar faces was noted as early as the 1860s but was not considered to be of special interest until Bodamer (1947) described it as an independent disability and gave it the name of "prosopagnosia."

Of these partial defects in visual recognition, prosopagnosia is the one which has been studied most intensively. The development of knowledge and concepts about the nature of this uncommon disability parallels in many respects the evolution of thought about agnosic disorders in general. Following the publication of Bodamer's paper, as well as that of Faust (1947), there was a significant surge of interest in prosopagnosia, an influential paper by Hécaen and Angelergues (1962) citing 12 studies on the topic published between 1950 and 1960. Reporting the clinical findings in 21 personally observed cases, Hécaen and Angelergues emphasized the association of the disability with diverse signs of right-hemisphere disease such as left visual field defect, constructional apraxia, dressing dyspraxia and left lateral inattention as well as its lack of association with aphasic disorder. They concluded that posterior right-hemisphere disease played a decisive role in the genesis of the disorder and, although expressing some reservations because of the lack of relevant anatomic data, they were inclined to believe that a lesion confined to the right hemisphere could produce prosopagnosia. The available anatomic information was brought forth by Meadows (1974) who showed that bilateral lesions were found in all seven cases that had come to autopsy as of that date. Nevertheless, he also ascribed a special significance to right posterior hemisphere disease, specifically involvement of the basal occipitotemporal region, and he pointed to the remarkably high frequency of left superior visual field defect (already noted by Faust, 1955) as indicative of this localization. In a thoughtful discussion, Meadows pointed out that the "lesion" of prosopagnosia, involving occipitotemporal cortex, underlying white matter, the inferior longitudinal fasciculus and often the lower fibers of the optic radiation, must impede the transmission of information between occipital cortex and the temporal lobe and limbic structures. Thus a restricted type of impairment in visual memory and recall might well ensue from such a breach in neural connections.

Since Meadows's (1974) review, several additional prosopagnosic cases have come to autopsy; all showed bilateral lesions (cf. Damasio et al., 1982a; Benton, 1985). CT scan findings have been less consistent. While the majority of scans of prosopagnosic patients have been indicative of bilateral disease, a number of cases with lesions apparently confined to the right hemisphere have been reported (cf. Whitely and Warrington, 1977; De Renzi, 1986; Landis et al., 1986).

Independently of the issue of lesional localization, the question of the nature of neuropsychological mechanisms underlying facial identification and its disturbances has received much attention. The observation that the prosopagnosic patient's failure in identification was apparently confined to faces and did not encompass objects or other attributes of persons, led to its classification as a "material-specific" or "stimulus-specific" defect of either perceptual integration or memory (cf. Benton and Van Allen, 1972). But this proved to be not completely accurate because many prosopagnosic patients also experience difficulty in identifying a particular automobile, building, street or animal (cf. Bornstein et al., 1969; Lhermitte et al., 1972; Damasio and Damasio, 1983). Hence a somewhat broader conception of prosopagnosia as a loss of the capacity to recognize individuality within a class of persons or objects was substituted for the face-specificity formulation and has been widely accepted. Damasio, Damasio, and Van Hoesen (1982) have proposed that the perception of a familiar face evokes historical information about the possessor of that face and this provides the basis for its identification. Visual inspection of a face by a prosopagnosic patient does not evoke this historical information and hence, while the face is recognized as such, its provenance cannot be identified. But other perceptions, e.g., stature, clothes, voice, can lead to identification. Thus it is specifically the visual evocation of facial memory which is defective and not a "store" of personal memories. That this process of evocation consists of a number of stages is indicated by the observations of Bauer (1984) and Tranel and Damasio (1985), which revealed that prosopagnosic patients who, by their verbal report, fail to recognize familiar faces nevertheless show a stronger electrodermal response to these faces than to unfamiliar faces. Evidently there is recognition on the autonomic level that does not reach the level of conscious awareness.

A significant effect of the increased concern with the problem of prosopagnosia was to provide an impetus to study the clinical and normative aspects of the discrimination of unfamiliar faces. Originally conceived as a means of assessing mild degrees of prosopagnosia, the tests that were contrived brought to light an essentially independent disability that had little relationship to the clinical complaint (cf. Warrington and James, 1967; Benton and Van Allen, 1968, 1972; De Renzi et al., 1968; Landis et al., 1986). Impairment in the discrimination of unfamiliar faces was found to be a far more frequent deficit than prosopagnosia and one that was shown not only by nonaphasic patients with right-hemisphere lesions but also by some aphasic patients (cf. Hamsher et al., 1979). Tachistoscopic studies of normal subjects generated findings in consonance with those of the clinical studies (cf. Hilliard, 1973; St. John, 1981).

Current Trends

A salient feature of present-day neuropsychology is the enormous expansion of activity as compared to 10–15 years ago. One reflection of this expansion is the proliferation of new journals (at least seven since 1977) devoted to the study of brain–behavior relationships in human subjects. The number of papers in the standard neurological journals dealing with neuropsychological issues has also increased significantly. (There were 13 papers of a neuropsychological nature in the 1975 volume of *Neurology*; in the 1985 volume there were 32.) This expansion has been accompanied by qualitative changes in the area and in its content. Neuroanatomy, neurophysiology, and linguistics are prominent components of the present effort and the focus of attention has shifted from topography (e.g., "right posterior," "angular gyrus") to a concern with underlying neural and cognitive mechanisms.

The Concept of Localization

Everyone accepts the broad principle of cerebral localization, i.e., that different regions of the brain participate in a distinctive way in the mediation of specific aspects of behavior and mentation. However, no one seems to be sure about what is localized or about the nature of the neural mechanisms involved in localization. The notion of cortical *centers* harboring (or controlling) specific capacities has still not entirely disappeared (perhaps reflecting the influence of practical medical thinking which, after all, is primarily concerned with the locus of lesions), but it has largely given way to that of *networks*, i.e., aggregates of interconnected neural loci, as the core concept in localization. For example, Babinski's (1918, 1923) center in the right hemisphere for the integration of somesthetic experience and somesthetic memory (to explain unilateral neglect and anosognosia) has been displaced by Mesulam's (1981) construct of a far more complicated "cortical network for directed attention and unilateral neglect."

The complexity of the mechanisms underlying behavioral performances has been compellingly demonstrated by neurophysiological and neurobehavioral study in animals. On the one hand, there is extreme specificity, as exemplified by the presence of cells in the temporal cortex of the monkey that respond preferentially to different wavelengths (Zeki, 1980, 1982) or to faces (Perret et al., 1982) and by cell columns in striate and prestriate cortex that respond preferentially to discrete stimulus features such as directional orientation, angles, edges and brightness (Hubel and Wiesel, 1965, 1968). On the other hand, it is obvious that these units are only elements of more extensive systems. A description of the neural mechanisms underlying visual object perception in the monkey by Ungerleider and Mishkin (1982) is derived from an integration of neuroanatomic and neurophysiologic data with ablation studies. It postulates both ipsilateral and crossed transmission of visual information from the striate to the prestriate to the inferior temporal area with many identifiable loci, and with the behavioral outcome being dependent upon the integrity of specific combinations of pathways rather than of one or more loci. Thus pattern discrimination remains undisturbed after lesions are made in both the striate area in one hemisphere and the inferior temporal area of the other hemisphere; but when these bilateral lesions are followed by transection of the corpus callosum, the animal shows complete and persisting failure on the pattern discrimination task.

Although necessarily more speculative, the same approach is now being applied to the problem of functional localization in the human subject. One example will be cited.

On the basis of a review of the pertinent experimental and clinical literature, Mesulam (1981) has formulated a detailed account of the neural mechanisms that may underlie normal and impaired attentional behavior. Very briefly stated, the formulation implicates four cerebral components—posterior parietal, cingulate, frontal and reticular—that form an integrated neural network mediating directed attention to events in external space. Mechanisms for sensory schemata are to be found in posterior parietal cortex (cf. Bisiach et al., 1979). Motivational significance is attached to sensory stimulation through mechanisms in the cingulate region. Frontal mechanisms provide the basis of the scanning, exploratory and manipulative components of attentional behavior (cf. Luria et al., 1966; Heilman and Valenstein, 1972, 1979). An adequate overall level of vigilance results from activity of the reticular system (cf. Heilman et al., 1978; Watson and Heilman, 1979).

Thus attentional behavior is seen as the consequence of the integrated operation of a complex network, rather than of a circumscribed cerebral region with distinctive functional properties. Mesulam discusses the implications of his formulation for clinically observed "types" of neglect, hemispheric asymmetry in directed attention and the relevance of earlier concepts of the nature of hemispatial neglect and sensory extinction. His comprehensive approach furnishes a model for analyses of the neuropsychological basis of the diverse behavioral impairments associated with brain disease.

Hemispheric Cerebral Dominance

Currently the theme of asymmetry of cerebral function is being as vigorously pursued as it has been during the past few decades. The enormous accumulation of data on diverse aspects of the question (e.g., specification of the performances that are "lateralized," relationship to hand preference, sex differences, influence of age) has yet to be integrated into a coherent body of knowledge. The morphologic approach to the problem, initiated by the pathbreaking study of Geschwind and Levitsky (1968), has enjoyed a limited degree of success; continued application of neuroradiologic methods may generate more precise and cogent information about the structural basis of functional asymmetry. Physiologic methods, such as positron emission tomography and cerebral blood flow determinations, may also be expected to contribute to the elucidation of the neural basis of "hemispheric dominance" (cf. Gur et al., 1983). What seems to be needed on the behavioral level at this time is the careful development of tests that will assess equally carefully defined cognitive and perceptual performances which are the focus of interest.

Although observations on the role of the right hemisphere in mediating speech and language extend over many decades, they are still quite sparse. The mélange of positive and negative findings to date have not provided a satisfying answer to the question, and the parameters that may determine the extent of right hemisphere participation in language behavior remain to be identified. It is highly probable that individual subject characteristics, such as sex, age, and family background for handedness, are important factors in this respect. Hence large-scale investigation is likely to provide a more fruitful approach at this time than the "illustrative" case reports that form such a large part of current knowledge.

Memory and Perception

As has been noted, the study of human memory and its disorders is a major concern of present-day neuropsychology. No doubt there will be further attempts to dissect memory processes into meaningful types and to relate these types to different lesional localizations and disease conditions. In addition, as with attentional behavior, the focus of interest in respect to lesion–behavior correlations is shifting from single structures (or simple combinations of structures, such as Ojemann's hippocampal–fornix–mammillary body system) to more complex networks (cf. Crosson, 1986).

The same trend is evident in recent efforts to specify the neural mechanisms underlying normal and impaired visual recognition. For example, Damasio (1985; Damasio et al., 1982a) proceeding from the studies of prosopagnosia described earlier in this chapter, views facial recognition as a multiple-step process, essential elements of which are accurate perceptual identification, discrimination between individual members of a class of very similar stimuli, and the evocation of relevant past experience. Thus his formulation integrates earlier single-factor explanations which emphasized one or another of these processes. While the perceptual and discriminative components of facial recognition may require the operation of mechanisms in striate and extrastriated cortex occipital regions, it is evident that the memory component must involve (at the very least) mesial temporal structures. Moreover, the demonstration of different levels of facial recognition (i.e., autonomic vs. verbal report) indicates that more than one process is involved in the specifically visual evocation of memories that make facial identification possible. Thus, this formulation of the mechanisms involved in a specific type of visual recognition implies the operation of a complex neural system that extends beyond the limits of the "visual area."

The Aphasic Disorders

One effect of the steadily increasing volume of linguistically oriented studies of aphasic performances has been to raise questions not only about the cogency of traditional classification, but also about the adequacy of current methods of clinical assessment. One example is the demonstration that "auditory comprehension" is a collective or multifaceted concept covering different types of impairment in function. Decades ago Kleist (1923, 1934) distinguished between "speech–sound deafness" and "speech–meaning" deafness. Adopting the same approach, both Hécaen (1969) and Luria (1970) proposed that the defects in oral language comprehension of some aphasic patients result from a specific disturbance in phonemic discrimination, while the disability of others is due either to failure to associate meaning with the speech percepts or to the inability to grasp sequences of speech sounds. Similarly, Goodglass and co-workers (1970) showed that a patient may be far more severely impaired in his understanding of messages consisting of successive items than of messages where meaning is conveyed by syntactic structures, or vice versa; further, there were indications that these patterns of performance are related to different aphasic symptom-complexes. It is clear then that, although undoubtedly useful for most clinical purposes, an aphasia test battery that includes only one or two tests of auditory comprehension cannot provide a full assessment of the capacity.

Naming performances furnish another example of the limitations of current aphasia test batteries. Presented with an object to be named, a patient may respond in one of a number of ways: he may say nothing or "don't know"; he may give a phonemic aphasic response; he may give a semantic paraphasic response; he may utter a neologism that has no recognizable phonetic or semantic relationship to the name of the object. The examiner will, of course, note the nature of the patient's responses but scoring of performance typically ignores these qualitative differences, which consequently are not reflected in the recorded performance profile of the patient. In part, this deficiency is due to a lack of clear idea of what a test of naming is supposed to disclose. At one extreme, it can be seen as a direct measure of communicative efficiency and, at the other extreme, as an analytic instrument to probe a patient's retrieval of names of diverse classes of stimuli (e.g., inanimate objects, animals, body parts), and even his capacity for conceptual thinking. In addition, investigative work has shown that there may be striking discrepancies in the capacity to name objects in the different sense modalities; a patient may show a predominantly visual anomia or a predominantly tactile anomia (cf. Spreen et al., 1966; Goodglass et al., 1968). But the assessment in most aphasia test batteries is limited to visual confrontation naming. Numerous tests of language performance have been devised in the course of linguistic research. Those with demonstrable neuropsychological significance deserve a place in the next generation of aphasia test batteries.

Under the impetus of newly developed neurodiagnostic techniques, clinicoanatomic investigation of the aphasic disorders will continue to be vigorously pursued. The implications of some recent findings have been noted. One further observation deserves mention. The newer procedures of magnetic resonance imaging and positron emission tomography very often disclose more widespread abnormality than is indicated by CT scanning (cf. Metter et al., 1981). For example, a hemispheric lesion demonstrated by CT scan may entail metabolic changes in the thalamus and a "thalamic" aphasia may entail metabolic changes in cortex or subcortex. These indications of more extensive pathology fit in well with the view that it is more useful to conceive of aphasic disorder as the product of defective neural circuity than of a focal abnormality.

Concluding Comment

This sketch of the history and present status of human neuropsychology suggests that we are in an era which promises to generate an incomparably deeper and more comprehensive knowledge than we now possess of how the brain functions to mediate cognitive and affective behavior. The more or less direct lesion–behavior correlational approach has provided the primary basis of our current knowledge of brain–behavior relations. No doubt it will continue to generate useful information. Now the far more demanding task of discovering and elucidating the cerebral mechanisms that operate on incoming information through diverse modes of processing and eventually transmute it into behavior, must be undertaken if this deeper knowledge is to be attained. To state that these mechanisms are extremely complex, and that at this time they are for the most part beyond our understanding, is to state a truism. However, an integrated effort involving the diverse disciplines that form the compound discipline of neuropsychology should be able to achieve this understanding.

References

Alajouanine T., and Lhermitte F. (1964). Non-verbal communication in aphasia. In Reuck A. V. S. O'Connor M. (ed.), *Disorders of Language*. Boston: Little, Brown and Co., pp. 168–177.

Albert M. L., Reches A., and Silverberg R. (1975). Associative visual agnosia. *Neurology* 25: 322–326.

Albert M. S., Butters N., Levin J. (1979). Temporal gradients in the retrograde amnesia of patients with alcoholic Korsakoff's disease. *Arch. Neurol. (Chicago)* 36: 211–216.

Andral G. (1840). *Clinique Médicale, 4th ed.* Paris: Fortin, Masson.

Angyal L. (1941). Thumb-mouth agnosia: special form of Gerstmann syndrome. *Confin. Neurol.* 3: 245–252.

Archibald Y. M., Wepman J. M., and Jones L. V. (1967) Nonverbal cognitive performance in aphasic and nonaphasic brain-damaged patients. *Cortex* 3: 275–294.

Arrigoni G. and De Renzi E. (1964) Constructional apraxia and hemispheric locus of lesion. *Cortex* 1: 170–197.

Babinski J. (1914). Contribution à l'étude des troubles mentaux dans l'hémiplégie organique cérébral (anosognosie). *Rev. Neurol.* 22: 845–848.

Babinski J. (1918). Anosognosie. *Rev. Neurol.* 25: 265–367.

Babinski J. (1923) Sur l'anosognosie. *Rev. Neurol.* 30: 500–503.

Bartholow R. (1874). Experimental investigations into the functions of the human brain. *Am. J. Med. Sci.* 67: 305–313.

Basso A. De Renzi E., Faglioni P., Scotti G., and Spinnler H. (1973). Neuropsychological evidence for the existence of cerebral areas critical to the performance of intelligence tests. *Brain* 96: 715–728.

Bastian H. C. (1898) *A Treatise on Aphasia and Other Speech Defects*. New York: Appleton.

Bauer R. M. (1984). Autonomic recognition of names and faces in prosopagnosia: a neuropsychological application of the Guilty Knowledge Test. *Neuropsychologia* 22: 457–469.

Bay E. (1953). Disturbances of visual perception and their examination. *Brain* 76: 173–186.

Bender M. B. and Feldman M. (1965). The so-called "visual agnosias." In *Proceedings, VIII International Congress of Neurology, Vienna*, pp. 153–156.

Benson D. F. (1967). Fluency in aphasia: correlation with radioactive scan localization. *Cortex* 3: 258–271.

Benson D. F., and Geschwind N. (1967). Shrinking retrograde amnesia. *J. Neurol. Neurosurg. Psychiatry* 30: 539–544.

Benson D. F., and Geschwind N. (1985). The aphasias and related disturbances. In Baker A. B., Joynt R. J. (eds.), *Clinical Neurology*. Hagerstown, MD: Harper & Row, Ch. 10, pp. 1–34.

Benson D. F., Sheremata W. A., Bouchard R., Segarra J. M., Price D. L., and Geschwind N. (1973). Conduction aphasia: a clinicopathological study. *Arch. Neurol. (Chicago)* 28: 339–346.

Benton A. L. (1964). Contributions to aphasia before Broca. *Cortex* 1: 40–52.

Benton A. L. (1967). Constructional apraxia and the minor hemisphere. *Confin. Neurol.* 29: 1–16.

Benton A. L. (1969). Disorders of spatial orientation. In Vinken P. J., Bruyn G. W. (eds.), *Handbook of Clinical Neurology, Vol. 3. Disorders of Higher Nervous Activity* Amsterdam: North-Holland Publishing Co., Ch. 12, pp. 212–228.

Benton A. L. (1972). The "minor" hemisphere. *J. Hist. Med. Allied Sci.* 27: 5–14.

Benton A. L. (1973). Visuoconstructive disability in patients with cerebral disease: its relationship to side of lesion and aphasic disorder. *Doc. Ophthalmol.* 34: 67–76.

Benton A. L. (1981). Aphasia: historical perspectives. In Sarno M. T. (ed.), *Acquired Aphasia*. New York: Academic Press, Ch. 1, pp. 1–25.

Benton A. L. (1985). Facial recognition 1984. In Costa L., Spreen O. (eds.), *Studies in Neuropsychology*. New York: Oxford University Press, Ch. 23, pp. 224–235.

Benton A. L., Joynt R. J. (1960). Early descriptions of aphasia. *Arch. Neurol. (Chicago)* 3: 205–222.

Benton A. L., Van Allen M. W. (1968). Impairment in facial recognition in patients with cerebral disease. *Cortex* 4: 344–358.

Benton A. L., Van Allen M. W. (1972). Prosopagnosia and facial discrimination. *J. Neurol. Sci.* 15: 167–172.

Berker E. A., Berker A. H., and Smith A. (1986). Translation of Broca's 1865 report: localization of speech in the third frontal convolution. *Arch. Neurol. (Chicago)* 43: 1065–1072.

Bianchi L. (1895). The functions of the frontal lobes. *Brain* 18: 497–522.

Bisiach E., Luzzati C., and Perani D. (1979). Unilateral neglect, representational schema and consciousness. *Brain* 102, 609–618.

Bodamer J. (1947). Die Prosop-Agnosie (die Agnosie des Physiognomieerkennungs). *Arch. Psychiatr. Nervenkr.* 179: 6–53.

Bogen J. E. (1985). The callosal syndromes. In Heilman K. M. and Valenstein E. (eds.), *Clinical Neuropsychology*, 2nd ed. New York: Oxford University Press, Ch. 11, pp. 295–338.

Bonhoeffer K. (1899). Pathologisch-anatomische Untersuchungen an Alkolholdeliranten. *Monatsschr. Psychiatr. Neurol.* 5: 265–284.

Bonhoeffer K. (1901). *Die akuten Geisteskrankheiten der Gewohnheitstrinker*. Jena: Fischer Verlag.

Boring E. G. (1950). *A History of Experimental Psychology*, 2nd ed. New York: Appleton-Century-Crofts.

Bornstein B., Sroka H., and Munitz H. (1969). Prosopagnosia with animal face agnosia. *Cortex* 5: 164–169.

Bradshaw J. L. and Nettleton N. C. (1981). The nature of hemispheric specialization in man. *Brain Behav. Sci.* 4: 51–91.

Brain W. R. (1941). Visual disorientation with special reference to lesions of the right cerebral hemisphere. *Brain* 64: 244–272.

Brierly J. B. (1966) The neuropathology of amnesic states. In Whitty C. W. M. and Zangwill O. L. (eds.), *Amnesia*. London: Butterworths, Ch. 7, pp. 150–180.

Brissaud E. (1894). Sur l'aphasie d' articulation et l'aphasie d'intonation. *Sem. Méd.* 14: 341–343.

Broca P. (1863). Localisation des fonctions cérébrales: siège du langage articulé. *Bull. Soc. Anthropol.* 4: 200–204.

Broca P. (1865). Sur la faculté du langage articulé. *Bull. Soc. Anthropol.* 6: 337–393.

Brooks D. N. and Baddeley A. D (1976). What can amnesic patients learn? *Neuropsychologia* 14: 111–122.

Bruce D. (1985). On the origin of the term 'neuropsychology'. *Neuropsychologia* 23: 813–814.

Bryden M. P. (1982). *Laterality: Functional Asymmetry in the Intact Brain*. New York: Academic Press.

Burkland C. W. and Smith A. (1977). Language and the cerebral hemispheres. *Neurology* 27: 627–633.

Cappa S. F. and Vignolo L. A. (1979). "Transcortical" features of aphasia following left thalamic hemorrhage. *Cortex* 15: 121–130.

Carmon A. and Benton A. L. (1969). Tactile perception of direction and number in patients with unilateral cerebral disease. *Neurology* 19: 525–532.

Cermak L. S. (1982). *Human Memory and Amnesia.* Hillsdale: Erlbaum.
Clarke B. and Zangwill O. L. (1965). A case of "crossed aphasia" in a dextral. *Neuropsychologia* 3: 81–86.
Clarke E. Dewhurst K. (1972). *An Illustrated History of Brain Function.* Berkeley and Los Angeles: University of California Press.
Clarke E. and O'Malley C. D. (1968). *The Human Brain and Spinal Cord.* Berkeley and Los Angeles: University of California Press.
Cohen N. (1984). Preserved learning capacity in amnesia: evidence for multiple memory systems. In Squire L. R., Butters N. (eds.), *Neuropsychology of Memory.* New York: Guilford Press, Ch. 10, pp. 83–103.
Cohen N. and Squire L. R. (1980). Preserved learning and retention of pattern analyzing skills in amnesia. *Science* 210: 207–210.
Conrad K. (1949). Über aphasische Sprachstörungen bei hirnverletzten Linkshändern. *Nervenarzt* 20: 148–154.
Critchley M. (1964). The problem of visual agnosia. *J. Neurol. Sci.* 1: 274–290.
Crosson B. (1986). On localization versus systemic effects in alcoholic Korsakoff's syndrome. *J. Clin. Exp. Neuropsychol.* 8: 744–748.
Czopf J. (1972). Ueber die Rolle der nicht dominanten Hemisphäre in der Restitution der Sprache der Aphasischen. *Arch. Psychiatr. Nervenkr.* 216, 162–171.
Damasio A. R. (1985). Prosopagnosia. *Trends Neurosci.* 8: 132–135.
Damasio A. R. and Damasio H. (1983). Localization of lesions in achromatopsia and prosopagnosia. In Kertesz A. (ed.), *Localization in Neuropsychology.* New York: Academic Press, Ch. 17, pp. 419–428.
Damasio A. R. Damasio H., and Van Hoesen G. W. (1982). Prosopagnosia: anatomic basis and behavioral mechanisms. *Neurology* 30: 1064–1071.
Damasio A. R. Damasio H., Rizzo M., Varney N., and Gersh F. (1982). Aphasia with nonhemorrhagic lesions in the basal ganglia and internal capsule. *Arch. Nuerol. (Chicago)*: 39: 15–20.
Damasio H., and Damasio A. R. (1980). The anatomical basis of conduction aphasia. *Brain* 103: 337–350.
Déjerine J. (1892). Contribution à l'étude anatomo-pathologique et clinique des différentes variétés de cécité verbale. *Mém. Soc. Biol.* 4: 61–90.
Déjerine J. (1914). *Sémiologie des Affections du Système Nerveux.* Paris: Masson.
De Renzi E. (1982). *Disorders of Space Exploration and Cognition.* New York: John Wiley.
De Renzi E. (1986). Prosopagnosia in two patients with CT scan evidence of damage confined to the right hemisphere. *Neuropsychologia* 24: 385–389.
De Renzi E., Faglioni P., and Spinnler H. (1968). The performance of patients with unilateral brain damage on face recognition tasks. *Cortex* 4: 17–34.
Douglas R. J. (1967). The hippocampus and behavior. *Psychol. Bull.* 67: 416–442.
Duffy R., Duffy J., and Pearson K. (1975). Pantomine recognition in aphasic patients. *J. Speech Hear. Res.* 18: 115–132.
Ebbinghaus H. (1885). *Ueber das Gedächtnis.* Leipzig: Duncker und Humbolt.
Ettlinger G., Jackson G. V., and Zangwill O. L. (1956). Cerebral dominance in sinistrals. *Brain* 79: 569–588.
Faust C. (1947). Partielle Seelenblindheit nach Occipitalverletzung mit besonderer Beeinträchtigung des Physiognomieerkennungs. *Nervenarzt* 18: 294–297.
Faust C. (1955). *Die zerebralen Herdstörungen bei Hinterhauptsverletzungen und ihre Beurteilung.* Stuttgart: George Thieme Verlag.
Freud S. (1891). *Zur Auffassung der Aphasien.* Leipzig und Wien: Deuticke.

Fritsch G. and Hitzig E. (1870). Ueber die elektrische Erregbarkeit des Grosshirns. *Arch. Anat. Physiol.* 37: 300–332.

Galper R. E. and Costa L. (1980). Hemispheric superiority for recognizing faces depends upon how they are learned. *Cortex* 16: 27–38.

Gamper E. (1928). Zur Frage der Polioencephalitis haemorrhagica der chronischen Alkoholiker: Anatomische Befunde beim alkoholischen Korsakoff und ihre Beziehungen zum klinischen Bild. *Dtsch. Z. Nervenheilkd.* 102: 122–129.

Gazzaniga M. S. (1970). *The Bisected Brain.* New York: Appleton-Century-Crofts.

Gelb A. and Goldstein K. (1920). *Psychologische Analysen hirnpathologischer Fälle.* Leipzig: Barth. 1920.

Gerstmann J. (1924). Fingeragnoise: eine umschriebene Störung der Orientierung am eigenen Körper. *Wien. Klin. Wochenschr.* 37: 1010–1012.

Gerstmann J. (1930). Zur Symptomatologie der Hirnläsionen im Uebergangsgebiet der unteren Parietal-und mittleren Occipital-windung. *Nervenarzt* 3: 691–695.

Geschwind N. (1965). Disconnexion syndromes in animals and man. *Brain* 88: 237–294, 585–644.

Geschwind N. (1967). Wernicke's contribution to the study of aphasia. *Cortex* 3: 449–463.

Geschwind J. and Levitsky W. (1968). Human brain: left-right asymmetries in temporal speech region. *Science* 161: 186–187.

Goldstein K. (1924). Das Wesen der amnestischen Aphasie. *Schweiz. Arch. Neurol. Psychiatr.* 15: 163–175.

Goodglass A., Barton M., and Kaplan E. (1968). Sensory modality and object naming in aphasia. *J. Speech Hear. Res.* 11: 488–496.

Goodglass H., Gleason J. B., Hyde M. (1970). Some dimensions of auditory language comprehension in aphasia. *J. Speech Hear. Res.* 13: 595–606.

Goodglass H., and Quadfasel F. A. (1954). Language literality in left-handed aphasics. *Brain*: 77, 521–548.

Goodglass H., Quadfasel F. A., and Timberlake W. H. (1964). Phrase length and type and severity of aphasia. *Cortex* 1: 133–153.

Graff-Radford H. R., Eslinger P. J., Damasio A. R., and Yamada T. (1984) Nonhemorrhagic infarction of the thalamus; behavioral anatomic and physiologic correlates. *Neurology* 34: 14–23.

Gudden H. (1896) Klinische und anatomische Beiträge zur Kenntnis der multiplen Alkoholneuritis nebst Bemerkungen über die Regenerationsvorgänge im peripheren Nervensystem. *Arch. Psychiatr. Nervenkr.* 28: 643–741.

Gur R. C., Gur R. E., Rosen A. D., Warach S., Alavi A., Greenberg J., and Reivich M. (1983). A cognitive-motor network demonstrated by positron emission tomography. *Neuropsychologia* 21: 601–606.

Hamsher K. (1981). Intelligence and aphasia. In Sarno M. T. (ed.), *Acquired Aphasia.* New York: Academic Press, Ch. 11, pp. 327–359.

Hamsher K. Levin H. S., Benton A. L. (1979). Facial recognition in patients with focal brain lesions. *Arch. Neurol. (Chicago)* 36: 837–839. 1979.

Harnad S. (1977). *Lateralization in the Nervous System.* New York: Academic Press.

Head H. (1926). *Aphasia and Kindred Disorders of Speech.* London: Cambridge University Press.

Hebb D. O. (1949). *The Organization of Behavior.* New York: Wiley.

Hécaen H. (1969). Essai de dissociation du syndrome de l'aphasie sensorielle. *Rev. Neurol. (Paris)* 120: 229–231. 1969.

Hécaen H., Ajuriaguerra J. (1945). L'apraxie de l'habillage. *Encéphale* 35: 113–143.

Hécaen H., and Angelergues R. (1962). Agnosia for faces (prosopagnosia). *Arch. Neurol. (Chicago)* 7: 92–100.

Hécaen H., Ajuriaguerra J., and Massonet J. (1951). Les troubles visuoconstructives par lésion pariéto-occipitale droite. *Encéphale* 40: 122–179.

Hécaen H. and Albert M. (1978). *Human Neuropsychology*. New York: John Wiley.

Hécaen H. and Consoli S. (1973). Analyse des troubles du langage au cours des lésions de l'aire de Broca. *Neuropsychologia*: 11, 377–388.

Hécaen H., Goldblum M. C., Masure M. C., and Ramier A. M. (1974). Une nouvelle observation d'agnosie d'objet: déficit de l'association ou de la catégorisation, spécifique de la modalité visuelle? *Neuropsychologia* 12: 447–464.

Heilman K. M. and Valenstein E. (1972). Frontal lobe neglect in man. *Neurology* 22: 660–664.

Heilman K. M. and Valenstein E. (1979). Mechanisms underlying hemispatial neglect. *Ann. Neurol.* 5: 166–170.

Heilman K. M., Schwartz and H. D., Watson R. T. Hypoarousal in patients with the neglect syndrome and emotional indifference. *Neurology* 28: 229–232.

Heilman K. M., Rothi L., Campanella D., and Wolfson S. (1979). Wernicke's and global aphasia without alexia. *Arch. Neurol. (Chicago)* 36: 129–133.

Hier D. B. and Mohr J P. (1977). Incongruous oral and written naming. *Brain Lang.* 4: 115–126.

Hilliard R. D. (1973). Hemispheric laterality effects on a facial recognition task in normal subjects. *Cortex* 9: 246–258.

Hoffmann H. (1885). Stereognostische Versuche. *Dtsch. Arch. Klin. Med.* 36: 398–426.

Hubel D. H. and Wiesel T. N. (1965). Receptive fields and functional architecture in two nonstriate visual areas (18 and 19) of the cat. *J. Neurophysiol.* 28: 229–289.

Hubel D. H. and Wiesel T. H. (1968). Receptive fields and functional architecture of monkey striate cortex. J. Physiol. 195: 215–243.

Humphrey M. E. and Zangwill O. L. (1952). Dysphasia in left-handed patients with unilateral brain lesions. *J. Neurol. Neurosurg. Psychiatry.* 15: 184–193.

Huppert F. A., and Piercy M. Recognition memory in amnesic patients. *Cortex* 12: 3–20.

Huppert F. A. and Piercy M. (1979). Normal and abnormal forgetting in amnesia: effect of locus of lesion. *Cortex* 15: 385–390.

Isserlin M. (1932). Ueber Sprache und Sprechen. *Nervenarzt* 5: 1–7.

Jackson H. J. (1878). On affections of speech from disease of the brain. *Brain* 1: 304–330.

Kennedy F. (1916). Stock-brainedness, the causation factor in the so-called "crossed aphasias." *Am. J. Med. Sci.* 6: 849–859.

Kerchensteiner M., Poeck K., and Brunner F. (1972). The fluency-nonfluency dimension in the classification of aphasic speech. *Cortex* 8: 233–247.

Kertesz A. (1983). *Localization in Neuropsychology*. New York: Academic Press.

Kertesz A., Harlock W., and Coates R. (1979). Computer tomographic localization, lesion size and prognosis in aphasia and nonverbal impairment. *Brain Lang.* 8: 34–50.

Kinsbourne M. (1971). The minor cerebral hemisphere as a source of aphasic speech. *Arch. Neurol. (Chicago)* 25: 302–306.

Kleist K. (1923). Kriegsverletzungen des Gehirns in ihrer Bedeutung für die Hirnlokalisation und Hirnpathologie. In Von Schjerning O (ed.), *Handbuch der ärtzlichen Erfahrung im Weltkriege, 1914/1918, Bd IV, Geistes-und Nervenkrankheiten*. Leipzig: Barth, pp. 1343–1369.

Kleist K. (1934). *Gehirnpathologie*. Leipzig: Barth.

Knopman D. S., Selnes O. A., and Niccum N., (1983). A longitudinal study of speech fluency in aphasia. *Neurology* 33: 1170–1178.

Landis T., Cummings J. L., Christen L., Bogen J. E., and Imhof H. G. (1986). Are unilateral right posterior cerebral lesions sufficient to cause prosopagnosia? Clinical and radiological findings in six additional patients. *Cortex* 22: 243–252.

Lashley K. S. (1950). In search of the engram. *Symp. Soc. Exp. Biol.* 4: 454–482.

Lebrun Y., and Hoops R. (1974). *Intelligence and Aphasia*. Amsterdam: Swets & Zeitlinger.

Levin H. S., Peters B. S. and Hulkonen D. A. (1983). Early concepts of anterograde and retrograde amnesia. *Cortex* 19: 427–440.

Levin H. S., High W. M., Meyers C. A., Von Laufen A., Hayden M. E. and Eisenberg H. M. (1985). Impairment of remote memory after closed head injury. *J. Neurol. Neurosurg. Psychiatry* 48: 556–563.

Levine D. N. and Mohr J. P. (1979). Language after bilateral cerebral infarctions: role of the minor hemisphere in speech. *Neurology* 29: 927–938.

Levine D. N., Warach J., and Farah M. (1985). Two visual systems in mental imagery: dissociation of "what" and "where" in imagery disorders due to bilateral posterior cerebral lesions. *Neurology* 35: 1010–1018.

Lewandowsky M. (1908). Ueber Abspaltung des Farbensinnes. *Monatschr. Psychiatr. Neurol.* 23: 488–510.

Lezak M. D. (1983). *Neuropsychological Assessment*, 2nd ed. New York: Oxford University Press.

Lhermitte F. and Signoret J-L. (1972). Analyse neuropsychologique et differciation des syndromes amnésiques. *Rev. Neurol. (Paris)* 126: 161–178.

Lhermitte F., Chain F., Escourolle R., Ducarne B., and Dillon B. (1972). Étude anatomicclinique d'un cas de prosopagnosie. *Rev. Neurol. (Paris)* 126: 329–346.

Lichtheim L. (1885). On aphasia. *Brain* 7: 433–485 [originally published in *Dtsch. Arch. Klin. Med.* 36: 204–268, 1885].

Liepmann H. (1900). Das Krankheitsbild der Apraxie (motorischen Asymbolie). *Monatsschr. Psychiatr. Neurol.* 8: 15–44, 102–132, 182–197.

Lissauer H. (1890). Ein Fall von Seelenblindheit nebst einen Beitrag zur Theorie derselben. *Arch. Psychiatr. Nervenkr.* 21: 222–270.

Loeb J. (1886). Beiträge zur Physiologie des Grosshirns. *Pflügers Arch. Gesamte Physiol. Menschen. Tiere.* 39: 265–346.

Lotmar F. (1933). Zur Pathophysiologie der erschwerten Wortfindung bei Aphasischen. *Schweiz. Arch. Neurol. Psychiatr.* 30, 86–158, 322–379.

Luria A. R. (1970). *Traumatic Aphasia*. The Hague: Mouton.

Luria A. R., Karpov B. A., and Yarbuss A. L. (1966). Disturbances of active visual perception with lesions of the frontal lobes. *Cortex* 2: 202–212.

Mack J. L. and Boller F. (1977). Associative visual agnosia and its related deficits: the role of the minor hemisphere in assigning meaning to visual perception. *Neuropsychologia* 15: 345–349.

Marie P. (1906). Revision de la question de l'aphasie. *Sem. Méd.* 26: 241–247, 493–500, 565–571.

Mazzocchi F. and Vignolo L. A. (1979). Localization of lesions in aphasia: clinical CT scan localization in stroke patients. *Cortex* 15: 627–654.

McFie J., Piercy M. F., and Zangwill O. L. (1950). Visual-spatial agnosia associated with lesions of the right cerebral hemisphere. *Brain* 73: 167–190.

McGlone J. (1980). Sex differences in human brain asymmetry: a critical survey. *Behav: Brain Sci.* 3: 215–263.

Meadows J. C. (1974). The anatomical basis of prosopagnosia. *J. Neurol. Neurosurg. Psychiatry* 37: 489–501.

Mendez M. F. and Benson D. F. (1985). Atypical conduction aphasia: a disconnection syndrome. *Arch. Neurol. (Chicago)* 42: 886–891.

Mesulam M. M. (1981). A cortical network for directed attention and unilateral neglect. *Ann. Neurol.* 10: 733–755.

Metter E. J. Wasterlain C. G., Kuhl D. E., Hanson W. R., Phelps M. E. (1981). FDG positron emission computed tomography in a study of aphasia. *Ann. Neurol.* 10: 173–183.

Meunier M. (1924). *Histoire de la Médicine*. Paris: LeFrancois.

Meyer A. (1971). *Historical Aspects of Cerebral Anatomy*. London: Oxford University Press.

Meyer J. S., Sakai M., Yamaguchi F., Yamamoto M., and Shaw T. (1980). Regional changes in cerebral blood flow during standard behavioral activation in patients with disorders of speech and mentation compared to normal volunteers. *Brain Lang.* 9: 61–77.

Meynert T. (1867). Der Bau der Grosshirnrinde und seine örtlichen Verschiedenheiten. *Vierteljahresschr. Psychiatr.* 1: 77–93, 126–170, 198–217.

Milner B. (1958). Psychological defects produced by temporal lobe excisions. *Proc. Assoc. Nerv. Ment. Dis.* 36: 244–257.

Milner. B. (1962). Laterality effects in audition. In Mountcastle V. B. (ed.), *Interhemispheric Relations and Cerebral Dominance*. Baltimore: John Hopkins Press, Ch. 9, pp. 171–195.

Milner B. (1973). Hemispheric specialization: scope and limits. In Schmidt F. O. and Worden F. G. (eds.), *The Neurosciences: Third Study Program*. Boston: MIT Press, Ch. 8, pp. 75–87.

Milner B., Branch C., and Rasmussen T. (1966). Evidence for bilateral speech representation in some non-righthanders. *Trans. Am. Neurol. Assoc.* 91: 306–308.

Mishkin M. (1982). A memory system in the monkey. *Philos. Trans. R. Soc. London Ser. B* 298: 85–95.

Mohr J. P. (1983). Thalamic lesions and syndromes. In Kertesz A. (ed.), *Localization in Neuropsychology*. New York: Academic Press, Ch. 11, p. 269–293.

Mohr J. P., Pessin M. S., Finkelstein S., Funkenstein H. H., Duncan G. W., and Davis K. R: Broca's aphasia: pathological and clinical aspects. *Neurology* 28: 311–324.

Monrad-Krohn G. H. (1947). Dysprosody or altered melody of language. *Brain* 70: 405–415.

Morlaas J. (1928). *Contribution à la Étude de l'Apraxie*. Thesis. Paris.

Moutier F. (1908). *L'Aphasie de Broca*. Paris: G. Steinheil.

Munk H. (1878). Weitere Mitteilungen zur Physiologie der Grosshirnrinde. *Arch. Anat. Physiol.* 2: 162–178.

Munk H. (1890). *Über die Funktionen der Grosshirnrinde*. Berlin: August Hirschwald.

Naeser M. A. (1983). CT scan lesion size and lesion locus in cortical and subcortical aphasias. In Kertesz A. (ed.), *Localization in Neuropsychology*. New York: Academic Press, Ch. 3, pp. 63–119.

Naeser M. A. and Hayward R. W. (1978). Correlation between CT scan findings and the Boston Diagnostic Aphasia Exam. *Neurology* 28: 545–551.

Newcombe F. (1969). *Missile Wounds of the Brain: A Study of Psychological Deficits*. London: Oxford University Press.

Nielsen J. M. (1962). *Agnosia, Apraxia, Agnosia: Their Value in Cerebral Localization, 2nd ed.* New York: Hafner Publishing Company.

Ojemann R. G. (1966). Correlation between specific brain lesions and memory changes. *Neurosci. Res. Program Bull.* 4, Suppl.: 1–51.

Pagel W. (1958). Medieval and Renaissance contributions to knowledge of the brain and its functions. In Poynter F. N. L. (ed.), *The Brain and its Functions.* Oxford: Blackwell, pp. 95–114.

Paterson A. and Zangwill O. L. (1944). Disorders of visual space perception associated with lesions of the right cerebral hemisphere. *Brain* 67: 331–358.

Pearson G. H. J, Alpers B. J., and Weisenburg T. (1928). Aphasia: a study of normal control cases. *Arch. Neurol. Psychiatry* 19: 281–295.

Perret D. I., Rolls E. T., and Caan A. W. (1982). Visual neurones responsive to faces in the monkey temporal cortex. *Exp. Brain Res.* 47: 329–342.

Pick A. (1908). *Ueber Störungen der Orientierung am eigenen Körper. Arb. Dtsch. Psychiatr. Univ. Klin. Prag.* Berlin: Karger.

Pitres A. (1895). Étude sur l'aphasie chez les polyglottes. *Rev. Méd.* 15: 873–899.

Pitres A. (1898). *L'Aphasie Amnésique et ses Variétés Cliniques.* Paris: Alcan.

Polyak S. (1955). *The Vertebrate Visual System.* Chicago: University of Chicago Press.

Poppelreuter W. (1923). Zur Psychologie und Pathologie der optischen Wahrnehmung. *Z. Gesamte Neurol. Psychiatr.* 83: 26–152.

Prins R., Snow C., and Wagenaar E. (1978). Recovery from aphasia: spontaneous speech versus language comprehension. *Brain Lang.* 6: 192–211.

Ribot T. (1882). *Diseases of Memory.* London: Kegan Paul, Trench.

Rubens A. B. (1976). Transcortical motor aphasia. In Whitaker H., Whitaker H. A. (eds.) *Studies in Neurolinguistics*, Vol. 1. New York: Academic Press, Ch. 9, pp. 293–303.

Rubens A. B. and Benson D. F.: Associative visual agnosia. *Arch. Neurol. (Chicago)* 24: 304–316.

Rubens A. B. and Kertesz A. (1983). The localization of the lesions in transcortical aphasias. In Kertesz A (ed.), *Localization in Neuropsychology.* New York: Academic Press, Ch. 10, pp. 245–268.

Russell W. R. and Nathan P. W. (1946). Traumatic amnesia. *Brain* 69: 183–187.

Schiller F. (1965). The rise of the "enteroid process" in the 19th century: some landmarks in cerebral nomenclature. *Bull. Hist. Med.* 39: 326–338.

Scoville W. B. and Milner B. (1957). Loss of recent memory after bilateral hippocampal lesions. *J. Neurol. Neurosurg. Psychiatry* 20: 11–21.

Seltzer B. and Benson D. F. (1974). The temporal pattern of retrograde amnesia in Korsakoff's disease. *Neurology* 24: 527–530.

Sittig O. (1921). Störungen im Verhalten gegenüber Farben bei Aphasischen. *Monatsschr. Psychiatr. Neurol.* 49: 63–68. 169–187.

Smith A. (1966). Speech and other functions after left (dominant) hemispherectomy. *J. Neurol. Neurosurg. Psychiatry* 29: 467–471.

Soury J. (1899). *Le Système Nerveux Central.* Paris: Carré et Naud,

Spreen O., Benton A. L., and Van Allen M. W. (1966). Dissociation of visual and tactile naming in amnesic aphasia. *Neurology* 16: 807–814.

Springer S. P. and Deutsch G. (1985). *Left Brain, Right Brain.* New York: W. H. Freeman.

Squire L. R. (1980). The anatomy of amnesia. *Trends Neurosci.* 3: 52–54.

Squire L. R. and Butters N. (1984). *Neuropsychology of Memory.* New York: Guilford Press.

St. John R. C. (1981). Lateral asymmetry in face perception. *Can. J. Psychol.* 35: 213–223.

Strauss H. (1924). Über konstruktive Apraxie. *Monatsschr. Psychiatr. Neurol.* 56: 65–124.

Taylor A. and Warrington E. K. (1971). Visual agnosia: a single case report. *Cortex* 7: 152–164.

Tonkonogy J. and Goodglass H. (1981). Language function, foot of the third frontal gyrus, and Rolandic operculum. *Arch. Neurol. (Chicago)* 38: 486–490.

Tranel D. and Damasio A. R. (1985). Knowledge without awareness: an autonomic index of facial recognition by prosopagnosics. *Science* 228: 1453–1454.

Tulving E. (1972). Episodic and semantic memory. In Tulving E, Donaldson W. (eds.), *Organization of Memory*. New York: Academic Press, pp. 382–403.

Ungerleider L. G. and Mishkin M. (1982). Two cortical visual systems. In Ingle D. J., Goodale M. A., and Mansfield M. A. (eds.), *Analysis of Visual Behavior*. Cambridge, MA: MIT Press, Ch. 18, pp. 549–586.

Varney N. R. (1978). Linguistic correlates of pantomime recognition. *J. Neurol. Neurosurg. Psychiatry* 41: 564–568.

Varney N. R. and Benton A. L. (1982). Qualitative aspects of pantomime recognition defects in aphasia. *Brain Cogn.* 1: 132–139.

Victor M. and Yakovlev P. I. (1955). S. S. Korsakoff's psychic disorder in conjunction with peripheral neuritis: a translation of Korsakoff's original contribution with brief comments on the author and his contribution to clinical medicine. *Neurology* 5: 394–406.

Vignolo L. A. (1969). Auditory agnosia: a review and report of recent evidence. In Benton A. L. (ed.), *Contributions to Clinical Neuropsychology*. Chicago: Aldine Publishing Co., Ch. 7, pp. 172–208.

Von Kuenberg M. (1930). Zuordnungsversuche bei Gesunden und Sprachgestörten. *Arch. Gesamte Psychol.* 76: 257–352.

Wagenaar E., Snow C., and Prins R. (1975). Spontaneous speech of aphasic patients: a psycholinguistic analysis. *Brain Lang.* 2: 281–303.

Walsh K. W. (1978). *Neuropsychology: A Clinical Approach. Edinburgh*: Churchill Livingstone.

Warrington E. K. and James M. (1967). An experimental investigation of facial recognition in patients with unilateral lesions. *Cortex* 3: 317–326.

Warrington E. K. and Sanders H. I. (1971). The fate of old memories. *Q. J. Exp. Psychol.* 23: 432–442.

Watson R. H. and Heilman K. M. (1979). Thalamic neglect. *Neurology* 29: 690–694.

Weisenburg T. and McBride K. E. (1935) *Aphasia: A Clinical and Psychological Study.* New York: Commonwealth Fund.

Wernicke C. (1874). *Der aphasische Symptomencomplex*. Breslau: Cohn und Weigert.

Wernicke C. (1866). Einige neuere Arbeiten über Aphasie. *Fortschr. Med.* 4: 371–377.

Wernicke C. (1895) Zwei Fälle von Rindenläsion. *Arb. Psychiatr. Klin. Breslau* 2: 33–53.

Whitely A. M. and Warrington E. K. (1977). Prosopagnosia: a clinical psychological and anatomical study of three patients. *J. Neurol. Neurosurg. Psychiatry* 40: 395–403.

Wilbrand H. (1887). *Die Seelenblindheit als Herderscheinung und ihre Beziehungen zur homonymen Hemianopsie*. Wiesbaden: JF Bergmann.

Wilbrand H. (1892). Ein Fail von Seelenblindheit und Hemianopsie mit Sektionsbefund. *Dtsch. Z. Nervenheilk.* 2: 361–387.

Winocur G. (1984). Memory localization in the brain. In Squire L. R. Butters N. (eds.), *Neuropsychology of Memory*. New York: Guilford Press, Ch. 13, pp. 122–133.

Young A. W. (1983). *Functions of Right Cerebral Hemisphere*. London: Academic Press.

Zaidel E. (1977). Unilateral auditory language comprehension on the Token Test following cerebral commissurotomy and hemispherectomy. *Neuropsychologia* 15: 1–18.

Zangwill O. L. (1964). Intelligence in aphasia. In Reuck. A. V. S. O'Conner M. (eds.) *Disorders of Language*. Boston: Little, Brown and Co., pp. 261–274.

Zangwill O. L. (1969). Intellectual status in aphasia. In Vinken P. J. and Bruyn G. W. (eds.), *Handbook of Clinical Neurology*, Vol. 4. *Disorders of Speech, Perception and Symbolic Behavior* Amsterdam: North-Holland Publishing Co., Ch. 6, pp. 105–111.

Zeki S. M. (1980). Representation of colours in the cerebral cortex. *Nature (London)* 284: 412–418.

Zeki S. M. (1982). Do wavelength cells in monkey striate cortex respond to colour? *J. Physiol. (London)* 330: 57–58.

Zola-Morgan S. (1984). Toward an animal model of human amnesia: some critical issues. In Squire L. R., Butters N. (eds.), *Neuropsychology of Memory*. New York: Guilford Press, Ch. 30, pp. 316--329.

2

Four Neuropsychologists

When Hal Kløve did me the honor of asking me to give a talk on some aspects of the history of neuropsychology at this anniversary meeting, I accepted his generous invitation with sincere appreciation and much pleasure. When I came to consider the choice of a topic, I thought that a sketch of the evolution of our discipline, charting the major achievements and the development of influential concepts since Broca made his momentous discovery in the 1860s, would be an appropriate theme. However, on further reflection, I concluded that this celebratory occasion called for an account that was more personal in nature and one that was closer to home. I therefore decided (not unwisely, I hope) to consider the achievements of four of our fellow neuropsychologists, each of whom made an enormously significant contribution to the form and content of the field of neuropsychology as we know it today. Their names are familiar to all of us. Many of us knew one or more of them personally. Some of us were their close friends. They are Henry Hécaen, Oliver Zangwill, Hans-Lukas Teuber, and Norman Geschwind. I intend to review their careers, evaluate their work and influence, and consider the debt that we owe to them.

Three of them (the exception being Geschwind) began their careers as neuropsychologists during the years of World War II. A brief look at the status of human and clinical neuropsychology in 1939 may be useful as a backdrop against which to assess their contributions.

It was a field that engaged the interest of only a few neurologists, psychiatrists, and psychologists. Kurt Goldstein had elaborated his distinctive concepts of the nature of brain–behavior relationships, and Karl Kleist had published his

---

Reprinted with permission from Kluwer Academic/Plenum Publishers, *Neuropsychology Review*, Vol. 4, No. 1, 1994.

Adapted from a lecture at the 1987 meeting of the International Neuropsychological Society, Washington, D.C., to commemorate the fifteenth anniversary of the emergence of the society as a major organization. The style of the original oral presentation has been retained.

monumental volume on wartime brain injuries. Goldstein's ideas had gained some currency abroad but were largely rejected in Germany. Kleist's localizationist approach was accepted in Germany but was practically unknown outside of that country. In any case, given the antilocalizationist bias generated by the findings and conclusions of Franz, Lashley, and Head, it probably would not have received a warm reception in the United States or Britain. Carlyle Jacobsen's observations on the effects of prefrontal ablation in monkeys and the introduction of prefrontal leucotomy by Moniz had aroused intense interest in the question of the behavioral significance of the frontal lobes. The field of aphasia was still dominated by the controversy between the "holists" (Jackson, Marie, Head) and the "diagram makers" (Wernicke, Bastian, Dejerine) about the nature and neurological basis of the aphasic disorders. In the United States and Britain, at least, there had been a definite waning of interest in the anatomic aspects of aphasia. The concept of complementary hemispheric specialization had yet to be taken seriously (cf. Benton, 1972). The men whose lives and achievements are the subject of this presentation made decisively important contributions to the enhanced understanding of each of these issues.

Henry Hécaen

Henry Hécaen was born in Brittany in 1912. He was a true Breton, independent, strong-willed, stubborn—traits that on more than one occasion caused him to be at odds with the French medical establishment. After taking the M.D. degree in Bordeaux, he went to Paris for training in neurology and psychiatry where his chief mentor was Jean Lhermitte, one of France's most distinguished neurologists of that period. A productive clinical researcher and prolific writer, Lhermitte himself had significant neuropsychological interests that were reflected in his studies of aphasia, constructional apraxia, disorders of the body image, and visuoperceptive disabilities. Hécaen always spoke of him with respect and admiration and no doubt Lhermitte's interest in brain–behavior relationships influenced the direction of Hécaen's future work as it did that of his fellow student, Julien de Ajuriaguerra, who later was his close collaborator.

An early paper (Cénac and Hécaen, 1943), written during the stressful years of World War II, when Hécaen was engaged in private practice and at the same time was also participating actively in the French Resistance against the Nazi occupation, dealt with the neuropsychological significance of systematic reversal of right–left orientation in children. It was a pioneer study of the topic that I discovered some 15 years later when I encountered the same phenomenon (Benton, 1958).

The end of World War II freed Hécaen to devote his energies to the practice

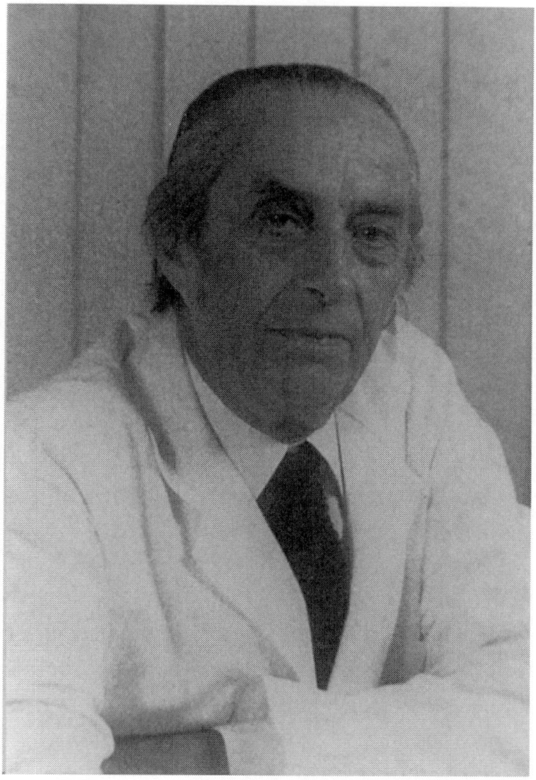

FIGURE **2.1.** Henry Hécaen, 1912–1983.

of neurology and to neuropsychological research. He and Ajuriaguerra set out to write a monumental volume on the cerebral cortex with major emphasis on the cognitive, perceptual, and emotional changes associated with brain disease (Ajuriaguerra and Hécaen, 1949). The book, which was dedicated to Jean Lhermitte, provided a comprehensive summary of what was then known about brain–behavior relationships in health and disease. Its influence on the direction of research in neurological centers in France was quite evident. As Martin Albert (1984) has written, "It opened the field of neuropsychology before the term existed" in that country. The book went through several printings and a second edition was published in 1960. Regrettably, it was not translated into English; an English version would have been of enormous value as a stimulus and a guide to American and British neurologists and psychologists in the 1950s as they embarked on research in neuropsychology. A monograph on disturbances of the body schema authored by Hécaen and Ajuriaguerra appeared in 1952. Presenting a detailed analysis of the diverse defects in perception and action associated with this concept, it provided a useful framework for further research. In 1956, Hécaen and Ajuriaguerra again collaborated in a study of the mental changes associated with brain tumors.

Valuable as these monographic contributions were, Hécaen's research on hemispheric cerebral dominance during this period surpassed them in importance. In the 1940s and 1950s, at a time when the prevailing concept of hemispheric dominance was that it meant simply the "dominance" of the left hemisphere in the mediation of language, praxis and abstract thought, he and his co-workers generated an irrefutable mass of evidence that the right, supposedly "minor," hemisphere played a crucial role in the mediation of visuoperceptual and visuoconstructional processes (Hécaen and Ajuriaguerra, 1945; Hécaen et al., 1951; Hécaen et al., 1956). As we shall see, Oliver Zangwill in Britain was concurrently pursuing the same line of research and advancing the same conclusion. In any case, if Hécaen had done nothing further in the field, his demonstrations of the functional properties of the right hemisphere would have earned him an enduring place in the history of neuropsychology for they left an indelible mark on subsequent formulations of the organization of cerebral function.

His work continued and steadily expanded in scope. With his co-workers and students, he explored almost every aspect of neuropsychology. He continued his investigations of hemispheric cerebral dominance, which resulted in a comprehensive definition of the distinctive constellation of deficits preferentially associated with disease of the right hemisphere. There followed a series of studies involving hundreds of patients with focal brain lesions that sought to identify the locus of the lesions associated with diverse cognitive and perceptuomotor defects such as topographical disorientation, dyspraxia for dressing, acalculia, body schema disturbances, constructional apraxia, and impairment in writing (cf. Galtier, 1984). His analyses led to useful classification of types of disability as, for example, his division of the acalculias into spatial, aphasic, and anarithmetic types, each type being predominantly associated with lesions at particular sites and having distinctive behavioral correlates (Hécaen et al., 1961).

Hécaen undertook many studies in the field of aphasia and he was a pioneer in the linguistic approach to the analysis of the aphasic disorders. For the most part, his work was published in various neurological, neuropsychological, and linguistic journals, but at least some of it was summarized in a monograph on language pathology (Hécaen and Angelergues, 1965) and in his book, *Human Neuropsychology*, co-authored with Martin Albert, which appeared in 1978. His paper on prosopagnosia (Hécaen and Angelergues, 1962) went a long way toward convincing American clinicians that this odd complaint reflected a genuine neuropsychological disability and was not, as some maintained, an hysterical phenomenon. Finally, one must mention his interest in laterality and the neuropsychological implications of left-handedness. He and Ajuriaguerra wrote a monograph on left-handedness (Hécaen and Ajuriaguerra, 1963), a theme to which he returned 20 years later (Hécaen, 1984).

One factor that permitted Hécaen to undertake so many large-scale studies was the circumstance that he was the attending neurologist at the large neurosurgical unit of the Hôpital Sainte-Anne in Paris and thus had access to the material from that unit as well as from the neurological clinic at Sainte-Anne. In addition, as his expertise became known, physicians throughout France and abroad referred patients to him for evaluation, and some of these proved to be particularly interesting for research purposes.

However, the beginning of his own unit was very modest indeed. In 1950, when he received a half-time appointment as a neurologist, in the neurosurgical clinic (the other half-time being taken up with private practice), he was a one-man show. But his unit grew steadily in size and importance, and in due course, he was able to give up private practice and devote almost full time to research, writing, and editing. As everyone knows, he was the founder and editor of *Neuropsychologia*. His research program attracted many students on both the predoctoral and postdoctoral levels, as well as many visiting scientists. He directed at least a score of doctoral dissertations. Among the neurologists who worked with him were Martin Albert, Gilbert Assal, Jason Brown, Carlos Mendilaharsu, and Athanase Tsavaras. Among the neuropsychologists who spent extended periods of time in his unit were Harold Goodglass, Malcolm Piercy, and myself.

Oliver Louis Zangwill

Oliver Zangwill was a quite different sort of person—quiet, gentle, and given to understatement. He was born in Sussex in 1913 and studied psychology under Frederic Bartlett at the University of Cambridge where he took the B.A. and M.A. degrees. Following the example of an older generation of English scholars (including Bartlett), he saw no necessity to work for the Ph.D. degree.

From 1935 to 1939, Zangwill held an appointment as a research student in the Cambridge laboratory. During this period, he published a number of detailed experimental studies on memory and learning designed to evaluate competing theories about the basic processes involved in recognition and reproduction. The reports disclose a first-rate mind at work as experimental findings are compared to different theoretical formulations, as well as a remarkably detailed knowledge of the history of psychological thought. This last characteristic was especially evident in his lengthy review in the *British Journal of Psychology* of Charles Spearman's two-volume history, *Psychology Down the Ages*, in which the young man showed a masterful grasp of the basic philosophic issues with which psychology has had to grapple over the centuries. That Bartlett, who was editior of

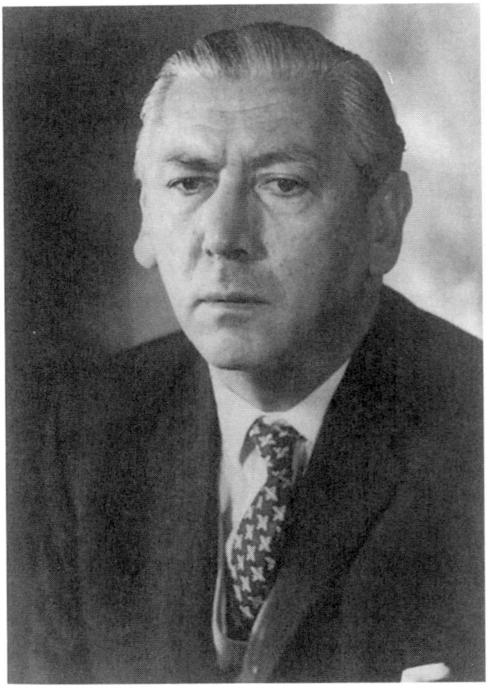

FIGURE **2.2.** Oliver Zangwill, 1913–1987.

the journal, entrusted this important and delicate assignment to a 24-year-old student indicates how highly he regarded Zangwill.

In these early years, Zangwill was concerned primarily with experimental-theoretical questions that had little bearing on neuropsychological issues. One exception was a lengthy critical analysis by Oldfield and Zangwill (1942–43 a, b) of the concept of schemata as applied by the neurologist, Henry Head, to somatosensory and somatoperceptual performances. R. C. Oldfield, a fellow student and close friend of Zangwill, was the senior author of this paper that pointed out the ambiguities inherent in the concept of schemata and its limited value for explaining the somatoperceptual deficits shown by patients with brain lesions. Frederic Bartlett had adopted Head's concept in his own studies and had postulated the operation of schemata in the processes of learning and remembering. Thus, to a degree, Oldfield and Zangwill were also criticizing the formulations of their mentor. But this was nothing new. As it happens, when, in his earlier experimental work, Zangwill had concluded that Bartlett's formulations were less than adequate, his mentor raised no objections. Later, Zangwill (1978) was to write about Bartlett's "strong, yet gentle, personality and his exceptional tolerance and modesty."

World War II transformed Zangwill into a clinical neuropsychologist. Working in the Edinburgh Brain Injury Unit of the British military services, he was called upon to evaluate hundreds of patients with traumatic brain lesions. It was here that he made his first contributions to the field. Finding that some patients with undoubted defects in learning and memory nevertheless performed adequately on the conventional digit span test, he devised a supraspan test requiring the patients to learn a series of digits longer than his span and found this test to be a more sensitive measure of short-term learning (Zangwill, 1943). Thus, he originated the serial digit learning procedure (supraspan) that was adopted by clinical investigators decades later (cf. Drachman and Arbit, 1966; Hamsher et al., 1980).

A second, more basic, contribution was his demonstration of the close association between visuospatial impairments and lesions in the posterior area of the right hemisphere (Paterson and Zangwill, 1944), a study that proved to be the precursor of a major program of clinical research undertaken after the war. Still another study described and evaluated the application of the Rey-Davis test of nonverbal learning in the assessment of brain-lesioned patients (Zangwill, 1946a). A final study dealt with verbal learning in some 200 patients with diseases or traumatic injury of the brain (Zangwill, 1946b). Once again, he found digit span performance to be generally adequate in nonaphasic patients, including those with frank amnesic syndromes. In contrast, digit span was impaired in apparently fully recovered aphasic patients. Confirming the World War I results of the German neurologist, Max Isserlin, he found defects in verbal learning to be extraordinarily frequent in nonaphasic patients and practically universal in those with a history of aphasic disorder. The paper concluded with a discussion of the implications of the results for both diagnostic evaluation and rehabilitation planning.

After the war, Zangwill went to Oxford as a lecturer and assistant director of the Psychological Laboratory. In 1952, he was called to Cambridge to succeed Bartlett as Professor of Psychology and Director of the Psychological Laboratory. At the same time, he established an association with the National Hospital for Nervous Disorders, Queen Square, where he served as a visiting psychologist. Working at Queen Square and other London hospitals, he initiated a series of studies of the cognitive defects associated with focal brain disease. In the 1950s and 1960s, the Zangwill group, which included George Ettlinger, John McFie, Malcolm Piercy, Elizabeth Warrington, and Maria Wyke, generated a substantial body of information on the nature of the perceptual and cognitive consequences of brain disease that significantly advanced the development of the emerging field of clinical neuropsychology.

Of course, his research extended beyond the issue of the deficits associated with unilateral brain disease. A persisting interest was the role of cerebral dominance and handedness in acquired aphasia and developmental learning disabilities. He was among the first investigators to show that hemispheric specialization for speech in left-handers did not conform to the then accepted rule of right hemisphere dominance. His 1960 monograph, *Cerebral Dominance and Its Relation to Psychological Function*, summarized his own observations, as well as the pertinent literature in the area. In it, he judiciously assessed the significance of left-handedness and incomplete hemispheric dominance as risk factors in developmental dyslexia. He investigated the role of familial left-handedness in the production of crossed aphasia in right-handed patients and from time to time presented critical analyses of the question (cf. Zangwill, 1981).

Still another area of interest was reflected in his studies of the amnesic syndromes, which perhaps can be viewed as the clinical application of his early experimental studies of memory processes. Finally, he was a sensitive and astute student of the aphasic disorders. For example, a 1964 paper demonstrated that some severely aphasic Wernicke patients who talked nonsense and whose understanding of oral speech was grossly defective were nevertheless, capable of abstract reasoning as reflected in their performances on the Raven Matrices. His superb scholarship was evident in his trenchant analyses of famous controversial cases in the literature that can still be read with profit (cf. Zangwill, 1967).

Oliver Zangwill was the founder of neuropsychology in Britain. His students, and now their students, carry on his work.

Hans-Lukas Teuber

Hans-Lukas Teuber was born in Berlin in 1916. After completing secondary school in Berlin, he studied at the University of Basel. He emigrated to the United States in 1941 and enrolled as a graduate student in psychology at Harvard University where his fellowship stipend was in the field of personality and social psychology and where his mentor was Gordon Allport. Entering the U.S. Navy in 1944, he had the good fortune to be assigned to the Naval Hospital in San Diego where he worked with the neurologist, Morris Bender. A productive collaboration in research on perceptual disorders in brain-diseased patients developed and continued for a number of years after the war. Teuber's bibliography includes 16 papers and a monograph by Bender and himself on a variety of topics, among them visual field defects and visual extinction, visuospatial disabilities, performances on complex visual tasks, disorders of the body schema, and impairment in weight discrimination.

In passing, it may be noted that Teuber was as responsible as anyone for the current usage of the term "neuropsychology," which was the title of a presentation he made at the 1948 APA convention. His presentation was subsequently published in a book on diagnostic psychological testing (cf. Teuber, 1950).

Having established a Psychophysiological Laboratory at New York's Bellevue Hospital in the late 1940s (where Bender was a senior neurologist), Teuber

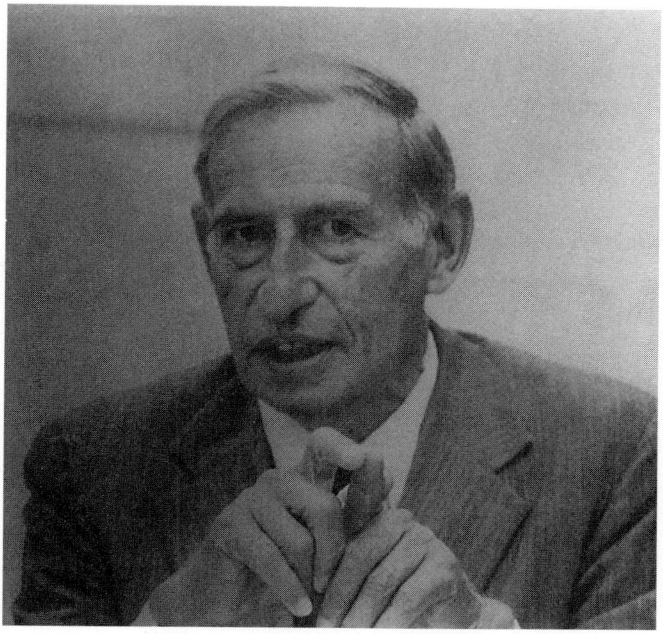

FIGURE **2.3.** Hans-Lukas Teuber, 1916–1977.

embarked on a large multifaceted study of the perceptual and cognitive defects caused by penetrating brain injury, the subjects being World War II and (later) Korean War veterans. He gathered round him a team of gifted young researchers and students, among them Lila Ghent, Mortimer Mishkin, Rita Rudel, Josephine Semmes, and Sidney Weinstein. Devising ingenious tests for the purpose, the team addressed a multitude of empirical and theoretical questions about the visuoperceptual, somatoperceptual and audioperceptual capacities, the learning abilities, and the intellectual status of the patients. Their studies offered analyses of the basic nature of the observed performance deficits, as well as dealing with questions of lesional localization.

Even a brief account of the contributions made to these several fields, e.g., Semmes et al. (1956, 1963) on spatial orientation, Weinstein's (1954, 1955) studies of tactile performances, and the Teuber–Mishkin (1954) investigation of patients' judgments of verticality, would consume too much time. I will mention only the monumental study of somatosensory impairments in patients with unilateral injuries that was described in a monograph by Semmes et al. in 1960. This study showed that bilateral and ipsilateral sensory defects were a fairly frequent consequence of unilateral brain disease; that these defects occurred more frequently after left hemisphere injury; that the cerebral representation of somatosensory function was more diffuse in the right hemisphere than in the left; and finally, that the patterns or combinations of sensory defect were different in the two hands. Thus the study modified traditional concepts of contralateral innervation, and at the same time, demonstrated hemispheric asymmetry in the mediation of somatosensory performance. These basic findings, which were in the main confirmed by later investigators, had a profound impact on thinking in this field.

In 1960 Teuber moved to the Massachusetts Institute of Technology as Professor of Psychology with the mandate to establish a Department of Psychology, a formidable task in view of MIT's history of unsuccessful past attempts to do so (cf. Held, 1979). Within a few years, he had organized a vigorous department with an active research program.

Teuber's research and scholarly work expanded in scope in the 1960s and 1970s, and in some respects, assumed a more theoretical character. Concerned with the problem of the true implications of the behavioral defects observed in association with focal brain lesions, he advanced the concept of double dissociation of symptoms as a reasonable methodological approach to interpretation. Wrestling with the unresolved question of the nature of the agnosic disorders, he invoked the principle of corollary discharge from central motor to central sensory systems as a mechanism underlying normal perception and disorders of which could lead to incomplete information processing and, hence, to faulty recognition. He once again turned his attention to developmental neuropsychological questions and, for example, studied the course of cognitive growth in children with congenital or early acquired unilateral brain lesions.

Possessing a prodigious knowledge of psychology, physiology, and clinical neurology, Hans-Lukas Teuber was, above all, a superb synthesizer. His review papers and chapters in handbooks were masterpieces of integration that brought together information from diverse areas to elucidate specific questions. He was an inspiring mentor of a generation of students at MIT. His untimely death in 1977 at the height of his career was a major tragedy.

Norman Geschwind

Norman Geschwind was born in 1926 in New York. After taking the M.D. degree at Harvard in 1951, he trained in neurology at the National Hospital, Queen Square, and at the Boston City Hospital under Derek Denny-Brown. He then spent 2 years in neurophysiological research at MIT. In 1958 he joined the staff of the neurological service of the Boston Veterans Administration Hospital. It was there that two older neurologists, Fred Quadfasel, who was chief of the service at the hospital, and Paul Jossmann, who was on the staff of the VA Mental Hygiene Clinic in Boston, introduced him to the concepts of the nature

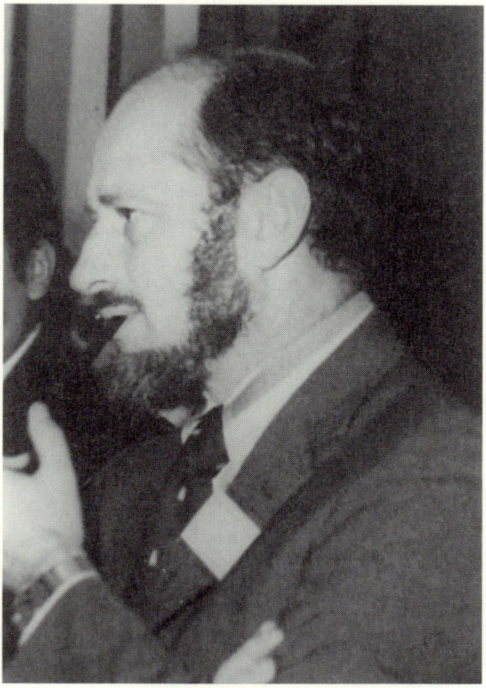

FIGURE **2.4.** Norman Geschwind, 1926–1984.

of aphasia and apraxia of the German neurological school, as exemplified in the work of its dominant representatives, Carl Wernicke and Hugo Liepmann. Geschwind wholeheartedly accepted their formulations as basically valid and proceeded to refine and modify them in the light of modern anatomical and psychological knowledge and as indicated by his own clinical observations (cf. Geschwind and Kaplan, 1962).

He presented his ideas in a now classic paper, "Disconnexion Syndromes in Animals and Man," which was published in 1965. This comprehensive analysis, some 100 pages in length, presented the concept of disconnection and illustrated its far-reaching implications. Its impact was immediate and far-reaching. In a real sense, it brought neuroanatomy back into the fields of aphasia, apraxia, and agnosia, and it provided a fruitful approach to the understanding of these types of disorder, as well as other behavioral manifestations of brain disease. Today, when we undertake to analyze the mechanisms underlying aphasic disorders, amnesic syndromes, perceptual defects, and visuomotor disabilities, we think in terms of disconnections—not simple disconnections, to be sure, but rather of disturbances of progression and interactions in information processing that are based on the destruction of specific pathways. This mode of approach is the legacy of Norman Geschwind.

In the 1960s, Geschwind's faith that anatomy had to play a central role in the description and operation of complex mental functions led him to an important discovery. Despite the traditional view that the cerebral hemispheres of the human brain were morphologically equivalent, he was convinced that asymmetry of hemispheric function, as reflected in the dominance of the left hemisphere for speech, must have an anatomic basis. He decided to reexamine the question. With a young colleague, Walter Levitsky, he studied the gross morphologic features of the left and right hemisphere of 100 brains and determined that indeed there was a strong trend toward a larger auditory association cortex in the left hemisphere, a finding that was in accord with theoretical expectations (Geschwind and Levitsky, 1968). Their findings were confirmed and led to a paradigmatic shift in thinking on the topic as well as to a continuing search for morphologic disparities that might be correlated with functional differences. This also is a legacy of Norman Geschwind.

In 1968 he was appointed Professor of Neurology at the Harvard Medical School and Chief of the Harvard Neurological Service at the Boston City Hospital. Subsequently, he moved the service to Beth Israel, where he established a Behavioral Neurology Unit. The broad scope of Geschwind's interests and investigative activity is indicated by his studies on diverse subjects: the neuropsychological and psychiatric aspects of temporal lobe epilepsy, linguistic aspects of aphasia, disturbances in attention, and the apraxic disorders. In addition, he made important contributions to mainstream neurology.

His last major effort was, by all criteria, the most original and daring. On the basis of his own observations and data in the literature, he postulated relationships between variations in brain development, uterine endocrine functions, and immunological disorders. In turn, the variations in brain development were linked to variations in hand preference, hemispheric cerebral dominance, and specific cognitive abilities. A detailed exposition of his hypotheses was published in 1985, some months after his sudden death in November 1984 (Geschwind and Galaburda, 1985).

Norman Geschwind was an enthusiastic teacher and a generous colleague who single-handedly founded the speciality of behavioral neurology in this country. Frank Benson, François Boller, Antonio Damasio, Martha Denckla, Albert Galaburda, Kenneth Heilman, Marcel Mesulam, and Alan Rubens were among his students. Harold Goodglass and Edith Kaplan were his close collaborators in research from the moment he joined the staff of the Boston VA Hospital in 1958. In the early 1960s, Davis Howes and Geschwind jointly pursued some pioneer linguistic studies of aphasia (cf. Howes and Geschwind, 1964). Thus, another link with clinical neuropsychology was forged. His premature death in 1984 deprived behavioral neurology of its preeminent figure.

A Summing-Up

We have reviewed the life and careers of four of our fellow neuropsychologists. They were very different from each other in respect to personal traits. Hécaen was direct, intense, and although unpretentious in manner, full of fierce pride. Zangwill was sensitive, considerate, attentive to the needs of others, and endowed with a keen sense of humor. Teuber was dynamic, even somewhat flamboyant, quick-thinking, and paternalistic toward his students and younger colleagues, somewhat in the manner of a prewar German professor. Geschwind was open, fun-loving, challenging, and passionate in defense of his ideas.

Obviously, our colleagues had four quite different personalities. What traits did they have in common? The first that comes to mind is their drive, their stamina, and their prodigious productivity. They had immense energy and worked very, very hard. This was quite evident for Hécaen, Teuber, and Geschwind, who were always on the move, who always had some neuropsychological issue on their minds, and who invariably took home a briefcase of material with them at the end of the day. On the other hand, Zangwill was perhaps a bit of a dissimulator in this regard. Quiet and apparently relaxed, he was always ready to talk about a variety of topics other than neuropsychology, to take tea, or to show one the sights of Cambridge. Yet there is no doubt that he spent many thousands of hours in the privacy of his study reading, writing, and analyzing research results.

Nevertheless, none of them could be classified as "workaholics" if that term describes a person who has no concerns other than with his work. Each of them had a set of quite serious outside interests. Hécaen was an ardent student of classical Greek art and he was active politically. Zangwill's conversation revealed that he had read everything, including contemporary French and German literature. Teuber was a true polymath whose historical knowledge was both broad and deep and who kept abreast of diverse developments in the neurosciences in astounding detail. Norman Geschwind had a passion for languages and had attained a level of proficiency in French, German, Spanish, and Italian that allowed him to lecture in these languages. Perhaps these extracurricular interests, activities, and accomplishments can be regarded as simply additional expressions of their immense drive and energy.

A second important characteristic that these men shared was simply that they were very, very bright. Their capacity to analyze and integrate information, to detect the significance of isolated observations, to get to the heart of a problem, and to do all this so quickly as to suggest multiple integrative processing was quite extraordinary. Clearly all of them possessed the prepared mind that Pasteur had specified as being the only kind that was likely to profit from chance observations.

A personal note: To sit with Norman Geschwind in one-to-one conversation of an evening was (at least to me) an exceptional experience. The first hour consisted of genuine conversation with an exchange of information and views. By the second and third hours, my own store of knowledge and insights having been depleted, Norman would carry on an instructive monologue at a rapid pace, making diverse observations bearing on a particular theme and integrating them to prove a particular point, to all of which I would react with bewildered admiration.

Epilogue

The debt we owe to our colleagues is incalculable. No doubt, neuropsychology would have progressed in due course without them. But its development would have been much slower and, I think, probably along less fruitful lines. Our sense of loss is keen and sometimes we feel that they are irreplaceable. But, in fact, their places have already been taken by gifted younger men and women, some of whom were their students. On this anniversary celebration, we pay tribute to our four colleagues and we welcome their successors.

References

Ajuriaguerra J. de and Hécaen H. (1949). *Le Cortex Cérébrale*. Paris: Masson (2nd ed., 1960).

Albert M. L. (1984). Henry Hécaen, MD: Neurologist-neuropsychologist. *Arch. Neurol.* 41: 457–459.

Benton A. L. (1958). Significance of systematic reversal in right-left discrimination. *Acta Psychiatr. Neurol. Scand.* 33: 129–137.

Benton A. L. (1972). The "minor" hemisphere. *J. Hist. Med. Allied Sci.* 27: 5–14.

Cénac M. and Hécaen H. (1943). Inversion systématique dans la designation droite-gauche chez certains enfants. *Ann. Med. Psychol.* 101: 415–419.

Drachman D. and Arbit J. (1966). Memory and the hippocampal complex. II. Is memory a multiple process? *Arch. Neurol.* 15: 52–61.

Galtier A. (1984). Publications de Henry Hécaen. *Neuropsychologia* 22: 647–659.

Geschwind N. (1965). Disconnexion syndromes in animal and man. *Brain* 88: 237–294, 585–644.

Geschwind N. and Galaburda A. (1985). Cerebral lateralization: Biological mechanisms, associations and pathology. *Arch. Neurol.* 42 : 428–259, 521–552.

Geschwind N. and Kaplan E. (1962). A human cerebral deconnection syndrome. *Neurology* 12: 675–685.

Geschwind N. and Levitsky W. (1968). Human brain: Left-right asymmetries in temporal speech region. *Science* 161: 186–187.

Hamsher K., Benton A. L., and Digre K. (1980). Serial digit learning: Normative and clinical aspects. *J. Clin. Neuropsychol.* 2: 39–50.

Hécaen H. (1984). *Les Gauchers: Etude Neuropsychologique*. Paris: Presses Universitaires de France.

Hécaen H. and Ajuriaguerra J. de. (1945). L'apraxie de l'habillage: Ses rapports avec la planotokinésie at les troubles de la somatoagnosie. *Encéphale* 35: 113–143.

Hécaen H. and Ajuriaguerra J. de. (1952). *Méconnaissances et Hallucinations Corporelles*. Paris: Masson.

Hécaen H. and Ajuriaguerra J. de. (1956). *Les Troubles Mentales au cours des Tumeurs Intracraniennes*. Paris: Masson.

Hécaen H. and Ajuriaguerra J. de. (1963). *Les Gauchers: Dominance Cérébrale et Prevalence Manuelle*. Paris: Presses Universitaires de France.

Hécaen H., Ajuriaguerra J. de., and Massonet J. (1951). Les troubles visuoconstructives par lésion pariéto-occipitale droite. *Encéphale* 40: 122–179.

Hécaen H. and Albert and M. L. (1978). *Human Neuropsychology*. New York: Wiley.

Hécaen H. and Angelergues R. (1962). Agnosia for faces (prosopagnosia). *Arch. Neurol.* 7: 92–100.

Hécaen H. and Angelergues R. (1965). *Pathologie du Langage*. Paris: Larousse.

Hécaen H., Angelergues R., and Houillier S. (1961). Les variétés des acalculies au cours des lésions retrorolandiques. *Rev. Neurol.* 105: 85–103.

Hécaen H., Penfield W., Bartrand C., and Malmo R. (1956). The syndrome of apractognosia due to lesions of the minor cerebral hemisphere. *Arch. Neurol. Psychiatry* 75: 400–434.

Held R. (1979). Hans-Lukas Teuber. *Neuropsychologia* 17: 117–118.

Howes D. and Geschwind N. (1964). Quantitative studies of aphasic language. In Rioch, D. and Weinstein E. (eds.), Disorders of communication, *Proceedings, Association for Research in Nervous and Mental Disease* (Vol. 42). Baltimore, MD: Williams and Wilkins, pp. 229–264.

Oldfield R. C. and Zangwill O. L. (1942–3a). Head's concept of the schema and its applications in contemporary British psychology. *Br. J. Psychol.* 32: 267–286.

Oldfield R. C. and Zangwill O. L. (1942–3b). Head's concept of the schema and its applications in contemporary British psychology. *Br. J. Psychol.* 33: 58–64, 113–129, 143–149.

Paterson A. and Zangwill O. L. (1944). Disorders of visual space perception associated with lesions of the right cerebral hemisphere. *Brain* 67: 331–358.

Semmes J., Weinstein S., Ghent L., and Teuber H.-L. (1956). Spatial orientation in man: I. Analysis by locus of lesion. *J. Psychol.* 42: 149–263.

Semmes J., Weinstein S., Ghent L., and Teuber H.-L. (1963). Correlates of impaired orientation in personal and extrapersonal space. *Brain* 86: 747–772.

Semmes J., Weinstein S., Ghent L., and Teuber H.-L. (1960). *Somatosensory Changes after Penetrating Brain Wounds in Man*. Cambridge, MA: Harvard University Press.

Teuber H.-L. (1950). Neuropsychology. In Harrower, M. R. (ed.), *Recent Advances in Diagnostic Psychological Testing*. Springfield, IL: C. C. Thomas, pp. 30–52.

Teuber H.-L. and Mishkin M. (1954) Judgment of visual and postural vertical after brain injury. *J. Psycho.* 38: 161–175.

Weinstein S. (1954). Weight judgment in somesthesis after penetrating injury to the brain. *J. Comp. Physiol. Psychol.* 47: 31–35.

Weinstein S. (1955). Tactile size judgment after penetrating brain injury. *J. Comp. Physiol. Psychol.* 48: 106–109.

Zangwill O. L. (1943). Clinical tests of memory impairment. *R. Soc. Med.* 36: 576–580.

Zangwill O. L. (1946a). Some clinical applications of the Rey-Davis performance test. *J. Ment. Sci.* 92: 19–34.

Zangwill O. L. (1946b). Some quatitative observations on verbal memory in cases of cerebral lesion. *Br. J. Psychol.* 37: 8–19.

Zangwill O. L. (1960). *Cerebral Dominance and its Relation to Psychological Function.* Edinburgh: Oliver and Boyd.

Zangwill O. L. (1964). Intelligence and aphasia. In Reuck A. V. S. de and O'Connor M. (eds.), *Disorders of Language*. London: Churchill, pp. 261–274.

Zangwill O. L. (1967). The Grünthal-Störring case of amnesic syndrome. *Br. J. Psychiatry* 20: 113–128.

Zangwill O. L. (1968). Frederick Bartlett. In Sills D. L. (ed.), *International Encyclopedia of the Social Sciences* (Vol. 2). New York: Macmillan and The Free Press, pp. 19–21.

Zangwill O. L. (1981). Crossed aphasia and its relation to cerebral lateralisation. In LeBrun Y. and Zangwill O. L. (eds.), *Lateralisation of Language in the Child.* Lisse: Swets and Zeitlinger, pp. 147–174.

3

The Fate of Some Neuropsychological Concepts: An Historical Inquiry

In some essays that appeared in the 1950s and early 1960s the historian, Edwin Boring (1961, 1963), discussed the influence of the *Zeitgeist* on the progress of science in general and on the development of psychology in particular. The term *zeitgeist*, which translates into English literally as the "spirit of the time" and more broadly as the "climate of opinion," is the label for the prevailing body of knowledge, beliefs, attitudes, and criteria of judgment that determines what observations and theories are evaluated as correct or incorrect, valid or invalid, credible or incredible, important or not important—in a word, what needs to be taken seriously and what need not to be taken seriously.

Boring (1961, p. 330) pointed out that the influence of the *Zeitgeist* on scientific progress is "sometimes helpful and sometimes hindering." It is helpful (indeed necessary) in that it provides the background of knowledge and experience that is required for sound judgment as new alleged facts and novel conceptions are advanced. Without it, all facts and conceptions, no matter how dubious or far-fetched, would have to receive equal consideration and this could result in a state of confusion resembling, let us say, the state of affairs in modern art or contemporary music. Moreover, the *Zeitgeist* is not immutable. It does change in the face of substantial empirical evidence and convincing argument that one or another aspect of it can no longer be maintained.

But the *Zeitgeist* can also be a hindrance to the progress of a science or discipline because by its very nature it offers at least initial resistance to facts

Reprinted with permission from E. Goldberg (Ed), *Contemporary Psychology and the Legacy of Luria*, Hillsdale, NJ: Lawrence Erlbaum, Publishers, 1990.

or conceptions that challenge it and that later prove to be valid. The history of science is full of examples of delayed recognition of the significance of discoveries and conceptions that were not congruent with the system of theories and beliefs prevailing at the time.

This chapter is a small excursion into the history of neuropsychology that deals with some early studies, each of which was in its way highly original in nature. Decades after their publication, these studies were seen to have provided information of considerable significance. However, at the time when they appeared, the observations contained in them were either ignored by the authors' contemporaries or at best judged to be of little importance. The studies will be described and the possible reasons why recognition of their significance was so long delayed will be explored.

We will deal with three studies, the first published in the 1840s, the second in the 1850s, the third in the 1860s. The paper by Puchelt (1844) offers the first description of what today is called "astereognosis," that is, inability to identify objects that have been palpated without the aid of vision, this failure in identification occurring within a setting of adequate tactile sensitivity. The second paper, by Panizza (1855), presents the first demonstration of the crucial role of the occipital lobes in vision. The third paper, by Quaglino and Borelli (1867), includes the first description of facial agnosia or prosopagnosia, that is, specific loss of the ability to identify the faces of familiar persons.

Astereognosis

Consider what was known about somesthesis when Puchelt published his paper on "partial paralysis of sensation" in 1844. Aristotle's designation of touch as one of the five primary senses was universally accepted as was his opinion that it was more complex than the other senses in that it probably represented a combination of different types of sensibility. Impairment in skin sensitivity associated with disease of the nervous system (including brain disease) was fairly commonly noted by physicians in early case reports (i.e., in the sixteenth and seventeenth centuries) where a patient might be described as having a "paralysis of touch," a "paralysis of feeling," a "paralysis of motion and feeling," or a "paralysis of motion but not feeling." (In those days and for a long time afterward, the term "paralysis" was applied to sensory processes as well as to movement.) In 1826 Charles Bell definitively established the "muscle sense" as a sixth sense whose effective stimulus was in the muscles rather than in the skin. He described what he called "the nervous circle which connects the voluntary muscles with the brain," in which muscular contraction itself sends information along the sensory nerves to the central nervous system, this information then serving as a guide to direct subsequent movements as well as a basis for judgments about weight, size and shape, hardness and softness.

On the other hand, although Ernst Heinrich Weber's Latin monograph which dealt in part with the sense of touch was published in 1834, his far more widely known *Der Tastsinn und das Gemeingefühl* appeared in 1846, that is, 2 years after Puchelt's paper (cf. Ross and Murray, 1978). Moreover, anatomical descriptions of encapsulated nerve endings in the skin, such as Meissner corpuscles. Ruffini cylinders, and the like, which were regarded as sensory end organs, began to appear only in the 1840s.

This was the background of knowledge against which Puchelt made his observations. Quite clearly he applied the term "partial paralysis" to two different phenomena. The first was what today is known as dissociated loss of sensitivity. Thus he described one patient who showed a specific loss of temperature sensitivity with preservation of sensitivity to touch as well as of the ability to identify objects by palpation without the aid of vision. Other patients with loss of pressure sensitivity and the loss of the ability to identify objects by palpation had preserved sensitivity to both pain and temperature. The second phenomenon noted by Puchelt was astereognosis or tactile agnosia. Thus one patient showed preserved sensitivity for all the tactile modalities (pressure, pain, and temperature) but was unable to identify palpated objects. Yet she could report accurately whether the object was warm or cold, large or small, and soft or hard.

Discussing the basis for these "partial paralyses," Puchelt concluded that "the cause of these partial paralyses of sensation is to be found neither in the lamed limb nor in the conducting pathways nor in the spinal cord but in the brain." This is as far as he was able to go, given the knowledge of neuroanatomy of the time.

It can be assumed, I think, that Puchelt's contemporaries were aware of his paper. But evidently they found his observations to be of little interest, because the next investigation of disturbances in tactile object perception did not appear until 39 years later, in 1883. This was reported in a monograph by H. Hoffman in Strassburg, who coined the term "stereognosis," and who fully confirmed Puchelt's contention that failure in tactile object identification could occur within a setting of intact basic tactile sensitivity. However, Hoffmann made the further point that stereognostic capacity was related to the muscle sense, that is, kinesthesis or proprioception. Patients with defective propioceptive sensitivity could identify objects but they did experience difficulty, often taking a long time before they succeeded in the task.

After Hoffmann paved the way, a number of further contributions appeared in the 1880s and 1890s, perhaps the most important of which was made by Wernicke in 1895, when he demonstrated astereognosis with intact tactile sensitivity in two patients with focal cortical lesions and implicated the postcentral gyrus as the locus of the underlying neural mechanism.

Why did it take 40 years before Puchelt's observations were looked into? A reasonable (perhaps oversimplified) explanation is that the time was not ripe. As we saw, sensory end-organs in the skin, muscles, and joints for the reception of somesthetic stimulation had just begun to be described. With respect to the central nervous system, all that Puchelt could say is that he believed that his "partial paralyses" were due to brain disease, possibly because he had not observed them in patients with lesions of the spinal cord or peripheral nerves. But, in the 1870s, physiologists such as Munk and Ferrier parcellated the cerebral cortex into sensory territories or spheres. The visual sphere was in the occipital lobes according to Munk; in the region of the angular gyrus, according to Ferrier. The auditory sphere was in the temporal lobes and the somesthetic sphere was in the parietal lobes. Now disturbances in tactile recognition began to acquire some degree of specific neurological significance and, as we saw, clinical studies on the topic in fact began in the 1880s.

A subsequent development in neuropsychological thought of at least equal importance retrospectively made Puchelt's observations of interest. What he had described was later to be called a form of "agnosia," that is, a failure in recognition or identification that cannot be entirely ascribed to basic sensory deficit. Of necessity, Puchelt and his contemporaries were not aware of this concept which was formulated only in the 1870s. It was then that the Berlin physiologist, Hermann Munk, described the consequences of partial ablation of the occipital lobes in dogs. Complete ablation of the lobes rendered the dog blind. But partial ablations led to a peculiar condition that Munk labeled "mind-blindness." The dog obviously was not blind in the ordinary meaning of the term. It could ambulate freely and would avoid obstacles placed in his path by walking around them or climbing over them or even crawling under them. But it behaved in an oddly stupid fashion. It showed no sign that it recognized his master. It did not react to threatening gestures or even to a flame until the flame was brought close enough so that it felt its warmth. The sight of food did not arouse it but, if the food were brought close enough so that it could smell it, then the animal would snap at it, as any normal dog would.

Munk explained the dog's disability by postulating that the animal had lost its store of visual memory images; in other words, that it had been reduced to the status of a puppy with no background of visual experience, and hence, had to learn the meaning of ongoing visual experience all over again. The fact that typically the "mind-blind" dog recovered from its disability over time was congruent with Munk's hypothesis of relearning. (But it was also congruent with the position of skeptics who believed that "mind-blindness" was nothing more than a partial impairment of vision from which the dog eventually recovered.)

However, in the 1880s ophthalmologists encountered and described patients who showed failure to recognize objects and persons despite seemingly adequate vision and they did not hesitate to classify these patients as cases of mindblindness or visual agnosia (cf. Lissauer, 1890: Wilbrand, 1887). Now astereognosis could be conceived as the tactile analogue of mind-blindness and cases such as those of Wernicke were designated as instances of tactile agnosia. Retrospectively, some of Puchelt's cases fell into this category.

In summary, the possible significance of Puchelt's observation was not grasped by his contemporaries, who probably regarded it as not a very exciting medical curiosity. This was not because they were particularly obtuse or unimaginative. It was rather a consequence of their ignorance of the neural underpinnings of tactile sensation and perception and the circumstance that the concept of agnosia had not yet been introduced into neuropsychological thought. Thus, they were not prepared to incorporate Puchelt's observations into the structure of their knowledge and understanding. Puchelt himself seems to have had only a vague awareness that there was something special about his "partial paralyses."

Vision and the Occipital Lobes

In 1854, the French anatomist and anthropologist Pierre Gratiolet, through careful dissection of fixed specimens, was able to demonstrate for the first time the optic radiations arising from the lateral geniculate nuclei and fanning out to the cortex of the occipital and posterior parietal lobes. In the following year (1855), Bartolomeo Panizza, who was professor of anatomy at Pavia, published a paper in which he confirmed the existence of the optic radiations. But Panizza went beyond this purely anatomical determination to investigate the functional significance of this extension from the thalamic level to the cortex. He did this experimentally by destroying the occipital lobes in dogs and finding that bilateral ablation resulted in complete blindness, as Munk was to report 20 years later. Panizza also reported that ablation of a single occipital lobe resulted in blindness in the opposite eye. (He was wrong, of course, and Munk later identified the deficit correctly as visual loss in the opposite half-field or a contralateral hemianopia.) Panizza also described visual loss in some patients with occipital lobe disease and these were the first clinical observations of this type.

It is clear enough that the thrust of Panizza's report was to establish the crucial role of the occipital lobes in the mediation of vision. However, his work was completely ignored. It was only after Munk's definitive studies in the late 1870s that a compatriot, Augusto Tamburini (1880), a neuropsychiatrist, called attention to Panizza's work.

There may have been some incidental reasons why Panizza's observations were ignored. First, it does not seem that he was particularly well-known internationally. Secondly, he published in Italian, which may have been a handicap.

Finally, his papers were published not in a major journal but in a provincial periodical, which perhaps was distributed as a matter of course to the major libraries of Europe but which probably did not find its way to the desks of the leading researchers of the period.

But there was a more basic reason why Panizza's contentions could have been ignored. The dominant neurological theory of vision at the time stipulated that the cerebral center for vision was at the level of the thalamus—in the lateral geniculate nuclei and in other nuclei (hence, the old term, the "optic thalamus"). Panizza's work was, of course, not congruent with this doctrine. Thus, if there were physiologists or physicians who did read his paper, they could well have dismissed it as being outlandish, that is, making no sense. In short, under the influence of prevailing dogma, they were not prepared to consider the implications of Panizza's findings.

Prosopagnosia

The paper by Antonio Quaglino (who was professor of ophthalmology at Pavia) and Giambattista Borelli (who was a practicing ophthalmologist in Turin) had to do with the appearance of a triad of symptoms—defective facial recognition, loss of color vision, and impairment in spatial orientation—in a 54-year-old man who had suffered a right-hemisphere stroke. Evidently Quaglino and Borelli considered that this was a very instructive case, since their paper is actually one of a series of three dealing with the same patient. Their primary interest was in the issue of cerebral localization. Here, while they acknowledge that Gall had been in error in a number of respects, such as postulating the existence of cortical centers for complex traits such as "cautiousness," "self-esteem," and "reverence," and assuming that the conformation of the skull coincided with the conformation of the surface of the brain, nevertheless they believed that his fundamental thesis that different parts of the brain mediated different simpler functions was correct. They believed that their case supported the thesis.

Immediately after his stroke this patient had a left hemiplegia and also an apparently complete loss of vision. The hemiplegia disappeared within a month and his vision gradually returned over the course of a few months. When he was first seen by Quaglino and Borelli a year after the stroke, he felt quite well and had no motor disability. His visual acuity was excellent by his own testimony and by examination. He read without difficulty. However, although central vision was intact, he did have a left visual field defect. His main complaints were those that have been mentioned:

First, a loss of color vision. All objects and faces looked pale, white, or gray, and devoid of color. Examination disclosed that he was unable to distinguish colors. In short, the patient showed a bilateral central achromatopsia. (Incidentally, "achromatopsia" is the term used by Quaglino and Borelli.)

Second, some loss of spatial orientation. He retained the concept of orientation and would confidently state that the window of his room faced east. Nevertheless he could no longer indicate the directional arrangements in his apartment, for example, where the east wall stood in relation to the south wall and so on.

Third, there was impairment in facial recognition:

> The patient no longer recognizes the faces of persons, even those familiar to him at home and he has lost his orientation. During the first year he still retained the memory of figures of certain people and he could recall them by listening to their voices. However, for some time now he cannot remember them at all. He sees the figure as in a photograph, but less clearly. . . .

In addition, the authors mention that the patient had forgotten the facades of houses. Whether or not this meant that he no longer could identify specific houses is not clear. In any case, it was this disability that was responsible for the phrase "loss of memory of the configuration of objects" in the title of their paper.

The authors concluded that Gall's postulation of a specific cerebral center for color perception was correct. They diagnosed their case as one of cerebral hemorrhage involving the right hemisphere primarily but possibly extending to parts of the left side of the brain.

Each of the defects noted by Quaglino and Borelli were taken up about 20 years later, in the 1880s, and it was only then that reference was made to their 1867 papers. A case of hemiachromatopsia, or loss of color vision in one visual half-field (in this instance, the right visual field), was described by the French ophthalmologist, Verrey, in 1888. In this case postmortem examination disclosed a lesion in the left occipital lobe. A patient with bilateral or complete achromatopsia, comparable with Quaglino and Borelli's case, was described by MacKay and Dunlop in 1899. In this instance, postmortem study showed infarcts in both occipital lobes. Thus, these case reports provided a more precise determination of the site of the lesions producing loss of color vision than Quaglino and Borelli were able to make.

In 1876 Hughlings Jackson described a patient with fairly serious disturbances in spatial orientation, as reflected in her losing her way as she walked the familiar route from her home to the place where she did her shopping. Sometimes she even became lost in her own house. Almost certainly Jackson was not aware of the Quaglino–Borelli papers. However, in the 1880s and 1890s the topic of loss of spatial orientation within a setting of intact visual acuity and object recognition in patients with brain disease became a topic of considerable interest to ophthalmologists and neurologists and it was then that the papers of

Quaglino and Borelli were cited. The site of the lesions producing disorientation were often identified by postmortem study in these later studies and they proved to be in the occipital-posterior temporal territory of the brain.

With respect to the facial agnosia or prosopagnosia that Quaglino and Borelli had noted in their patient, this also was observed some years later. Indeed Jackson's patient who had marked visual disorientation also must have had significant facial agnosia since on occasion she would mistake her niece for her daughter. Jackson considered the defect to be one aspect of a more widespread disability that he called "imperception" and that included visual disorientation and impairment in visual recognition.

As has been mentioned, in the 1880s ophthalmologists described patients with visual object agnosia that was roughly comparable with Munk's mind-blindness. Typically these patients also had lost the ability to identify persons by inspection of their faces. But little was made of the deficit since it seemed reasonable to expect that a patient who could not recognize a familiar object would also have difficulty in identifying a specific face.

The Quaglino–Borelli papers were not completely ignored—at least, not in the sense that Panizza's report was ignored. They were cited as early as 1881 in a book on the brain and vision by a German ophthalmologist, Mauthner. In any case, their description of their patient's facial agnosia was rather sparse and, without postmortem examination, they could only guess at the locus and extent of the underlying pathology.

Yet, despite the limitations of their report, Quaglino and Borelli did think of their patient's failure as representing a specific disability in the identification of individual objects—in contrast to the more general concept of visual object agnosia that was developed a decade later. And this their contemporaries seemed to have missed. Moreover, they related the disability (as well as the accompanying achromatopsia) not to some ocular condition (as they might well have, since they were ophthalmologists) but to brain disease.

It was only in the 1930s that facial agnosia was conceived to be a more or less specific disorder of visual recognition. Two complementary reasons why it was not singled out for special study earlier suggest themselves. On the one hand, facial agnosia was typically observed within a setting of other disabilities—with color blindness and some degree of spatial disorientation, as in the Quaglino–Borelli case, and with pronounced spatial disorientation, as in Jackson's patient. Thus it seemed to be only a number of expressions of a pervasive visual disability, "imperception," as Jackson called it. On the other hand, when facial agnosia presented in more or less isolated form without other obvious signs of cerebral dysfunction, it must have appeared to be such a bizarre complaint that many physicians would have been inclined to regard it as an hysterical phenomenon.

Concluding Comment

This has been the story of three neuropsychological studies whose significance was grasped only decades after they were reported. Apart from incidental factors, the major reason for their neglect would seem to be that the corpus of knowledge and climate of belief at the time of their appearance hindered appreciation of their potential importance.

Can a moral be drawn from this story? One cannot be sure. Of necessity all of us are more or less prisoners of the *Zeitgeist*. But perhaps we can resolve to be rather "less" than "more" by consciously guarding against the tendency to reject out of hand data and concepts that are not in accord with established doctrine and by giving them a critical but fair reception.

References

Bell C. (1826). On the nervious circle which connects the voluntary muscles with the brain. *Philos. Trans.*, 116 (Pt. 2): 163–173.

Boring E. G. (1961). *Psychologist at Large: An Autobiography and Selected Essays*. New York: Basic Books.

Boring E. G. (1963). *History, Psychology, and Science: Selected Papers*. New York: Wiley.

Gratiolet P. (1854). Note sur les expansions des racines cérébrales du nerf optique et sur leur terminaison dans une région determinée de l'écore des hémisphères. *Comptes Rendus de l'Academie des Sciences* 29: 274–278.

Hoffmann H. (1883). *Stereognostische Versuche*. Dissertation. Strassburg.

Jackson J. H. (1876). Case of large cerebral tumour without optic neuritis and with left hemiplegia and imperception. *Royal London Hospital Reports* 8: 434–444.

Lissauer H. (1890). Ein Fall von Seelenblindheit nebst einem Beitrag zur Theorie derselben. *Archiv für Psychiatrie und Nervenkrankheiten* 21: 222–270.

MacKay G. and Dunlop J. C. (1899). The cerebral lesions in a case of complete acquired colour-blindness. *Scott. Med. J.* 5: 503–512.

Mauthner L. (1881). *Gehirn und Auge*. Wiesbaden, Germany: Bergmann.

Munk H. (1878). Weitere Mittheilungen zur Physiologie der Grosshirnrinde. *Archiv für Anatomie und Physiologie* 2: 162–178.

Panizza B. (1855). Osserzioni sul nervo ottico. *Giornale, Istituto Lombardo di Scienze e Lettere* 7: 237–252.

Puchelt B. (1844). Über partielle Empfindungslähmung. *Medicinische Annalen* 10: 485–495.

Quaglino A. and Borelli G. (1867). Emiplegia sinistra con amaurosi; guaragione; perdita totale della percezione dei colori e della memoria della congigurazione degli oggetti. *Giornale d'Oftalmologia Italiano* 10: 106–117.

Ross H. E. and Murray D. J (1978). *E. H. Weber: The Sense of Touch*. London: Academic Press.

Tamburini A. (1880). Rivendicazione al Panizza della scoperta del centro visivo corticale. *Revista Sperimentale di Freniatria e medicina Legale* 6: 152–154.

Verrey D. (1888). Hémiachromatopise droite absolue. *Archives d' Ophthalmologie* 8: 289–300.

Wernicke C. (1895). Zwei Fällen von Rindenläsion. *Arbeiten aus der Psychiatrischen Klinik Breslau* 2: 33–53.

Wilbrand H. (1887). Die Seelenblindheit als Herderscheinung und ihre Beziehungen zur homonymen Hemianopsie. Wiesbaden, Germany: Bergmann.

4

The Prefrontal Region: Its Early History

This historical sketch deals with the early development of knowledge and concepts about the structure and functions of the prefrontal region, i.e., the region anterior and mesial to those areas of frontal cortex having to do with motor functions (motor cortex and frontal eye fields) and speech (Broca's area). The greater part of the prefrontal region has a characteristic cellular structure, frontal granular cortex, and within the region a number of areas are differentiated from each other on architectonic grounds. However, it is not yet clear that, apart from different afferent and efferent connections with other parts of the brain, this partition into sectors on an architectonic basis in itself possesses basic functional implications. The prefrontal region is simply a topographic concept and, indeed, one whose boundaries vary slightly in the descriptions of different anatomists. It differs from other regions of the cerebral cortex in that its destruction is not associated with loss of basic sensory or motor capacities or with obvious impairment of speech.

What gave the prefrontal region a special significance was the conviction that it provides the neural substrate of complex mental processes such as abstract reasoning, foresight, planning capacity, self-awareness, empathy, and the elaboration and modulation of emotional reactions. Different authors singled out one or another of these defects as the core disability generating the other defects. At the same time the ensemble of defects came to be known as the "frontal lobe syndrome."

This chapter describes, in a necessarily sketchy and fragmentary way, the evolution of ideas about these functions of the prefrontal region from the sixteenth century, when the frontal lobes were first clearly identified, to 1947, the

Reprinted from H. S. Levin, H. M. Eisenberg, A. L. Benton (Eds.) *Frontal Lobe Function and Dysfunction*. New York: Oxford University Press. © 1991.

date of a landmark conference in which knowledge and conceptions of frontal lobe function were discussed, particularly as they related to prefrontal leukotomy. More detailed accounts of specific aspects of the broad topic can be found in the monographs of Soury (1899), Kleist (1934), Rylander (1939), Ajuriaguerra and Hécaen (1949), Sanides (1962), Clarke and O'Malley (1968), Meyer (1971), Fuster (1980/1989), and Spillane (1981).

Earliest Conceptions

Gross Morphology

The frontal lobes make their first appearance in the scientific literature as one of three "prominences" (anterior, medial-inferior, posterior) into which Varolio (1573, 1591) divided the cerebral hemispheres. Willis (1664) was the first to apply the term "lobes" to these prominences, and Chaussier (1807) proposed the names "frontal," "temporal," and "occipital" to take the place of anterior, medial-inferior, and posterior, respectively. Arnold (1838) introduced the term "parietal lobe," thus forming the modern fourfold classification.

The division of the frontal lobe into component gyri and sulci had to wait until opinion about the significance of the cerebral convolutions underwent a change. Before 1820 anatomists held the pleats and creases of the cerebral cortex in very low esteem indeed (see Schiller, 1965). Called "enteroid processes" by Malacarne and Rolando, they were regarded either as reflecting the manner in which the pia mater succeeded in penetrating into the depth of the brain or as containing minute glands that discharged phlegm or animal spirits into the ventricles. In either case, there seemed to be as little reason to assign names to these bulges and creases as there would be to specify every fold in the intestines. No great care was exercised to depict them accurately, and early illustrations of the convexity of the hemispheres led Rolando to write that they reflected artistic skill more than scientific observation. Later these illustrations provoked Ecker's derisive comment that they reminded him of a bowl of macaroni (Fig. 4–1). No doubt a number of factors—the very limited opportunity to study fresh brains before decomposition, faulty communication between the anatomist and his artist (perhaps combined with the latter's creative imagination), and interindividual differences in the external morphology of the hemispheres—all contributed to this failure to depict any constancy in pattern.

Nevertheless, some major structures attracted sufficient attention to lead to specific identification. Bartholin, Sylvius, and Vicq d'Azyr described the Sylvian fissure (see Baker, 1909), and Reil provided a detailed description of the oval mass at the base of the Sylvian fissure that came to be known as the insula or the island of Reil. By the third decade of the nineteenth century the cortical

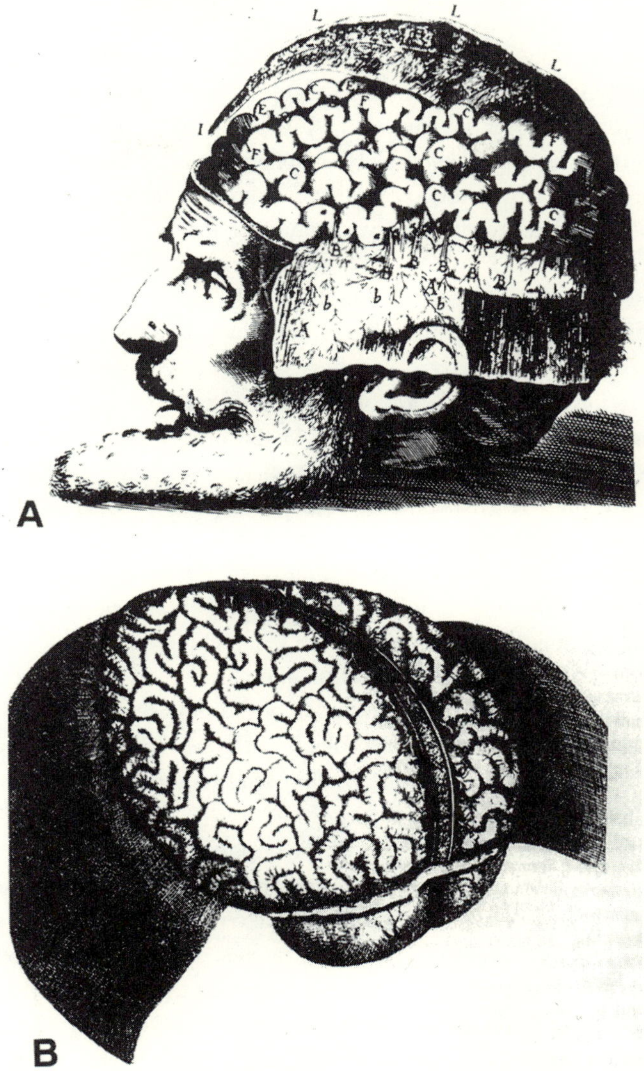

FIGURE **4.1.** **A.** An enteroid process? Illustration by Giulio Casserio in Adrian Van de Spiegel's *De Humanis Corporis Fabrica* (Venice, 1627). **B.** A bowl of macaroni? Illustration in Vieussens's *Nevrographia Universalis* (Leiden, 1685). (From the Martin Rare Book Room, Hardin Library for the Health Sciences, University of Iowa.)

gyri appeared to some anatomists to be sufficiently constant, in that they formed a recognizable pattern and therefore, to warrant identification. There is no doubt that Gall's placement of his "faculties" in the cortical gyri provided a strong impetus to closer examination. Rolando (1831) himself wrote a paper, "On the Structure of the Cerebral Hemispheres," in which he emphasized the importance of describing the cerebral convolutions and in which he identified the precentral and postcentral gyri surrounding the fissure that now bears his name.

The description of the external surface of the hemispheres in terms of four major lobes and the subdivision of each lobe into its constituent gyri and sulci were then carried forward by anatomists in France, Germany, and Britain, among them Leuret, Foville, Gratiolet, Broca, and Ecker. The work was essentially completed by the middle decades of the nineteenth century. Figure 4–2 reproduces Ecker's illustration of the lateral and superior aspects of the left hemisphere in his *Die Hirnwindungen des Menschen* (1869/1873). As will be seen, the three gyri of the convexity of the frontal lobe and their corresponding sulci are clearly shown and labeled. Similarly, the major convolutions of the parietal, temporal, and occipital lobes as well as transitional ridges such as the supramarginal and angular gyri are accurately depicted.

The landmarks on the inferior and medial surfaces of the frontal lobes also were described during the middle decades of the nineteenth century. The gyrus rectus was identified and named by Valentin in 1841. The other orbital and mesial gyri were described by Foville, Leuret, and Gratiolet as well as by Valentin.

Although later workers described many important details (see Meyer, 1971), by 1870 the gross morphology of the cerebral hemispheres was essentially as well known as it is today; Ecker's 1869 sketch could well find a place in a modern textbook of anatomy. Thereafter, interest in the external configuration of the hemispheres waned somewhat as it appeared that the gyri and sulci were merely convenient landmarks that bore no necessary correspondence either to underlying structure as disclosed by neurohistology or to functional properties inferred from animal experimentation and clinical observation.

Functional Aspects

From the earliest periods and extending to the nineteenth century there were two opposing points of view about the functional significance of the cerebral hemispheres. Aristotle was a "cardiocentrist," maintaining that the brain merely served the function of cooling the body heat generated by the heart, which was itself the seat of mentation. However, many "cerebrocentric" theorists regarded the brain as a secretory organ also, their basic concept being that perceptual and cognitive processes took place in the ventricles.

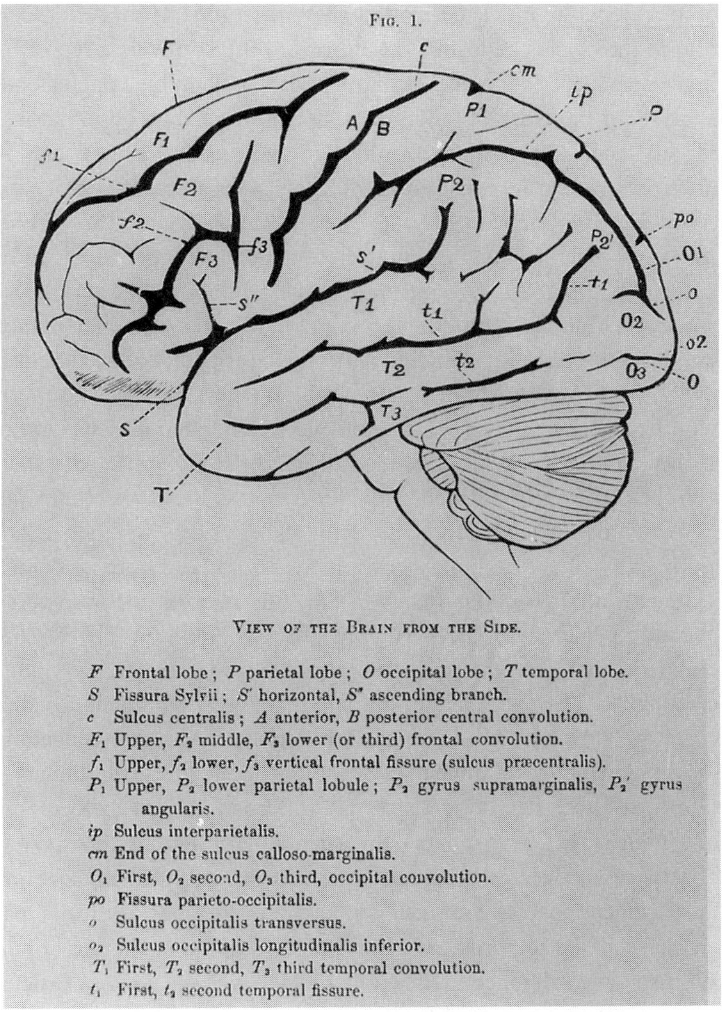

FIGURE **4.2.** Lateral view of left cerebral hemisphere (Ecker, 1869/1873).

Localization of mental functions in the substance of the brain largely displaced ventricular localization in the seventeenth and eighteenth centuries when the corpus callosum and the corpus striatum were identified as the seat of intellect. The choice of these organs was probably dictated in part on theoretic grounds because of their central location. However, empirical observations, such as those of the eighteenth-century French surgeon La Peyronie, that various parts of the cerebral hemispheres could be damaged without apparent impairment of intellectual function must also have played a role in the localization.

However, in due course, the cerebral hemispheres were accorded some degree of functional significance. Although Willis (1664/1681/1965) localized perception in the corpus callosum, he did regard the cortex as a repository of memory images and not as a mere secretory organ. Basing his conclusions on a detailed analysis of the work of others rather than on his own observations. Swedenborg placed the higher mental faculties in the cerebral cortex and suggested that different cortical regions served different modalities of sensory experience (see Akert and Hammond, 1962; Spillane, 1981). Rolando (1828) believed that consciousness and voluntary action are dependent on the integrity of the cerebral cortex. By the 1830s the concept that the cerebral cortex was the seat of intellect was almost universally accepted. Thus the French clinician–pathologists of that era, in their studies of patients with "general paralysis of the insane," reasoned that lesions of the white matter produced the characteristic motor disabilities, while cortical lesions were responsible for the mental deterioration (see Soury, 1899). Similarly, in his famous *Lehrbuch der Nervenkrankheiten* (1840–1846, 1853), Romberg implicated cortical disease as the basis of mental impairment.

A related question of equally long standing was whether or not the size and complexity of the cerebral hemispheres could be related to "intelligence." Beginning with Herophilus (ca. 400 B.C.), the majority of observers answered the question positively. Others, such as Thomas Bartholin (1616–1680), voiced an emphatic negative opinion, pointing out that the cerebral convolutions were exceedingly complex in some animals that were not noted for their intellectual capacity. However, when nineteenth century comparative anatomy established the systematic development of the brain along the evolutionary scale, a relationship of the size, complexity, and differentiation of the cerebral hemispheres to "intelligence" was universally accepted. The finding that the most impressive differences between the human brain and that of infrahuman primates consisted in a tremendous development of the prefrontal and posterior parietal regions emphasized the importance of these regions in the mediation of human behavior. With specific reference to the frontal lobes, workers such as Broca and Rüdinger pointed out that the third frontal gyrus, the "organ of speech," reached its full development only in the human brain (see Meyer, 1971).

Intrahemispheric Localization

The early nineteenth century controversy over localization of function within the hemispheres has been recounted many times (e.g., Benton, 1976, 1981; Clarke and Jacyna, 1987; Clarke and O'Malley, 1968; Gibson, 1962; Krech, 1964; Riese and Hoff, 1950; Swazey, 1970; Walker, 1957). A few representative examples illustrating the major trends in thought will be mentioned.

By his placement of "faculties" in discrete parts of the cerebral cortex and his insistence that the brain was an assemblage of organs, each of which subserved a specific intellectual capacity or trait of character, Franz Joseph Gall

(Gall and Spurzheim, 1809) made localization of function a central issue in neurophysiology and neuropsychology. Predictably, his radical thesis engendered a mixed reception and a rancorous controversy. It was rejected by many physiologists and clinicians for a variety of reasons, among them the conviction that Flourens was essentially correct in his view that the hemispheres acted as a unit as well as a rejection of Gall's far-reaching claims, materialistic position, and absurd phrenology. In addition, numerous clinical reports of patients with documented hemispheric lesions but with no observable impairment of function fitted in well with Flourens's "mass action" hypothesis, which stipulated that the amount of loss of brain tissue had to reach a critical level before any noticeable symptoms appeared. Most of these reports concerned patients with frontal lobe injuries.

However, clinical observation did impel many clinicians to embrace the basic concept of localization of cerebral function, whatever their attitudes toward Gall's claims might be. Pointing to the discrete deficits, such as monoplegia of an arm or leg, sensory defect without paralysis, and hemiplegia with or without sensory defect, that were produced by stroke, traumatic injury, or tumor, they concluded that specific cerebral centers governing these functions must exist. Postmortem findings disclosing limited areas of loss of tissue supported the conclusion. Nevertheless, no agreement about the precise locus of the crucial lesions could be reached. The state of affairs was well summarized by Andral (1823–1827) as follows: "We cannot yet assign in the brain a distinct seat to the motions of the upper and lower limbs. No doubt such distinct seat exists, since each of these limbs may be paralysed separately, but we do not know it yet" (cited by Spillane, 1981).

The most spirited disagreement over hemispheric localization revolved around Gall's placement of two centers, one for speech articulation and the other for the "memory of words" in the orbital area of the frontal lobes. Bouillaud (1825) expanded the crucial locus to encompass the whole of the "anterior" lobes and for 40 years argued strenuously that a frontal lobe lesion would be found in every patient who had exhibited an "alalia" or an "amnesia for words" during life. The contradictory evidence (i.e., aphasic disorder produced by lesions in the temporal or parietal lobe), which was brought forth by Andral and others, failed to shake Bouillaud, who continually fueled a controversy that was resolved only in the 1860s and 1870s (Benton, 1964).

Thus, by the close of the first half of the nineteenth century there was still uncertainty about whether or not there was differentiation of function within the cerebral hemispheres of the human brain as opposed to the holistic concept that the hemispheres operated as a unit as envisioned by Flourens. The observation that brain-diseased patients showed discrete deficits of different types persuaded clinicians that almost certainly such differentiation was the case, but consistent correlations between these defects and the locus of the presumably causative lesions could not be established. The evidence was particularly ambiguous with respect to the frontal lobes. Case reports describing asymptomatic patients with fairly extensive frontal lesions were not difficult to find, and this led to the concept that from a clinical standpoint the prefrontal region was a "silent area" of no recognizable functional significance. But countering this nihilistic conclusion was not only the conviction that the massive development of the frontal lobes in the human animal must possess some significance but also the indisputable evidence that disease of the region could cause disturbances in the characteristically human capacity of speech.

In 1850 Bigelow published his account of the famous "crowbar case," originally described by Harlow (1848). The young man had sustained the passage of an iron bar (1.25 inches in diameter at the larger end, 3.5 feet in length and 13.5 pounds in weight), which had entered the left frontal lobe and emerged from the right frontal bone near the sagittal suture, leaving a circular opening of about 3.5 inches in diameter and destroying the left frontal lobe and anterior temporal pole, as well in all probability some right frontal tissue. Interest at the time of publication of Bigelow's paper was focused on the patient's survival from such a massive brain injury. Bigelow himself characterized it as "perhaps unprecedented in the history of surgery," and one distinguished surgeon suspected that it was a "Yankee invention" (see Steegman, 1962).

The implications of the "crowbar case" for frontal lobe function were appreciated only in later years after the publication of Harlow's (1868) follow-up report describing the patient's status until his death 13 years after the accident. Phineas Gage did not appear to have suffered intellectual impairment in the narrow sense of the term. His memory and temporal orientation were intact and he was sufficiently competent to secure employment. Four years after his injury he went to South America where he worked for 8 years before returning to the United States a year before his death. Apparently he was self-supporting during all of this period. However, beginning about one month after his injury, he exhibited a remarkable change in personality. Before the injury he was considered to be an honest, reliable, deliberate person and a good businessman. He was now "childish, capricious and obstinate," showed poor judgment, used profane language, and was inconsiderate of others (Macmillan, 1986: Steegman, 1962). In short, he showed a distinctive type of personality change that later authors such as Welt (1888) associated with prefrontal lobe disease.

The Late Nineteenth Century

The closing decades of the nineteenth century, i.e., the 1870s, 1880s, and 1890s, witnessed an extraordinary growth in knowledge of the central nervous system. The discoveries of Broca and of Fritsch and Hitzig, the introduction of antisepsis, and the advances in the development of neurohistologic techniques led to a surge of activity on the part of experimentalists and clinicians on all fronts—anatomic, physiologic, and behavioral—the fruits of which were a deeper and more detailed understanding of the structure and functions of the brain and spinal cord. Among the topics that were pursued most vigorously was the issue of localization of function in the brain. The aspects of this development dealing with the structure and functions of the frontal lobes will be considered.

Anatomy and Physiology

The structure of the upper brain stem and the limbic regions was reasonably well delineated by the early decades of the nineteenth century (see Lewy, 1942; Meyer, 1971). For example, the basal ganglia had been described in detail by Willis (1664), Vieussens (1684), Vicq d'Azyr (1786), and Burdach (1826), the thalamus by Burdach (1826), and the hippocampus by Treviranus (1820). The interests of these early anatomists were not always confined to gross structure but also, at least on occasion, included consideration of the functional significance of the organs, although their pronouncements were necessarily rather vague. Thus Willis wrote that "the corpus striatum represents an exchange between brainstem and cortex" (cited by Lewy, 1942). And Treviranus (1820), having noted the connections between the hippocampus and the olfactory nerve, corpus striatum, and the fornix and having commented that no other convolution is so closely connected with other regions of the brain, drew the following remarkably prescient conclusion: "Therefore, the hippocampus is probably involved with a higher mental function, perhaps that of memory, which is so greatly aroused by olfactory sensations" (cited by Meyer, 1971).

An event of capital importance in fostering the evolution of thought about cerebral structure and function was the discovery by Gratiolet (1854) of the optic radiations arising from the lateral geniculate nuclei and fanning out to the parietal and occipital lobes. His demonstration that there was in fact a cortical terminus for vision above the thalamic level reinforced the nascent idea that the cerebral cortex was indeed the end-station for sensory information. A year later Panizza (1855) established a rough correspondence between lesions in the occipitoparietal region and impairment of vision in both human cases and in dogs subjected to experimental ablations. But his observations, published in a provincial journal with a limited circulation, remained unknown until resurrected some 25 years later and hence they had no influence on contemporary thought (Benton, 1978).

During the latter decades of the nineteenth century many gifted neuroanatomists, among them Betz, Broca, Cunningham, the Dejerines, Edinger, Flechsig, Golgi, Meynert, Nissl, Ramon y Cajal, and Retzius, utilized both gross dissection and newly developed histologic techniques to investigate the central nervous system. Their studies established the basis for modern concepts of the structure and functions of the human brain. In this regard, the work of the Viennese neuroanatomist, Theodor Meynert (1867, 1869, 1877, 1884/1885), was perhaps most influential in shaping the ideas of neurologists and psychiatrists about brain–behavior relationships. Meynert presented a thorough account of brain structures and their possible functional significance with detailed descriptions of the thalamus and its cortical connections, the hypothalamus, the hippocampus, the lateral geniculate nucleus, and the cerebral cortex. He demonstrated the significance of the corpus striatum as a relay station between brain stem and cortex, thus empirically validating the early speculation of Willis. He was the first to describe the nucleus basalis (nbM), which has figured so prominently in current discussions of the neuropathology of Alzheimer's disease and other dementing illnesses. He identified commissural, projection, and cortico-cortical pathways (later called association tracts) and contributed to knowledge of regional differences in the cellular architecture of the cortex. Overall, his researches proved to be a powerful stimulus to the formulation of concepts about the nature of the neural mechanisms underlying cognitive behavior such as those advanced by Wernicke (1874) and Liepmann (1900).

The Experimental Physiologists

The major feature of the "golden age of cerebral localization" (1870–1890) consisted of the attempts of physiologists to assign specific sensory, motor, perceptual, and cognitive capacities to specific regions of the cerebral cortex through ablation and stimulation experiments. Their findings, conclusions, and disagreements about the functional properties of the frontal lobes will be reviewed by sketching the positions of some of the leading investigators of the period.

Friedrich Goltz (1834–1902), still remembered for his remarkable demonstrations of the behavioral characteristics of dogs deprived of both cerebral hemispheres, is generally regarded as having been a thoroughgoing holist, carrying forth and defending the tradition of Flourens against the accumulating evidence in favor of specialization of function in the cerebral hemispheres. Indeed, he did argue that the size rather than the locus of lesions was the prime determinant of the sensory, motor, and cognitive deficits observed in brain-injured animals and humans. Moreover, using a water-jet technique that destroyed tissue with minimal bleeding but with poor control of extent of lesion, he reported finding that ablation of loci alleged to be the exclusive cortical centers for one or another function did not have the specific effects ascribed to them by the "localizationists" (Goltz, 1888).

In fact, Goltz was far from being a Flourensian antilocalizationist. He expressed himself as being in principle not at all opposed to the concept of localization of function within the cerebral hemispheres, but he did insist that adequate techniques of experimentation and careful observation are required to clarify the issue (Goltz, 1892). For example, he found that a complete unilateral hemispherectomy did lead to disturbances in a dog's motor behavior but not to the hemiplegia predicted by many investigators. His able assistant, Jacques Loeb (1885, 1886), reported that unilateral destruction of Munk's visual cortical area did not produce a contralateral hemianopia but rather a "hemiamblyopia," i.e., a lateralized weakness in visual attention that could be elicited by double simultaneous stimulation, a method that Loeb himself had devised. Moreover, more anterior unilateral lesions could also produce a comparable hemiamblyopia.

With respect to the question of the locus of intelligence, Goltz insisted that it was a property of the whole cerebral cortex and could not be localized in a particular region. Only extensive bilateral lesions produced a reduction in intelligence. The dog with a complete unilateral hemispherectomy was essentially as intelligent as he had been before the operation, although he might suffer from specific motor or perceptual defects. The degree of intellectual impairment was proportional to the amount of bilateral tissue loss. Extensive bilateral lesions, anterior or posterior, produced significant impairment in intelligence with the qualitative characteristics of the impairment differing according to whether the bilateral ablation was anterior or posterior. Smaller lesions had little or no effect.

Goltz reported that bilateral removal of the frontal lobes produced awkwardness in movement, hyperactivity, hyperreflexia, and some diminution in tactile sensitivity. In addition, he noted that the operated dogs very often showed an alteration in character. They were irritable, restless, and aggressive, they had less to do with other dogs, and their intelligence was somewhat impaired. But ablations of smaller size restricted to the prefrontal region did not produce these effects, and this led Goltz and Loeb (1902) to deny that neural mechanisms underlying intelligence or personality traits were situated there.

The Berlin physiologist Hermann Munk (1839–1912), an indefatigable worker, was a dominant figure in the golden age of localization. Through ablation studies on the dog he identified the visual center in the occipital lobes and maintained that incomplete destruction of that region produced a condition that he designated as "mindblindness" and that was later given the name of visual agnosia (Munk, 1878, 1879). His discoveries, initially disputed by some of his fellow physiologists, had a direct influence on the thinking of clinicians who soon published case reports describing cortical blindness and mindblindness that confirmed his conclusions (Benton, 1978). Munk went on to localize cortical centers for somesthesis and audition in the parietofrontal and temporal regions, respectively. He also confirmed the existence of motor (or sensorimotor) centers in the frontal lobes. As for the prefrontal region, he had relatively little to say. He denied that the area was either exclusively or preferentially associated with the exercise of intelligence or any specific mental capacity such as attention, remarking that intelligence was a functional property of the whole cerbral cortex (Munk, 1890). In this respect at least he was in agreement with Goltz.

David Ferrier (1843–1928) was a pioneer localizationist of great prominence whose stimulation and ablation experiments, primarily on monkeys but also on dogs and cats, generated a comprehensive map of the major sensory and motor centers of the cerebral cortex (Ferrier, 1876, 1878/1886). Although some of his own observations would have suggested caution, he placed the cortical visual center in the angular gyrus in opposition to the occipital localization of Munk and others. How Ferrier came to make this unusual inference is not exactly clear; it is possible that either he inadvertently cut the underlying optic radiations in the course of his operations (Starr, 1884; Schäfer, 1888) or he misinterpreted visuomotor disability as absolute blindness (Glickstein, 1985). In any case, in due course he did acknowledge the participation of the occipital lobes in vision and concluded that the visual center occupied the territory of both the angular gyrus and the occipital lobe. His localization of somesthesis in the cerebral cortex was an unusual one. Finding no impairment of tactile sensitivity after extensive lesions of the convex surface of the hemispheres, he reported that experimentally produced lesions in the hippocampal region produced significant loss of response to pressure and pain. The auditory center was localized in the superior temporal cortex and the motor center in the rolandic region. He was one of the few investigators of the period to call attention to species differences, pointing out that the consequences of destruction of the motor area were far less severe in the dog and cat than in the monkey. He found that stimulation of the frontal cortex anterior to the motor area produced no overt responses.

Ferrier made careful observations on monkeys subjected to ablations of the prefrontal region and concluded that the consequences were a "decided alteration in the animals' character and behavior" but one that was "difficult to describe precisely." An observer who had not known the animals before operation might well judge them to be normal, since no sensory, perceptual, or motor defects were evident. But the animals were apathetic, not interested in their surroundings, and they responded only to momentary stimulation. Thus, "while not absolutely demented, they had lost, to all appearances, the faculty of attention and intelligent observation." Ferrier added that these behavioral changes did not appear in every monkey subjected to bilateral prefrontal ablation; in some animals the operation appeared to have no effect, perhaps because of incomplete removal of tissue.

The functional significance of the frontal lobes was the primary concern of the Italian neuropsychiatrist and physiologist Leonardo Bianchi (1848–1927). Beginning in the 1880s he undertook experimental studies extending over three decades on monkeys and dogs subjected to prefrontal ablations (Bianchi, 1895, 1920/1922). Having noted that unilateral ablations were without effect, he described the changes he had observed after bilateral removals. The animals showed no sensory or motor defects but there were profound changes in character. They no longer showed affection for people whom they used to caress, and when approached they were likely to be fearful. They were no longer sociable with other monkeys nor did they engage in play. At the same time they did groom themselves. They were impulsive and when frustrated they became violent. Bianchi offered a broad interpretation of these changes. Bilateral prefrontal ablation "does not so much interfere with the perceptions taken singly as it does disaggregate the personality." The animal is no longer capable of "serializing and synthesizing groups of representations." Their displays of fear and their agitation are direct consequences of this inability to integrate experiences and of their "defective sense of personality." Thus Bianchi saw frontal lobe changes as reflecting disintegration of the total personality rather than a loss of "general intelligence" or of a specific ability.

Comment

Experimental ablations of prefrontal cortex had generated positive results but nevertheless were somewhat ambiguous in that the predicted effects were not always obtained. The possibility of species differences in outcome was largely ignored, a circumstance that itself favored variation in findings. What had been reasonably well established was that whatever behavioral changes were observed came from bilateral destruction, with unilateral ablations usually being without effect. The prefrontal region was still only a unitary topographic landmark to these investigators. Its connections with other regions of the brain were scarcely known nor were there any indications that the region might consist of functional subdivisions. Unlike motor cortex, it was a silent area that was not responsive to electric stimulation.

In spite of their own observations that at least some of their frontally injured animals were hyperactive, irritable, aggressive, and asocial, Goltz and Loeb finally concluded that the region was a silent area. Perhaps, in their view, it was a question of the size of the lesion. In contrast, Ferrier had made some perceptive observations leading him to believe that prefrontally injured monkeys were partially demented and showed personality changes that he found difficult to describe. His observations were significantly extended by Bianchi, who gave a detailed account of these changes and interpreted them as reflecting a profound alteration of personality.

The Clinicians

By 1880 the associations between disease involving the territory of the precentral gyrus and motor disability and between aphasia and lesions of the foot of the left third frontal gyrus and its surround were universally recognized. The existence of the frontal eye fields and the supplementary motor area was to be brought to light only decades later. Three influential contributions in the late 1880s followed Harlow's 1868 paper describing the features of what came to be known as the "frontal lobe syndrome."

The first paper by Moritz Jastrowitz (1888) dealt with the clinical aspects of cerebral localization. In discussing frontal lobe symptomatology, he stated that he had seen a specific form of dementia, characterized by an oddly cheerful agitation, in patients with tumors of the frontal lobe, which he referred to as "so-called moria." He remarked that he had seen several such cases but had not called attention to them because of the difficulty in describing the peculiar condition and because of its inconstant presentation. But he emphasized that moria is found only in some frontal lobe patients and not necessarily only in tumors. "This peculiar disease picture is seen in many general paretics at the beginning of their illness, in senile dementia, in many alcoholics where certainly frontal lobe atrophy also occurs."

Later that year Leonore Welt (1888) wrote a lengthy paper in which she reported a personally observed case and presented a detailed review of earlier literature. Her patient, a 37-year-old man, had sustained a severe penetrating frontal fracture after a fall from a fourth story window. Presumably he had been trying to close the window but being drunk he lost his balance and fell. Physical recovery was swift and uneventful after an operation for removal of bone from the brain. However, beginning about 5 days after the traumatic event the patient showed a remarkable change in personality. He had always been an honest, industrious, cheerful man, skilled in his occupation as a furrier but somewhat given to boasting and a heavy drinker. There was now a complete change in his character. He was aggressive and malicious and given to making bad jokes. He teased other patients unmercifully and played mean tricks on the hospital personnel. He showed no respect for the physicians and threatened to "expose" them in the daily press. His behavior, which became increasingly intolerable, was the subject of almost daily complaints by the hospital personnel.

He exhibited this objectionable behavior for about a month at which time his behavior gradually improved. He was quieter, cleaner, no longer quarreled with everyone, and in a few days he was his old self. He was quite aware of how he had behaved and was genuinely remorseful. He could not explain what had happened to him. After discharge from the hospital he returned to work as a furrier but continued his heavy drinking. Some months later he died from a pleuritic infection. Autopsy disclosed destruction of the gyrus rectus in both hemispheres as well as the mesial sector of the right inferior frontal gyrus.

Having observed that the findings in her patient were consistent with the observations of Goltz and Ferrier as well as with Harlow's case, Welt pointed out that the number of such cases is very small and that far more often prefrontal injury does not produce these peculiar alterations in character. She discussed and tabulated the numerous negative cases of tumor, abscess, trauma, and atrophy of the frontal lobes in the literature that showed no personality changes although a diminution of intelligence was often apparent. Analyzing the eight autopsied cases showing personality change, she found that invariably there was involvement of the orbital gyri. Orbital pathology was also highly probable in two additional cases that had not come to autopsy. At the same time there were cases in the literature in which demonstrated orbital injury had not produced these personality changes. Welt concluded that the presentation of these character changes warrants the inference of orbital pathology. However, the converse was not true; the absence of such changes did not mean that the orbital area was intact.

In 1890 Hermann Oppenheim wrote a comprehensive paper on the clinical manifestations of brain tumors. In the section dealing with frontal lobe neoplasms he called attention to "a psychic anomaly which is perhaps of focal diagnostic value." Referring to Jastrowitz's concept of moria, he remarked that Bernhardt, Wernicke, and Westphal had made similar observations of childishness and inappropriate joking in patients with brain tumors but were unwilling to assign a lesional localization to this peculiar behavior. Hence, he was initially surprised at Jastrowitz's frontal lobe localization but his review of his own cases in fact confirmed it. However, he would not designate the condition as moria or silliness but rather a peculiar addiction to trivial joking of a predominantly sarcastic nature that was in sharp contrast to the patient's prevailing mood. Four patients who exhibited *Witzelsucht* proved to have tumors of the right frontal lobe, three of which had invaded the mesial and basal area. Nevertheless, this type of behavior can be observed in other conditions, as in a patient with chronic uremia whom Oppenheim had seen. This psychic anomaly appears predominantly in frontal lobe tumors. Future observation should be directed to the specific question of how frequently and under what circumstances it may be useful for focal diagnostic inference.

Comment

The studies of Jastrowitz, Welt, and Oppenheim established that distinctive changes in personality and behavior could be related to disease of the prefrontal region, and Welt specifically implicated involvement of the orbital and mesial sectors of that region. The terms moria (stupidity) and Witzelsucht (addiction to joking) are linguistic residues of their observations. Each of these clinicians called attention to a somewhat different combination of behaviors. Welt described a pattern of aggression, bad temper, and viciousness that she compared to Harlow's crowbar case and to the behavior of Goltz's dogs. Jastrowitz emphasized the inappropriate cheerfulness and lack of concern of his patients. Oppenheim was dubious about the reality of the patients' alleged cheerfulness and pointed to the sarcastic, latently hostile nature of the patients' compulsive joking. The frontal (really prefrontal) lobe syndrome is the legacy of these authors' descriptions.

Although this assemblage of behaviors was observed for the most part in patients with tumor of the frontal lobes, all three clinicians maintained that they could occur in other conditions involving frontal lobe pathology such as general paresis and trauma. Bilateral disease seemed to be the rule but this point was not emphasized. Instead the observation was made that involvement of the mesial-orbital area of the right frontal lobe might be of particular importance in the production of the symptoms.

The Twentieth Century: The First Fifty Years

Anatomy and Physiology

A major development in the early decades of the twentieth century was the rise of cytoarchitectonics, i.e., the systematic study of the cellular structure of the cerebral cortex. Some nineteenth century anatomists had described the internal structure of specific cortical areas and identified four to six layers in them. Cytoarchitectonics represented an extension of their observations and the mapping of all the areas. The major investigators in this ambitious and arduous enterprise (which was carried out on the brains of monkeys for the most part) were Campbell (1905), Brodmann (1909), Cécile and Oskar Vogt (1919), and Von Economo (1925) whose maps showed a basic similarity but nevertheless differed considerably in important details such as the number of areas that were identified. No doubt differences in investigative techniques were one determinant of these discrepant findings (Fleischhauer, 1978), and the unreliability of the more elaborate maps was the target of a harsh critique by Lashley and Clark (1946) who pointed out that significant individual differences were ignored and the boundaries between adjacent areas often could not be ascertained with any confidence. In the event, Brodmann's scheme, designating six layers and some 50 areas, was the one generally adopted by anatomists and neurologists. Although there was disagreement about the number and boundaries of these areas, the frontal pole was generally considered to occupy Brodmann areas 9–10, the mesial surface to occupy areas 24 and 32, the orbital surface to occupy areas 11–14 and 47, and the lateral convex surface to occupy areas 45–46. With some exceptions (e.g., area 24), these areas proved to be of the granular type with a clearly identifiable granular layer IV, in contrast to agranular motor cortex in which layer IV is obscured by layers III and V with their dense concentration of pyramidal cells. In any case, these studies demonstrated that the prefrontal region was far from being a homogeneous structure with the implication that its different parts might well have different functional properties.

Opinions differed with respect to the general question of the functional significance of these variations in internal structure of the cerebral cortex. It seemed reasonable to some students that the associations of pyramidal cell layers with efferent or motor functions and of granular layer IV with afferent or receptive functions must have functional implications. But there were so many exceptions to these rules that no strong generalizations could be made. Consequently, Brodmann's areas came to serve simply as topographic landmarks, primarily for the purpose of lesional localization, in the same way as did the cortical gyri and sulci. Only later was evidence adduced that the boundaries of the architectonic areas bore a relationship to the undersurface of the cortical sulci (Sanides, 1962).

At the same time the establishment of the neuron doctrine with its emphasis on directed (as opposed to diffuse) conduction, coupled with continued improvement in techniques of neurohistologic study, spurred investigation of the specific connections between the cerebral cortex (including prefrontal cortex) and other parts of the brain, most notably the thalamus. Many later nineteenth century anatomists, among them Gudden (1870), Monakow (1882, 1895), and the Dejerines (1895–1901), had already shown that experimentally produced lesions in the cortex led to degeneration in diverse subcortical structures. However, the reported findings were conflicting, the mechanisms and pathways involved were not clear, and the possibility that the observed effects had been produced by extraneous factors such as interference to the vascular supply of the subcortical structures had not been excluded. Experimental investigation during the early decades of the century, mainly on the monkey, identified these connections more precisely. Although the bulk of the work was concerned with motor cortex and the temporal, parietal, and occipital lobes, observations on the afferent and efferent connections of the prefrontal regions were also made. Some studies illustrative of the trend of results are reviewed below.

An early study by Beevor and Horsley (1902) found a striking degeneration of frontothalamic fibers in monkeys subjected to limited lesions in the prefrontal region. The only other area to which fibers could be traced from the inexcitable frontal cortex was the upper part of the substantia nigra. Minkowski (1922), describing his own results on monkeys in combination with some observations of his mentor, Monakow, inferred that there were projections from the dorsomedial nuclei of the thalamus to most of the prefrontal region extending to the frontal pole as well as to the prefrontal mesial surface. (In 1934 Pfeiffer reported the complementary observation that the dorsomedial nuclei formed the main termination of fibers from the anterior limb of the capsule.) In addition, Minkowski found that some projections from the anterior part of the globus pallidus reached the prefrontal region. Efferent connections included projections from the frontal pole to the internal capsule and the red nucleus and from the superior frontal gyrus to the rolandic area.

Levin (1936) made almost complete lesions of the prefrontal region of the right frontal lobe in two monkeys and traced the course of degeneration 2 weeks after the intervention. An extensive projection system, most of the fibers of which entered the rostral thalamus, was identified. The origin of these fibers appeared to be area 9 on the convexity of the frontal lobe. In addition, a bundle of fine fibers, apparently arising from the anterior part of the third frontal gyrus, descended to the midbrain (substantia nigra) and pons (dorsomedial pontine nuclei). Walker (1935, 1938) demonstrated that in monkeys the dorsomedial nucleus of the thalamus provides a spatially organized afferent projection system to the prefrontal region, the lateral part going to the upper frontal pole (area 9) and the mesial part going to the orbital area. He pointed out that this nuclear mass and cortical area attain their greatest development in the human brain. Correspondingly, motor cortex is connected in a definite spatial arrangement with lateral thalamic nuclei. Walker also described degenerative changes in the dorsomedial nucleus following ablation of prefrontal cortex, thus confirming Levin's finding of efferent connections between this region and the thalamus.

The introduction of prefrontal leukotomy and allied procedures in the late 1930s provided the opportunity to study the retrograde degeneration and glial proliferation in the brains of patients who had died after operation either as a result of the intervention or from intercurrent disease. The series of reports by Meyer et al. (1947; et al., 1950; McLardy, 1950) can serve to illustrate the tenor of results on this material. Degeneration of prefrontal-thalamic connections was found in every case, specifically retrograde degeneration in the dorsomedial nucleus. The findings of Walker (1938) of a spatially organized projection from the dorsomedial nucleus to prefrontal cortex in the monkey, e.g., the pars magnocellularis to orbital cortex and the pars parvicellularis to the dorsal convexity, were largely confirmed. And the point was made that a direct hypothalamic-prefrontal connection is probable in view of the established projection of hypothalamic nuclei to the pars magnocellularis, thus providing an anatomic basis for physiologic observations implicating the participation of the mesial orbital prefrontal cortex in emotional and autonomic changes. Lesions of the cingulate gyrus resulted in degeneration of anterior thalamic nuclei and degeneration of prefrontal-pontine pathways was demonstrable although it was not possible to identify the precise origin of these pathways.

Thus the outcome of these and other studies of the period in monkeys and human subjects was to establish definitively that the prefrontal region had rich afferent, efferent, and intracortical ("association") connections. The most prominent of these were the spatially organized links with the dorsal nuclei of the thalamus pointing to differentiation of function within the region. Connections to the basal ganglia, midbrain, and pons were also clearly demonstrable.

Studies of Animal Behavior

The rise of objective animal psychology, exemplified in the behavioral observations of C. Lloyd Morgan (1900), the puzzle box experiments of E. L. Thorndike (1898), and Jacques Loeb's (1902) studies of associative learning, provided a model for subsequent controlled assessment of the behavioral capacities and characteristics of animals with experimentally produced prefrontal lesions. Two series of studies, one by Shepherd Ivory Franz (1902, 1907, 1912) and the other by Carlyle Jacobsen and his co-workers (Crawford et al., 1948; Fulton and Jacobsen, 1935; Jacobsen and Nissen, 1937; 1931, 1935; Jacobsen et al., 1935), had a major influence on the evolution of thought about the role of the frontal lobes in the mediation of primate behavior.

Franz gave learning tasks, including the Thorndike puzzle box, to monkeys (and also cats) who had been subjected to unilateral and bilateral prefrontal ablations. Having learned the tasks preoperatively, the animals were tested for retention of the habits. Unilateral ablation had no significant effect, the operated animals retaining the habits almost as well as controls. Bilateral ablation produced loss of the habits in most of the animals; a few showed normal retention. However, those animals who had suffered loss of the recently acquired habits relearned them fairly readily. Franz's studies had the effect of including an attitude of skepticism on the part of students of animal behavior toward assigning any "higher-level" functions to the prefrontal region. It remained a "silent area" without identifiable behavioral significance.

Jacobsen's ingenious experiments with chimpanzees and monkeys, undertaken some 25 years later, effectively counteracted this rather nihilistic position. In essence he found that prefrontally injured animals exhibited a characteristic pattern of performances on a set of diverse learning tasks. They were not impaired on tasks, such as visual discrimination learning, in which all elements of the stimulus configuration are continuously in full view and that make no demands on short-term memory. In contrast, delayed response tasks, in which the animal is required to keep in mind an environmental event for 10 to 30 seconds in order to respond appropriately, were consistently failed by the animal who had been subjected to a bilateral prefrontal ablation. Jacobsen's findings in primates were readily confirmed and later work (e.g., Finan, 1939; Harlow and Settlage, 1948; Malmo, 1942) was devoted to the task of identifying basic factors, such as hyperactivity and distractibility, perseverative tendencies, and right–left confusion, that might underlie the failure in performance.

This defect in maintaining a set (in behavioristic terms) or carrying a representation of an environment event in mind over time (in mentalistic terms) was found in varying degrees in other prefrontally injured animals, such as dogs and cats, and rather less consistently in human subjects (see Hebb, 1945; Hebb and Penfield, 1940). Despite the negative findings reported for some patients, the demonstration of a specific type of cognitive defect associated with injury to the region weakened the cogency of "mass action" theories of cerebral functioning and offered promising clues to the understanding of the behavioral changes associated with frontal lobe disease.

The classic description by Jacobsen and his co-workers of a remarkable change in personality and behavior in one animal after a bilateral prefrontal ablation had a more direct and immediate impact on clinical thinking and practice. This female chimpanzee was a sociable, highly emotional animal who was eager to be tested in experimental tasks that brought her food rewards. Preoperatively she became greatly upset when she made errors on a very difficult task and often would fly into a temper tantrum. After a few errors in the course of training she refused to participate further and eventually had to be dragged from her cage to the experimental set-up, a condition that Jacobsen compared to a Pavlovian "experimental neurosis." She was gradually brought back to active participation in the experiments through feeding and play around the apparatus and was given an easy learning task with minimal possibility of failure. After left prefrontal lobectomy she was once again given the difficult task and once again developed an "experimental neurosis." However, after right frontal lobectomy her behavior changed profoundly. She showed a remarkable equanimity in the face of repeated failures on both the difficult and easy tasks. Jacobsen and his coworkers were sufficiently impressed by this postoperative change in the chimpanzee to make it a main point in their summary. "The basic disturbance is also manifest in the affective reactions. An 'experimental neurosis' was established by continued training on a problem situation too difficult for the animal to master. After bilateral extirpation of the frontal areas, the animal no longer had 'temper tantrums' when it made mistakes, and continued training on difficult problems did not evoke an 'experimental neurosis.' On the other hand, behavior suggestive of Witzelsucht which characterizes human cases with similar lesions, was noted" (Jacobsen et al., 1935, p. 14).

This series of experimental studies was reported by Fulton and Jacobsen in a major symposium on the frontal lobes at the 1935 International Congress of Neurology in London. The report included a description by Jacobsen of the disappearance of his chimpanzee's "experimental neurosis" following bilateral prefrontal lobotomy. After the presentation the Lisbon neurologist Egas Moniz, who was attending the symposium, raised the question of whether it ought not to be possible to alleviate anxiety states in human patients by a comparable surgical procedure (Valenstein, 1986). Since Moniz embarked on the operation of prefrontal leukotomy immediately after his return from London it has been generally assumed that the Fulton–Jacobsen report provided the impetus for his pioneering effort.

Clinical Studies

Clinical investigation during the first two decades of the century generated findings that were not always consistent but that did serve to document the diverse behavioral disorders observed in association with prefrontal injury. Early reports included that of Zacher (1901) who described a 54-year-old man with an illness of undetermined origin (however, he was diabetic with optic neuritis) that was characterized by lengthy periods of poor attention, fatigability, and apathy interspersed with periods during which he exhibited nearly normal behavior. At no time were there indications of speech disorder. However, gross visual impairment referable to the optic neuritis was evident. An outstanding feature of his condition was his lack of concern about his visual disability and hospitalization. Some years later Campbell (1909) also placed special emphasis on the lack of concern shown by his patient with a frontal lobe tumor. A second feature of Zacher's case was his patient's addiction to joking, which was evident even during his better periods. Zacher concluded by making two points: first, that Witzelsucht is a symptom of focal diagnostic significance; second, that his patient did not show the gross personality changes associated with prefrontal disease that had been described by Welt. On the other hand, Quensel (1914) reported a patient with prefrontal traumatic injury who showed no demonstrable intellectual impairment on either clinical observation or a comprehensive battery of psychologic tests. Yet he was impulsive and aggressive and showed grossly inappropriate conduct. In Quensel's view, the clinical picture presented by his patient was quite comparable to that of Welt's patient.

Both Schuster (1902) and Bernhardt (Bernhardt and Borchardt, 1909) discussed at some length the question of whether the childishness, moria, and Witzelsucht shown by some tumor patients were in fact a specific sign of frontal lobe disease. They agreed that, while the syndrome was seen in patients with tumors in other locations, it was shown with considerably greater frequency by those with frontal lobe tumors. Hence, in the absence of other symptoms indicative of a lesion in other locations, the appearance of these curious behavioral features was suggestive of frontal lobe disease. Bernhardt also noted that patients with right frontal involvement showed these features more frequently than did those with left frontal disease but, pointing out that aphasic disorder in left-hemisphere–damaged patients might mask the symptoms, he declined to draw a firm conclusion.

World War I produced thousands of cases of penetrating brain injuries including many with wounds more or less restricted to the frontal lobes. The carnage afforded ample opportunity for postwar study of these patients, and attempts were made to formulate a cogent definition of the "frontal lobe syndrome" as well as to relate different types of impairment to specific areas of the prefrontal region.

Feuchtwanger (1923) devoted a comprehensive monograph to his findings and interpretations of the behavioral changes seen in patients with prefrontal injuries. A comparison of frontal and nonfrontal cases showed contrasting patterns of performance. As compared to nonfrontal patients, mood disorders, apathy, attentional disturbance, impulsivity, and Witzelsucht were more frequently manifested, while sensorimotor defects, speech disorders, and memory impairment were less frequently manifested by the frontal patients. Individual patients showed distinctive clinical pictures, e.g., some were depressed or apathetic, others were euphoric, and still others "psychopathic" or "hysteroid." Feuchtwanger ascribed great importance to the patient's premorbid personality as a determinant of his clinical picture. No important differences between predominantly left and predominantly right prefrontal patients were apparent and Witzelsucht was not a frequent occurrence. Feuchtwanger saw his findings as indicating that, although basic cognitive functions such as perceptual capacity, memory, and ideation are not impaired in frontal patients, they show profound disturbances of affect and of the capacity to control or integrate behavior, which he considered to be a change in the total personality. His more detailed theoretic interpretation, fraught with unfamiliar terms and vague concepts, is difficult to understand. Nevertheless his contribution was of considerable value in showing the variety of changes that can follow prefrontal damage and in his demonstration that a simplistic concept of a single "frontal lobe syndrome" is quite untenable.

In the 1920s Kurt Goldstein (1927, 1936 a,b, 1944, 1948; Goldstein and Katz, 1937) advanced a theory of neuropsychologic function that was based on his conception of the "abstract attitude." This extremely broad concept incorporated not only the capacity for abstract reasoning but also a variety of other behavioral functions such as initiative, foresight, resistance to suggestion, self-awareness, flexibility in behavior, and the capacity to analyze a complex situation into its constituent components. In fact, his specifications could well serve as a broad definition of "general intelligence." Goldstein interpreted the diverse behavioral defects shown by patients with brain disease, and particularly those with prefrontal injury, as expressions of this single capacity. Given the breadth of the concept, it was easy enough to demonstrate that every patient was defective in one or another aspect of the abstract attitude. In the 1930s and 1940s the approach was widely adopted by clinical psychologists who were searching for signs of prefrontal dysfunction. In due course, however, this "single principle" approach lost popularity as it became evident that the concept of the abstract attitude was too broad and multifaceted to be useful.

Goldstein's more valuable contribution was his insightful interpretation of certain symptoms as defensive reactions on the part of the patient to protect him from failure, confusion, and loss of self-esteem. Thus, at least under some circumstances, the patient who shows apathy, rigidity, lack of concern, or facetiousness may be exhibiting these behaviors in order to cope with his disabilities and avoid painful awareness of his mental incompetence. This approach to the understanding of some of the peculiar behaviors encountered in brain-damaged patients, especially those with frontal lobe disease, was also adopted by Golla (1931) and Brickner (1936).

In a monograph of over 1000 pages, Karl Kleist (1934) reported his findings on some hundreds of patients who had sustained penetrating brain wounds during World War I. An old-fashioned localizationist who did not hesitate to infer functions from symptoms, he developed a detailed map of the brain in which diverse capacities were assigned to specific cortical areas (see Benton, 1976, p. 39; Kleist, 1934, pp. 1365–6). However, Kleist was also a careful examiner and a cautious interpreter who compared his findings with earlier observations. He laid great stress on the lack of drive or initiative (Antrieb) associated with orbital lesions and on the personality changes seen in prefrontally injured patients, which he related to deficiencies in self-perception. He also described impoverishment of verbal ideation and expression in the absence of frank aphasic disorder in patients with left prefrontal involvement, an observation that was amply confirmed in later decades (see Benton, 1968; Milner, 1964; Zangwill, 1966). Moreover, he was perhaps the first clinician to emphasize the significance of the close connections between the prefrontal orbital area and structures of the limbic system and to regard them as a neural network subserving self-perception and "egofunctions" (Kleist, 1931). His ideas, in contrast to those of Goldstein, had little influence outside of Germany, probably because his monumental volume was not translated into English or French.

Brickner's (1934, 1936) case report of a patient with practically total excision of the prefrontal region in the course of removal of a large meningioma aroused great interest because of its detailed and vivid account of the patient's social behavior and intellectual and personality characteristics over the course of several years. This 42-year-old businessman of high average intelligence first came under observation 1 year after surgery. During casual interactions of short duration he could appear to be entirely normal even to professional observers. His everyday behavior was quite different. He was obstinate, verbally aggressive, boastful, abusive to his caretakers, and addicted to poor joking. At times he was capable of simple abstract reasoning but usually was unable to maintain or follow a logical train of thought. Psychologic testing yielded IQs of 95–100, indicating a significant decline from premorbid "general intelligence." His Rorschach test performance reflected extreme ideational impoverishment with a predominance of color-naming responses. Brickner viewed his patient's behavior as an exaggerated expression of certain premorbid personality traits rather than as representing a qualitative personality change. Almost echoing Bianchi, he thought that the fundamental disability was a defect in the synthesis of essentially intact cognitive processes that rendered the patient incapable of engaging in complex or temporally integrated conduct.

Ackerly (1937) described unusual findings in a 37-year-old woman in whom the mesial sector of the left prefrontal region had been destroyed by the growth of a large meningioma and the entire right prefrontal region had been amputated in the course of removal of the tumor. Psychometric testing gave no indication of a decline in "general intelligence" or of diminished energy in carrying out household duties or engaging in social functions. Moreover, relatives and friends found her to be the same sociable, likable, kindhearted person that she was before her illness. Nevertheless there were some striking changes in her behavior. For example, once having begun a task (e.g., house cleaning or preparing a meal) she could not be made to abandon it, even momentarily, until it was completed. There were other conspicuous findings in this patient. She actually showed an increased capacity for work and physical exercise and she made remarkable progress in speaking and reading English, which was her second language. Ackerly interpreted his patient's behavior as reflecting an abnormal "lack of distractibility" that was based on an inability to handle more than one environmental event at the same time. The case once again illustrated the diversity of behavioral changes that are encountered in patients with prefrontal disease and in addition offered promising clues to the understanding of frontal lobe function.

A radically different note was sounded by the neurosurgeon Clovis Vincent (1936); on the basis of his clinical experience, he insisted that partial or even complete removal of the prefrontal region was not accompanied by the diverse mental symptoms traditionally associated with frontal lobe disease. Vincent pointed out that the prefrontal region is neither a simple nor an autonomous structure. Its activity is regulated by the other parts of the brain with which it is connected and hence pathologic alteration of these parts could disrupt prefrontal functioning.

Vincent presented his paper in the same symposium on the frontal lobes at the 1935 London International Neurological Congress in which Fulton and Jacobsen reported their findings on chimpanzees. With its emphasis on the lack of any major disruptive effects of prefrontal removals in human patients, Vincent's presentation may well have had a more significant effect on the thinking of Egas Moniz than did the Fulton-Jacobsen report, which dealt in the main with the cognitive defects produced by prefrontal lobotomy. However, Moniz himself denied that either presentation had had any such influence (see Valenstein, 1986).

The same theme was taken up in greater detail by Hebb (1945), who attacked the "almost universal belief that surgical removals from this area (the frontal lobes) must produce serious psychologic defects." The impetus for the critique was his study of a patient (Hebb and Penfield, 1940) who at the age of 16 had sustained a severe head injury that had injured both frontal poles. A 10-year period of convulsive disorder, violent behavior, and impairment of memory led to surgical intervention in which a large part of both prefrontal regions (almost all of Brodmann areas 9–12 and 46–47) was excised in the course of removal of scar tissue. Recovery following the operation was remarkable. He was considered by his relatives and friends to have once again become his old self, i.e., before the head injury. He served successfully in the Canadian army during World War II. The only "prefrontal" trait that he showed was a rather happy-go-lucky attitude with a penchant for changing jobs every few months and with no concern about the future. His test performance improved to a normal level from a preoperative subnormal level.

From the findings in this case, as well a critical review of the literature and an analysis of the methodologic difficulties in interpreting the symptoms of frontal lobe disease, Hebb argued that uncomplicated loss of prefrontal tissue did not have the major deleterious consequences encountered in cases of tumor, atrophy, or trauma where in all probability dysfunction of other parts of the brain was present. His trenchant critique aroused considerable discussion and no doubt encouraged surgical interventions including frontal leukotomy.

Summary

As a perusal of the list of references will show, not a single contribution before 1947 contained the adjective "prefrontal" in its title. Early investigators of the prefrontal region invariably employed the term "frontal" to indicate their field of study. This usage persists in large part today along with the more limiting designations, "prefrontal cortex" and "frontal granular cortex." In any case, the content of these early contributions leaves no doubt that they were dealing specifically with the prefrontal region.

A major achievement of the first three decades of the twentieth century was the description of the distinctive cellular composition of the prefrontal region and its parcellation into architectonic areas. Brodmann's maps, in common use as topographic landmarks today, are a lasting legacy of this monumental effort. Campbell, Brodmann, the Vogts, and Economo produced maps that differed from one another in not unimportant details, a circumstance that inevitably raised questions about their reliability. The negative findings of replicative studies reinforced this skepticism, particularly in regard to the cortical areas delimited by Brodmann. Nevertheless, the fundamental fact of areal cellular differentiation in the prefrontal region, as in other regions of the brain, was firmly established and provided the basis for the more searching studies of Sanides and Fleischhauer.

Of greater significance were the investigations of the connections between the prefrontal region and other parts of the brain that were instituted in the late nineteenth century and continued through the early decades of the twentieth.

The most important afferent and efferent connections were determined to be with the dorsomedial nucleus of the thalamus. As Walker and others demonstrated, the connections followed a definite spatial arrangement with the magnocellular sector of the nucleus projecting to the orbital and the parvocellular sector to the dorsolateral area of the prefrontal region. Other connections of the prefrontal region that were brought to light involved the basal ganglia, midbrain, and pons. It was an awareness of these multiple connections that would lead Vincent to the conclusion that prefrontal symptomatology reflected a disruption in the interrelations of the region with other centers rather than a mere loss of tissue.

Animal experimentation, exemplified by the studies of Bianchi and Jacobsen, indicated that prefrontally injured monkeys and dogs did indeed exhibit distinctive cognitive defects and peculiar alterations of personality that an experienced observer could readily detect but which were not easily described. Diverse verbal labels, e.g., "apathy," "agitation," "partial dementia," were employed to characterize the behavioral changes, and tentative hypotheses such as the incapacity to "serialize groups of impressions" and impairment in "recent memory" were advanced to explain them. But neither the behavioral descriptions nor the explanations that were proposed to account for them were felt to be altogether satisfactory and none received wide acceptance.

By 1947 a vast array of diverse behavior deficits of a cognitive, affective, and interpersonal nature had been described in association with disease of the prefrontal region. This mixture of deficits was far too variegated to permit the formulation of a satisfactory description in terms of one or two basic disabilities. Nevertheless, the term "frontal lobe syndrome" was adopted to refer to this aggregation of deficits, perhaps as much as a convenient label as from any conviction that it represented a true syndrome, i.e., a conjunction of inherently related symptoms.

Descriptions of the consequences of prefrontal disease and surgical removals ranged from thoroughgoing dementia to the absence of observable deficits. Between the extremes were reports of highly specific deficits and personality changes that more often than not seriously impaired overall behavioral competence. Still other reports, such as that of Ackerly, described pronounced personality changes that complicated but did not have a devastating effect on a patient's life adjustment. A number of observers related personality changes specifically to orbital-mesial injury, and a few raised the question of whether right hemisphere involvement might be a particularly important factor. The frequent descriptions of personality change in the direction of equanimity, lack of concern, and diminution of anxiety provided some rationale for surgical intervention to alleviate agitation, depression, and anxiety in psychiatric patients.

Thus in 1950 researchers were presented with an embarrassment of riches. They faced a number of formidable challenges. They had to sort out the diverse deficits that had been associated with lesions of the prefrontal region to determine which were primary and which were secondary or adventitious. They had to gain insight into the nature of the primary deficits as derangements of normal neuropsychologic functioning. Mindful of the fact that the prefrontal region is simply a topographic landmark encompassing a number of distinctive anatomic–functional areas, they had to identify the neural mechanisms that mediated the behavioral operations of each of these areas.

While everyone would agree that current factual knowledge is still incomplete and conceptual formulations still not entirely satisfying, researchers have achieved notable success in meeting these challenges at every level—anatomic, physiologic, and behavioral. Indeed the advances in understanding that have been made since 1950 (and particularly since 1970) are so radical and far-reaching as to justify the designation of developments up to 1950 as "early history." The results of this impressive recent progress are epitomized in the contributions to this volume.

Acknowledgments

I am indebted to Ms. Jan Carter for her help in the preparation of the manuscript.

References

Ackerly S. (1937). Instinctive, emotional and mental changes following prefrontal lobe extirpation. *Am. J. Psychiatry* 92: 717–729.

Ajuriaguerra J. and Hécaen H. (1949). *Le Cortex Cérébral*. Paris: Masson.

Akert K. and Hammond H. P. (1962). Emanuel Swedenborg and his contribution to neurology. *Med. Hist.* 6: 255–256.

Andral G. (1823–1827). *Clinique Médicale*. Paris: Fortin Masson.

Arnold F. (1838). *Bemerkungen über den Bau des Hirns und Rückenmarks*. Zurich: S. Hohr (cited by Clarke and Dewhurst, 1972).

Baker F. (1909). The two Sylviuses: an historical study. *Bulletin of the Johns Hopkins Hospital* 20: 329–339.

Beck E., McLardy T., and Meyer A. (1950). Anatomical comments on psychosurgical procedures. *J. Ment. Sci.* 96: 157–167.

Beevor C. E. and Horsley V. (1902). On the pallio-tectal or cortico-mesencepalic system of fibres. *Brain* 25: 436–443.

Benton A. L. (1964). Contributions to aphasia before Broca. *Cortex:* 314–327.

Benton A. L. (1968). Differential behavioral effects on frontal lobe disease. *Neuropsychologia* 6: 53–60.

Benton A. L. (1976). Historical development of the concept of hemispheric cerebral dominance. In Spicker S. F., Engelhardt H. T. (eds.), *Philosophical Dimensions of the Neuromedical Sciences*. Dordrecht, the Netherlands: Reidel.

Benton A. L. (1978). The interplay of experimental and clinical approaches in brain lesion research. In Finger S. (ed.), *Recovery from Brain Damage: Research and Theory*. New York: Plenum Press, pp. 49–68.

Benton A. L. (1981). Focal brain damage and the concept of localization. In Loeb C. (ed.), *Studies in Cerebrovascular Disease*. Milano: Masson Italia Editore.

Bernhardt M. and Borchardt M. (1909). Zur Klinik der Stirnhirntumoren nebst Bemerkungen über Hirnpunktion. *Berliner Klinische Wochenschrift* 46: 1341–1347.

Bianchi L. (1845). The functions of the frontal lobes. *Brain* 18: 497–522.

Bianchi L. (1920). *La Meccanica del Cervello e la Funzione dei Lobi Frontali*. Turin: Bocca; English translation by Macdonald J. H. (1922). *The Mechanisms of the Brain and the Functions of the Frontal Lobes*. Edinburgh: Livingstone.

Bigelow H. J. (1850) Dr. Harlow's case of recovery from the passage of an iron bar through the head. *Am. J. Med. Sci.* 39: 13–22.

Bouillaud J-B. (1825). *Traité Clinique et Physiologique de l'Encéphalite*. Paris: Baillière.

Brickner R. M. (1934). An interpretation of frontal lobe function based upon the study of a case of partial bilateral frontal lobectomy. In Orton S. T., Fulton J. F., Davis T. K. (eds.), *Localization of Function in the Cerebral Cortex*. Baltimore: Williams & Wilkins, pp. 259–351.

Brickner R. M. (1936). *The Intellectual Functions of the Frontal Lobes*. New York: Macmillan.

Brodmann K. (1909). *Vergleichende Lokalisationslehre der Grosshirnrinde*. Leipzig: Barth.

Campbell A. W. (1905). Histological Studies on the Localisation of Cerebral Function. Cambridge: Cambridge University Press.

Campbell D. (1909). Störungen der Merkfähigkeit und fehlendes Krankheitsgefühl bei einem Fall von Stirnhirntumor. *Monatsschrift für Psychiatrie* 26: 33–41.

Chaussier F. (1807). Exposition Sommaire de la Structure et des Différentes Parties de l'Encéphale ou Cerveau. Paris: Théophile Barrois, 1807 (cited by McHenry, 1969 and Meyer, 1971).

Clarke E. and Dewhurst K. (1972). *An Illustrated History of Brain Function*. Berkeley: University of California Press.

Clarke E. and Jacyna L. S. (1987). *Nineteenth-Century Origins of Neuroscientific Concepts*. Berkeley: University of California Press.

Clarke E. and O'Malley C. D. (1968). *The Human Brain and Spinal Cord*. Berkeley: University of California Press.

Crawford M. P., Fulton J. F., Jacobsen C. F., and Wolfe S. B. (1948). Frontal lobe ablation in chimpanzee: a résumé of 'Becky' and 'Lucy.' *Res. Publ. Assoc. Nerv. Ment. Dis.* 27: 3–58.

Dejerine J. and Dejerine-Klumpke A. (1895–1901). *Anatomie des Centres Nerveux*. Paris: Rueff.

Ecker A. (1869). *Die Hirnwindungen des Menschen nach eigenen Untersuchungen*. Braunschweig: Vieweg.

Ecker A. (1875). *The Cerebral Convolutions of Man Represented According to Original Observations*. Translated by R. T. Edes. New York: Appleton.

Economo C., and Koskinas G. N. (1925). *Die Cytoarchitektonik der Hirnrinde des Erwachsenen Menschen*. Vienna: Springer.

Ferrier D. (1876). *The Functions of the Brain*. London: Smith, Elder (2nd ed., 1886).

Ferrier D. (1878) *The Localisation of Cerebral Disease*. London: Smith, Elder.

Feuchtwanger E. (1923). *Die Funktionen des Stirnhirns*. Berlin: Springer.

Finan J. L. (1939). Effects of frontal lobe lesions on temporally organized behavior in monkeys. *J. Neurophysiol.* 2: 208–226.

Fleischhauer K. (1978). Cortical architectonics: the last 50 years and some problems of today. In Brazier M. A. and Petsche H. (eds.), *Architectonics of the Cerebral Cortex*. New York: Raven Press.

Franz S. I. (1902). On the functions of the cerebrum. *Am. J. Physiol.* 8: 1–22.

Franz S. I. (1907). On the functions of the cerebrum: The frontal lobes. *Arch. Psycho.* 1: 1–64.

Franz S. I. (1912). New phrenology. *Science* 35: 321–328.

Fulton J. F. and Jacobsen C. F. (1935). The functions of the frontal lobes: a comparative study in monkeys, chimpanzees and man. *Abstracts. International Second Neurological Congress*. Vol. 2, 70–71. London.

Fuster J. M. (1980). *The Prefrontal Cortex: Anatomy, Physiology and Neuropsychology of The Frontal Lobe*. New York: Raven Press (2nd ed., 1989).

Gall F. J., and Suprzheim G. (1809). *Recherches sur le système Nerveux en Général et sur Celui de Cerveau en Particulier*. Paris: F. Schoell. (Reprint. Amsterdam: Bonsel, 1967).

Gibson W. C. (1962). Pioneers in localization in the brain. *JAMA* 180: 944–957.

Glickstein M. (1985). Ferrier's mistake. *Trends Neurosci.* 8: 341–344.

Goldstein K. (1927). Die Lokalisation in der Grosshirnrinde. In Bethe A. (ed.), *Handbuch der Normalen und Pathologischen Physiologie,* Vol. 10, pp. 600–842. Berlin: Springer. 1927.

Goldstein K. (1936a). The significance of the frontal lobes for mental performance. *J. Neuro. Psychopathol.* 17: 27–40.

Goldstein K. (1936b). The modifications of behavior consequent to cerebral lesions. *Psychiatr. Q.* 10: 586–610.

Goldstein K. 1944). The mental changes due of frontal lobe damage. *J. Psychol.* 17: 187–208.

Goldstein K. (1948). *Language and Language Disturbances*. New York: Grune & Stratton.

Goldstein K., and Katz S. (1937). The psychopathology of Pick's disease. *Arch. Neurol. Psychiatry* 38: 473–490.

Golla F. (1931). Discussion on the mental symptoms associated with cerebral tumours. *Proc. Rov. Soc. Med.* 24: 1000–1001.

Goltz F. (1888). Über die Verrichtungen des Grosshirns. Pfüger's Archiv fur die gesamte Physiologie 42: 419–467. Translation by G. Von Bonin. *On the Functions of the Hemispheres*. In Von Bonin G. (ed.), (1960) *Some Papers on the Cerebral Cortex*. Springfield, IL: CC Thomas, pp. 118–158.

Goltz F. (1892). Der Hund ohne Grosshirn: Siebente Abteilung über die Verrichtungen des Grosshirns. *Pfluger's Archiv für die gesamte Physiologie* 51: 570–614.

Gratiolet P. (1854). Note sur les expansions des racines cérébrales du nerf optique et sur leur terminaison dan une région determinée de l'écorce des hémisphères. *Comptes Rendus de l'Académie des Sciences* (Paris), 29: 274–278.

Grünthal E. (1957). Geschichte der makroskopischen Morphologie des menschlichen Grosshirnsreliefs nebst Beiträgen zur Entwicklung der Idee einer Lokalisierung psychischer Funktionen. *Bibliotheca Psychiatrica et Neurologica, Fasc.* 100: 94–128.

Gudden B. (1870). Experimental untersuchungen uber das peripherische und centrale Nerven-system. *Archiv für Psychiatrie* 2: 693–723.

Harlow H. F. and Settlage P. H. (1948). Effect of extirpation of frontal areas upon learning performance of monkeys. *Res. Pub. Assoc. Res. Ner. Ment. Dis.* 27: 446–459.

Harlow J. M. (1848). Passage of an iron bar through the head. *Boston Medical and Surgical Journal* 39: 389–393.

Harlow J. M. (1868). Recovery from the passage of an iron bar through the head. *Publications of the Massachusetts Medical Society* 2: 327–347.

Hebb D. O. (1945). Man's frontal lobes: a critical review. *Arch. Neurol. Psychiatry* 54: 10–24.

Hebb D. O. and Penfield W. (1940) Human behavior after extensive bilateral removal from the frontal lobes. *Arch. Neurol. Psychiatry* 44: 421–438.

Jacobsen C. F. (1931). A study of cerebral function in learning: The frontal lobes. *J. Comp. Neurol.* 52: 271–340.

Jacobsen C. F. (1935). Functions of frontal association areas in primates. *Arch. Neurol. Psychiatry* 33: 558–569.

Jacobsen C. F. and Nissen H. W. (1937) Studies of cerebral function in primates. IV. The effects of frontal lobe lesions on the delayed alternation habit in monkeys. *J. Comp. Physiol. Psychol.* 23: 101–112.

Jacobsen C. F., Wolfe J. B., and Jackson T. A. (1935) An experimental analysis of the functions of the frontal association areas in primates. *J. Nerv. Ment. Dis.* 82: 1–14.

Jastrowitz M. (1888). Beiträge zur Localisation im Grosshirn und über deren praktische Verwerthung. *Dtsch Med Wochenschr* 14: 81–83, 108–112, 125–128, 151–153, 172–175, 188–192, 209–211.

Kleist K. (1931). Die Störungen der Ich-Leistungen und ihre Lokalisation im Orbital-Innen und Zwischenhirn. *Monatsschrift für Psychiatrie* 71: 338–350.

Kleist K. (1934). *Gehirnpathologie*. Leipzig: Barth.

Krech D. (1964). Cortical localization of function. In Postman L. (ed.), *Psychology in the Making: Histories of Selected Research Problems*. New York: Knopf.

Lashley K. S. and Clark G. (1946). The cytoarchitecture of the cerebral cortex of Ateles: a critical examination of architectonic studies. *J. Comp. Neurol.* 85: 223–305.

Levin P. M. (1936). The efferent fibers of the frontal lobe of the monkey, macaca mulatta. *J. Comp. Neurol.* 63: 369–419.

Lewy F. H. (1942). Historical introduction: the basal ganglia and their diseases. In Putnam T. J. Frantz A. M. and Ranson S. W. (eds.), *The Diseases of the Basal Ganglia*. Baltimore: Williams & Wilkins, pp. 1–20.

Liepmann H. (1900). *Das Krankheitsbild der Apraxie*. Berlin: Karger.

Loeb J. (1885). Die elementaren Störungen einfacher Funktionen nach oberflächlicher, umschriebene Verletzung des Grosshirns. *Pflüger's Archiv für die gesamte Physiologie* 37: 51–56.

Loeb J. (1886). Beiträge zur Physiologie des Grosshirns. *Pflüger's Archiv für die gesamte Physiologie* 39: 265–346.

Loeb J. (1902). *Comparative Physiology of the Brain and Comparative Psychology*. New York: Putnam.

Macmillan M. B. (1986). A wonderful journey through skull and brains: the travels of Mr. Gage's tamping iron. *Brain Cogn.* 5: 67–102.

Malmo R. B. (1942). Interference factors in delayed response in monkeys after removal of frontal lobes. *J. Neurophysiol.* 5: 295–308.

McLardy T. (1950). Thalamic projection to frontal cortex in man. *J. Neurol. Neurosurg. Psychiatry* 13: 198–202.

Meyer A. (1971). *Historical Aspects of Cerebral Anatomy*. New York: Oxford University Press.

Meyer A., Beck E. and McLardy T. (1947). Prefrontal leucotomy: a neuro-anatomical report. *Brain* 70: 18–49.

Meynert T. (1867). Der Bau der Gross-Hirnrinde und seine Örtlichen Verschiedenheiten.

Vierteljahresschrift für Psychiartrie 1: 77–93, 198–217 (cited by Clarke and O'Malley, 1968).

Meynert T. (1869). Beiträge zur Kenntnis der centralen Projection der Sinnesoberflächen. *Sitzungsberichte der Kaiserlichen Akademie der Wissenchaften. Mathematisch-Naturwissenschaftliche Classe* (Wein) 60: 547–566.

Meynert T. (1877). Die Windungen der Convexen Oberfläche des Vorderhirns bei Menschen. Affen und Raubtieren. *Archiv für Psychiatrie und Nervenkrankheiten* 7: 275–286.

Meynert T. (1884). *Psychiatrie: Klinik der Erkrankungen des Vorderhirns*. Vienna: Braunmüller. (Translation by B. Sachs. Psychiatry: *A Clinical Treatise on Diseases of the Fore-Brain*. New York: Putnam, 1885; reprinted, New York: Hafner, 1968.)

Milner B. (1964). Some effects of frontal lobectomy in man. In Warren J. M. and Akert K. (eds.), *The Frontal Granular Cortex and Behavior*. New York: McGraw-Hill. pp. 313–331.

Minkowski M. (1923, 1924). Etude sur les connexions anatomiques des circonvolutions rolandiques, pariétales et frontales. *Schweizer Archiv für Neurologie und Psychiatrie* 12: 71–104, 227–268 (1923); 14: 255–278, 15: 97–132 (1924).

Monakow C. (1882). Ueber einige durch circumscripter Hirdrindenregion bedingte Entwickelungshemmungen des Kaninchengehirns. *Archiv für Psychiatrie* 12: 141–156.

Monakow C. (1895). Experimentelle und pathologisch-anatomische Untersuchungen über die Haubenregion, den Sehhügel und die Region subthalamica. *Archiv für Psychiatrie* 27: 1–128, 386–479.

Morgan C. L. (1990) *Animal Behavior*. London: Scott.

Munk H. (1878). Weitere Mittheilungen zur Physiologie der Grosshirnrinde. *Archiv für Anatomie und Physiologie* 2: 162–178.

Munk H. (1879). Weiteres zur Physiologie der Sehsphäre der Grosshirnrinde. *Archiv für Anatomie und Physiologie* 3: 581–592.

Munk H. (1890). *Über die Functionen der Grosshirnrinde*. berlin: Hirschwald.

Neuburger M. (1897). *Historische Entwicklung der Experimentellen Gehirn-und Rückenmarks pysiologie vor Flourens*. Stuttgart: Enke, English translation and edition by. Clarke (1981). *The Historical Development of Experimental Brain and Spinal Cord Physiology before Flourens*. Baltimore: Johns Hopkins Press.

Oppenheim H. (1890). Zur Pathologie der Gehirngeschwulste. *Archiv für Psychiatrie* 21: 560–578, 705–745; 22: 27–72.

Panizza B. (1855). Osservazioni sul nervo ottico. *Giornale, Istituto Lombardo di Scienze Lettere* 7: 237–252.

Pfeiffer R. A. (1934). Myelogenetisch-anatomische Untersuchungen über den zentralen Abschnitt der Taststrahlung, der Pyramidenbahn, der Hirnnerven und zusätzlicher motorischer Bahnen. *Nova Acta Leopoldina* 1: 341–473.

Quensel F. (1914). Stirnhirnverletzung mit Charakterveränderung. *Muenchener Medizinische Wochenschrift* 61: 1761–1763.

Riese W and Hoff E. C. (1950). A history of the doctrine of cerebral localization. *J. Hist. Med.* 5: 50–71.

Rolando L. (1831). Della struttura degli emisferi cerebrali. *Memorie della Reale Academia di Scienze di Torino* 35: 103–146 (cited by Meyer, 1971).

Romberg M. H. (1840–46). *Lehrbuch der Nervenkrankheiten des Menschen*. Berlin: Duncker. 1840–1846. English translation by E. H. Sieveking. *A Manual of the Nervous Diseases of Man*. London: The New Sydenham Society.

Rylander G. (1939). *Personality Changes after Operations on the Frontal Lobes*. Copenhagen: Munksgaard.

Sanides F. (1962). Die *Architektonik des Menschlichen Stirnhirns*. Berlin: Springer.

Schäfer E. A. (1888). Experiments on special sense localisation in the cortex cerebri of the monkey. *Brain* 10: 362–380.

Schiller F. (1965). The rise of the "enteroid process" in the 19th century: some landmarks in cerebral nomenclature.*Bull. Hist. Med.* 39: 326–338.

Schuster P. (1902). *Psychische Störungen bei Hirntumoren*. Stuttgart: Enke.

Soury J. (1899). *Le Système Nerveux Central*. Paris: Carré et Naud.

Spillane J. D. (1981). *The Doctrine of the Nerves: Chapters in the History of Neurology*. New York: Oxford University Press.

Starr M. A. (1884). The visual area in the brain determined by a study of hemianopsia. *Am. J. Med. Sci.* 87: 65–83.

Steegman A. T. (1962). Dr. Harlow's famous case: the "impossible" accident of Phineas P. Gage. *Surgery* 52: 952–958.

Stookey B. (1954). A note on the early history of cerebral localization. *Bull. N.Y. Acad. Med.* 30: 559–578.

Swazey J. P. (1970). Action propre and action commune: the localization of cerebral function. *J. Hist. Biol.* 3: 213–234.

Thorndike E. L. (1898). Animal intelligence. *Psychological Review Monographs,* Supplement No. 8.

Valenstein E. S. (1986). *Great and Desperate Cures*. New York: Basic Books.

Varolio C. (1573). *De Nervis Opticis*. Padua: Meitti (cited by Clarke and O'Malley, 1968; Meyer, 1971).

Varolio C. (1591). *Anatomiae sive de Resolutione Corporis Humani*. Frankfurt: Wechel and Fischer (cited by Clarke and O'Malley, 1968; Meyer, 1971).

Vincent C. (1936). Neurochirurgische Betrachtungen über die Funktionen des Frontallappens. *Dtsche. Med. Wochenschr.* 62: 41–45.

Vogt O. and Vogt C. (1919). Allgemeine Ergebnisse unserer Hirnforschung. *Journal für Psychologie und Neurologie* 25: 273–462.

Walker A. E. (1935). The retrograde cell degeneration in the thalamus of macacus rhesus following hemidecortication. *J. Comp. Neurol.* 62: 407–419.

Walker A. E. (1938). *The Primate Thalamus*. Chicago: University of Chicago Press.

Walker A. E. (1957). The development of the concept of cerebral localization in the nineteenth century. *Bull. Hist. Med.* 31: 99–121.

Welt L. (1888) Über Charakterveranderungen des Menschen infolge von Läsionen des Stirnhirns. *Deutsche Archiv für Klinische Medizin* 42: 339–390.

Wernicke C. (1874). *Der aphasische Symptomenkomplex*. Breslau: Cohn und Weigert.

Willis T. (1964). *Cerebri Anatome*. London: Martyn & Allestry. Translation by S. Pordage. *On the Anatomy of the Brain*. London: Dring, 1681. Feindel W. (ed.), Thomas Willis *The Anatomy of the Brain and Nerves*. Montreal: McGill University Press. 1965.

Zacher W. (1901). Ueber ein Fall von doppelseitigem, symmetrisch gelegenem Erweichungsherd im Stirnhirn und Neuritis optica. *Neurologisches Zentralblatt* 20: 1074–1083.

Zangwill O. L. (1966). Psychological deficits associated with frontal lobe lesions. *Int. J. Neurol* 5: 395–402.

5

Cerebrovascular Disease in the History of Clinical Neuropsychology

> From the theoretical point of view, it is important to stress that it is the patient with the ischemic infarct who is the most important source of knowledge concerning the clinical syndromes of the aphasias and their localizations. Thrombotic cerebrovascular disease is by far the most important cause of aphasia in the adult. These patients can be studied over long periods of stability. At postmortem examination the lesions found are often well defined and can be mapped precisely together with the resultant secondary degenerations.
>
> Geschwind, 1970, p. 30

Few would dispute the soundness of Geschwind's assertion, and indeed it holds for other specific cognitive disabilities as well as the aphasic disorders. Nor is it any longer necessary to wait for the results of an autopsy study to identify the locus and extent of a focal brain lesion.

A detailed account of how developments in cerebrovascular anatomy and physiology, neurodiagnostic techniques, and clinical observation interacted with each other to effect progress in the understanding of brain–behavior relations would require a treatment of monographic length. The more modest aim of this chapter is to provide some indications of this progress by citing representative examples of observations and discoveries that reflect developments over the centuries. These examples should make it clear that the observed behavioral effects of cerebrovascular disease have played a significant role in fostering the

---

Reprinted from R. A. Bornstein and G. Brown (Eds.). *Neurobehavioral Aspects of Cerebrovascular Disease*. New York: Oxford University Press. © 1991.

growth of knowledge and thought about brain–behavior relations, particularly with respect to the issue of cerebral localization of function.

From Hippocrates to Morgagni

Apoplexy must have been known since time immemorial. In line with their concepts of humoral pathology, Greek physicians variously ascribed this disorder to excessively dry, cool, or phlegmatic states of the brain, to the flow of black bile to the veins, or to excessive filling of the veins (Creutz, 1934; Clarke, 1963). Galen implicated excessive phlegm as the cause. "Apoplexy and epilepsy arise from the accumulation of phlegmatic humors in the ventricles of the brain" (Siegel, 1968, p. 306). Although there were at times vague references to the circulatory system over the course of the following centuries, the association between stroke and cerebrovascular disease was tenuous until the appearance of Johann Jakob Wepfer's *Observationes Anatomicae* in 1658 (Donley, 1909; Major, 1945, pp. 429–443; Hoessly, 1965; Gawel, 1982).

Wepfer's contribution was truly epoch-making. An accomplished anatomist, he demolished the Galenic concept of the *rete mirabile* and instead showed that the internal carotid arteries penetrated the dura and entered the brain where it divided into its branches. He was the first to demonstrate through postmortem study that stroke was caused by intracranial hemorrhage, both intracerebral and subdural. He differentiated between hemorrhage and occlusion and indicated that each could produce stroke. He presented a description of the circle of Willis that, however, was somewhat less complete than the description of Thomas Willis (1664). More importantly, Willis was the first to point out the functional significance of these anastamoses, or "material conjoinings," in providing protective compensation for the effects of occlusion of a single vessel (Meyer and Hierons, 1962; Gawel, 1982).

Giovanni Battista Morgagni's (1769) great compilation of clinicopathologic correlations included many descriptions of cases of apoplexy. One of his major concerns was to emphasize the relation between paralysis on one side of the body and disease in the opposite cerebral hemisphere, i.e., to affirm the soundness of the doctrine of contralateral innervation. He also described speechlessness in combination with stroke-produced unilateral paralysis; and, in fact, analysis of his brief case reports discloses a definite trend toward a preferential association between speechlessness and *right* hemiplegia (Benton, 1984).

Early Observations

From the beginning it was obvious that apoplexy could produce gross mental changes such as confusion, obtundity, and speechlessness as well as motor and sensory disabilities. Wepfer himself suggested that the occurrence of mental changes was contingent on the part of the brain that was affected.

Cerebrovascular disease furnished the setting for the first analyses of specific behavioral disabilities that appeared during the seventeenth century, when it was noted that stroke could produce distinctive aphasic syndromes of medical and psychological interest. Johann Schmidt in 1673 described pure alexia without agraphia as a permanent residual of a stroke-produced aphasia. Peter Rommel in 1683 described a "rare aphonia" resulting from stroke in which a patient with practically complete loss of expressive speech nevertheless retained the capacity for rote recitation of prayers. Later, in 1745, Olof Dalin called attention to still another distinctive clinical picture, i.e., complete loss of expressive speech with retention of the ability to sing (Benton and Joynt, 1960).

Stroke also provided the opportunity for the first unequivocal description of pure anomic aphasia by Gerard Van Swieten in 1742–46. "I have seen many patients whose cerebral functions were quite sound after recovery from apoplexy, except for this one deficit: In designating objects, they could not find the correct names for them" (Benton and Joynt, 1960). In passing, it may be noted that Van Swieten was the first clinician to add embolic occlusion to the causes of stroke (McHenry, 1969).

The earliest descriptions of aphasic disorder that would be considered comprehensive and detailed by modern standards appeared during the second half of the nineteenth century. Johann A. P. Gesner (1770) wrote a chapter about 7000 words in length in which he analyzed the behavior of a patient who manifested a florid jargon aphasia after a stroke (Benton, 1965). Crichton (1798) described a striking case of stroke-produced paraphasia and invoked association theory to explain the patient's disability.

These early descriptions of diverse types and patterns of language disability enriched knowledge of aphasic symptomatology, but they contributed almost nothing to an understanding of brain-behavior relations. By the end of the eighteenth century the course of the major cerebral arteries had been described, at least in a sketchy way; but in all probability the findings were not widely known and were of major interest only to anatomists. The cerebral hemispheres were generally seen as a homogeneous structure to which different authors assigned different functions and only a few parts of which had been assigned names. Functional abnormality was ascribed to dryness, rigidity, or congestion of the brain substance. On the behavioral side, apart from the detailed descriptions of aphasic disability that have been cited, there was little behavioral analysis beyond the traditional division of mind into perception, reasoning, and memory. Thus there was little possibility of establishing meaningful correlations between behavior and the status of the brain.

Nineteenth Century

The first half of the nineteenth century was a period of significant advance along all fronts. Gall's (Gall and Spurzheim, 1809/1967) conception of the brain as a collection of organs, each of which subserved a specific mental faculty or disposition, as well as his emphasis on the cerebral hemispheres, generated a rancorous controversy and made localization of function in the brain a topic of major concern. The investigations of Rolando, Burdach, Cruveilhier, Leuret, and other anatomists established the basis for modern descriptions of the cerebral hemispheres and their convulutions. At the same time, histologic study of nerve fibers and their functional properties effectively displaced humoral doctrine and established the concept of neural transmission (Clark and O'Malley, 1968; Meyer, 1971).

The dispute over cerebral localization took two forms. There was first the broad issue of whether there was specialization of function in the brain. The influential physiologist Flourens insisted that the cerebral hemispheres operated as a unit, that each region subserved the same functions, and that the severity of behavioral impairment after brain insult was related to the quantity of tissue destroyed and not to its locus (Soury, 1899, pp. 518–527; Clark and O'Malley, 1968, pp. 483–488). His concept of a hemispheric *action commune* (later Lashley's laws of equipotentiality and mass action) was accepted by many clinicians who regarded Gall's system as absurd and who, in any case, were not able to find consistent relations between specific types of disability and lesions in specific areas of the brain. However, Flourens's position (derived from ablation studies on pigeons and chickens!) was contested by other clinicians, more on logical grounds than on established correlations between observed defects and identified lesion sites. For example, the physicians of the Salpetrière and the Pitié pointed to the discrete deficits produced by stroke—e.g., monoplegia of an arm or of a leg, hemiplegia with or without sensory impairment without paralysis—as evidence that specific cerebral centers governing these functions must exist. Postmortem examination did indeed disclose limited areas of hemorrhage or infarction in these patients. Nevertheless, it was not possible to achieve agreement about the precise location of the presumed centers.

Broca's Discovery

The second aspect of the dispute centered around the specific placement of centers for speech and the "memory of words" in the frontal lobes by Gall and his ardent champion, Bouillaud (1825). The acrimonious debate was resolved only during the 1860s when Paul Broca brought forth convincing autopsy evidence of an association between nonfluent aphasic disorder and frontal lobe disease. Of his first two patients, reported in 1861 (Broca, 1861a,b,c), the first (probably) and the second (certainly) had suffered from strokes. The first patient (Leborgne) had an extensive lesion in the posterior region of the left frontal lobe implicating the third and second gyri as well as generalized softening throughout the hemisphere. Broca interpreted the findings as supportive of the Gall-Bouillaud thesis that the center for speech was in the frontal lobes. However, he noted that the primary lesion was in the third frontal gyrus, and he raised the question of whether a more precise localization might be possible. When his second patient (Lelong) proved to have a deep well demarcated lesion in the third and second frontal gyri of the left hemisphere, Broca could not help but be forcibly impressed by the fact that the same area was implicated in both cases.

By early 1863 Broca had collected eight cases of "aphemia" resulting from lesions of probable vascular etiology in the third frontal gyrus of the left hemisphere. At the same time about a dozen confirmatory cases of varying etiology—stroke, abscess, tumor, trauma—had been reported by others. Subsequently, he himself described a number of cases of traumatic aphasia, all referable to injury of the third frontal gyrus of the left hemisphere (Broca, 1864a, b). He therefore identified this area (in either hemisphere) as the cerebral center for articulated speech. He was also convinced that the crucial lesion was in the left frontal gyrus but at the time hesitated to advance a conclusion that was so much at variance with preconceptions about the essential equivalence of the two hemispheres. However, by 1865 steadily accumulating observations on the consequences of unilateral strokes emboldened him to announce that "we speak with the left hemisphere" (Broca, 1865, p. 384).

Prosopagnosia and Achromatopsia

A stroke probably involving bilateral occlusion of the posterior cerebral artery provided the setting for the first description of a patient with prosopagnosia and its frequent accompaniment, achromatopsia. In 1867 Antonio Quaglino and Giambattista Borelli (ophthalmologists in Pavia and Turin, respectively) reported the case of a 54-year-old man who was seen 1 year after his stroke. He had a left visual field defect, but central visual acuity was excellent: he read without difficulty and had no motor deficits. His chief complaints were that he no longer recognized the faces of familiar persons and that objects in the environment looked pale and devoid of color. Quaglino and Borelli argued that their case supported the basic thesis of localization of function in the brain.

Some 20 years later prosopagnosia and achromatopsia, either singly or in combination, were again described and now correlated with focal brain disease. For example, Wilbrand's (1892) prosopagnosic patient showed bilateral inferior occipitotemporal infarction on postmortem examination, as did Heidenhain's (1927) patient. This lesional localization (almost always bilateral but occasionally rightsided) has been repeatedly confirmed in vascular and neoplastic cases (Meadows, 1974b; Damasio et al., 1982; Benton, 1985). Similarly, both complete achromatopsia and hemiachromatopsia were reported and related to focal brain disease. In 1888 Verrey described right hemiachromatopsia in a stroke patient resulting from a hemorrhagic cyst in the left inferior occipital lobe. Mackay and Dunlop (1899) described a patient with a complete achromatopsia who had bilateral inferior occipital lobe infarctions. This strikingly specific lesional localization has also been repeatedly confirmed (Meadows, 1974a; Damasio et al., 1980).

Dejerine and Pure Alexia

As has been noted, during the seventeenth century Schmidt called attention to the rather striking phenomenon of loss of reading ability with preservation of the capacity to write as a sequela of stroke. Many descriptions of the condition, which was by then called "pure wordblindness" and which was often attributed on theoretical grounds to destruction or dysfunction of a "reading center" in the angular gyrus, appeared during the 1870s and 1880s. No clinicopathologic correlations were made, however, until 1892, when Dejerine published his famous postmortem study of a case of pure alexia following a stroke. His patient, and educated man and accomplished musician, suddenly lost the ability to read musical scores as well as conventional written material. Yet he could write, perform music from memory, and showed no difficulty in the expression or understanding of oral speech. He had a right visual field defect—in all probability a hemiachromatopsia, not a hemianopia (Damasio, 1983).

Autopsy study disclosed infarctions in the territory of the left posterior cerebral artery, specifically, the mesial occipital area and the splenium of the corpus callosum. Dejerine inferred that the lesions had the effect of preventing the transmission of visual information to the language centers of the left hemisphere, thus making reading impossible while leaving the interpretation of nonverbal visual stimuli intact. His concept of pure wordblindness as a disconnection symptom, and not the result of destruction of a "reading center," was validated by later investigators who showed that variations in the clinical picture (e.g., with or without right visual field defect) could be related to varying locations of the infarcts produced by occlusion of the left posterior cerebral artery (Geschwind, 1965; Geschwind and Fusillo, 1966; Benson and Geschwind, 1969; Greenblatt, 1973; Ajax et al., 1977; Vincent et al., 1977).

Twentieth Century

Detailed knowledge of the distribution of the cerebral arteries, their anastomoses, functional interrelations and variations, and the cortical and subcortical areas served by their branches was achieved through a long series of studies beginning with those of Duret (1874) and Heubner (1874) and followed by, among others, those of Beevor (1908), Shellshear (1920); Foix and Levy (1927) and Pfeiffer (1928). Given this firm anatomic basis, clinicians were encouraged to attempt to identify the characteristic symptomatic manifestations of specific vascular abnormalities, in effect establishing a vascular system of cerebral localization.

Charles Foix was the pioneer worker in this endeavor. In a remarkable series of papers based on thorough anatomic study of the cerebrovascular system, he and his coworkers described the symptomatic features associated with occlusion of the vessels at various points along their course as well as of occlusion of individual branches. For example, Foix and Hillemand (1925) presented a detailed description of the "syndromes" of the anterior cerebral artery, a topic that was later taken up by the Critchley (1930). A more or less specific combination of symptoms resulted from alterations in specific branches of the artery, e.g., monoplegia, particularly of the leg, from involvement of the predominantly cortical-subcortical distribution. Of particular interest is their observation that defective vascular supply to the corpus callosum, mainly through occlusion of the pericallosal artery, produced unilateral ideomotor apraxia of the left hand. When explaining the disability, Foix and Hilleman accepted the model of Liepmann and Maas (1907), postulating a break in the connection between a "command center" in the left supramarginal territory and the right motor area. In his equally detailed exposition, Critchley (1930) also called attention to left ideomotor apraxia as a consequence of callosal infarction; in addition, he emphasized that some degree of general mental impairment is invariably present. He noted that transitory expressive speech disorder may occur with left-sided lesions.

Subsequently Foix (1926; Foix and Levy, 1927) dealt with the pathologic anatomy of the aphasic disorders and the syndromes of the middle cerebral artery and its branches. He introduced the first topic with the statement that:

> Aphasia is above all dependent upon cerebral softening. Not that one cannot encounter aphasic syndromes caused by tumors, hemorrhages and abscesses, but the great majority of cases, more than nine out of ten, depend upon cerebral softening. . . . Hence this study is devoted largely to cerebral softening, first the pathologic anatomy of Wernicke aphasia, then Broca aphasia and finally the so-called pure forms. [Foix, 1926, p. 787]

Under the heading of Wernicke aphasia, various forms of fluent aphasic disorder were discussed, e.g., *grand aphasie de Wernicke*; fluent aphasia with particularly severe impairment in reading (referable to involvement of the angular gyrus): amnesic aphasia (which he regarded as a forme fruste of Wernicke aphasia). He identified the posterior temporal artery with its distribution to the hinder parts of the first and second temporal gyri as the principal artery of aphasia. *Grande aphasie de Wernicke.* i.e., the combination of fluent aphasia with ideational apraxia and right hemianopia, is referable to involvement of the posterior parietal and occipitoparietal arteries in addition to that of the posterior temporal.

Occlusion of the posterior parietal and occipitotemporal arteries produces a fluent aphasia of moderate degree with severe alexia.

Similarly, under the heading of Broca aphasia. Foix discussed various forms of nonfluent speech disorder, ranging from apraxia of speech to global aphasia, and their correlations with the site, extent, and depth of cerebral softenings. Among other observations, he noted that the alexia shown by some Broca patients appeared to be associated with occlusion of the precentral artery. The report of Foix and Levy (1927) regarding the syndromes produced by lesions of the middle cerebral artery and its branches also dealt in large part with the aphasic disorders but in a complementary way, i.e., proceeding from the pathology to the symptom.

The topic was again addressed by Davidson and colleagues (1934) in a systematic study based on a sample of 48 patients with a single vascular lesion selected from a pool of about 200 cases. Their findings generally confirmed earlier observations (e.g., Critchley on the occurrence of general mental impairment in disease of the anterior cerebral artery) and in many instances indicated that localized vascular abnormality produces distinctive clinical pictures. Their conclusion was that "cerebral localization on the basis of vascular supply, although difficult and necessitating caution in interpretation, can still be definitely established. We were able, on the basis of our study of 48 cases, to demonstrate definite syndromes accompanying occlusion of the anterior and middle cerebral arteries or their branches" (Davidson et al., 1934, p. 465).

Critchley (1930), and indeed earlier observers, had noted that transient disturbances of speech could be produced by infarction of the left anterior cerebral artery. One form of disturbance was identified by Rubens (1975) in two patients as transcortical motor aphasia, i.e., the symptom complex of impoverished conversational speech, preserved capacity for repetition, echolalia, and relative preservation of understanding of speech. One of his patients had persisting apraxia and tactile anomia in the left hand pointing to involvement of the corpus callosum. The thrust of Rubens's contribution was to emphasize the importance of the left mesial and superior premotor region in the mediation of speech and language, a finding in accord with observations on surgical, epileptic, and traumatically injured patients. Later reports discussed the anatomic and clinical significance of transcortical motor aphasia as a component of the syndrome of the anterior cerebral artery (Damasio and Kassel, 1978; Alexander and Schmitt, 1980).

Disease of the anterior cerebral artery has also been related to the complex syndrome of akinetic mutism and a variety of behavioral deviations, including attentional disturbances, memory defects, and personality changes in the affected patients. Detailed study of these patients has given rise to a deeper understanding of the functional properties of different sectors of the frontal lobes (Damasio and Van Hoesen, 1983; Damasio, 1985; Stuss and Benson, 1986).

Epilogue

This chapter has presented some examples of how cerebrovascular disease brought to light certain specific defects in mentation and behavior and how in due time it was possible to relate these defects to specific abnormalities of the cerebral circulation. Strokes producing infarcts in a limited cerebral territory provided the opportunity for a variety of observations, such as those of Schmidt on pure alexia, Van Swieten on anomia, and Quaglino and Borelli on prosopagnosia and achromatopsia. Although it was not possible to identify the pathologic basis for the defects, these observations not only enriched clinical knowledge but also carried implications for localization theory. Broca's revolutionary correlation of nonfluent aphasic disorder with left frontal lobe disease ushered in an era of clinicopathologic study designed to elucidate brain–behavior relations. With progress in knowledge of the cerebrovascular system, attention was focused on the distinctive syndromes associated with abnormalities at various loci of the system.

Trauma, surgical intervention, tumor, and degenerative disease can also produce the same symptoms and symptom complexes as those resulting from stroke, either by a direct effect on the parenchyma or through injury to a blood vessel. Some examples that may be cited are pure alexia after surgical resection (Levin and Rose, 1979), prosopagnosia associated with tumor or surgical resection (Hécaen and Angelergues, 1962; Meadows, 1974b), and traumatic transcortical motor aphasia (Kleist, 1934; Rubens, 1976). Although these cases are less common than those of vascular etiology, they can provide information as useful as that derived from vascular cases. Moreover, individual variation as well as overlapping in the distributions of the vascular supply of the brain may complicate diagnostic inference (H. Damasio, 1983). Nevertheless, as Geschwind noted and the contributions in this volume illustrate, the ischemic infarct is the most valuable experiment of nature available for the clinical study of brain–behavior associations.

References

Ajax E. T., Schenkenberg T., and Kostaljanetz M. (1977). Alexia without agraphia and inferior splenium. *Neurology* 27: 685–688.

Alexander M. and Schmitt M. A. (1980). The aphasia syndrome of stroke in the left anterior cerebral artery territory. *Arch. Neurol.* 37: 97–100.

Beevor C. E. (1908). On the distribution of the different arteries supplying the human brain. *Philos. Transact. R. Soc.* B200: 1–55.

Benson D. F. and Geschwind N. (1969). The alexias. In Vinken P. J. and Bruyn G. W. (eds.), *Handbook of Clinical Nerology*. Vol. 4. Amsterdam: North Holland.

Benton A. L. (1965). Johann A. P. Gesner on aphasia. *Med. Hist.* 9: 54–60.

Benton A. L. (1984). Hemispheric dominance before Broca. *Neuropsychologia* 22: 807–811.

Benton A. L. (1985). Visuoperceptual, visuospatial and visuoconstructive disorders. In Heilman K. S., Valenstein E. (eds.), *Clinical Neuropsychology*. New York: Oxford University Press, pp. 151–185.

Benton A. L. and Joynt R. J. (1960). Early descriptions of aphasia. *Arch. Neurol.* 3: 205–222.

Bouillaud J. B. (1825). Recherches cliniques propres à démontrer que la perte de la parole correspond à la lésion des lobules antérieurs du cerveau. *Arch. Gén. Méd.* 8: 25–45.

Broca P. (1861a). Nouvelle observation d'aphémie produite de la moitié postérieure des deuxième et troisième circonvolutions frontales gauches. *Bull. Soc. Anat.* 36: 398–407.

Broca P. (1861b). Perte de la parole, ramollissement chronique et destruction partielle du lobe antérieur gauche. *Bull. Soc. Anthropol.* 2: 235–238.

Broca P. (1861c). Remarques sur le siège de la faculté du langage articulé, suives d'une observation d'aphémie. *Bull. Soc. Anat.* 36: 330–357.

Broca P. (1864a). Deux cas d'aphémie traumatique produite par des lésions de la troisième circonvolution frontale gauche. *Bull. Soc. Chir.* 5: 51–54.

Broca P. (1864b). Sur le siège du langage articulé: aphémie traumatique; lésion de la troisième circonvolution frontale. *Bull. Soc. Anthropol.* 5: 362–365.

Broca P. (1865). Sur le siège de la faculté du langage articulé. *Bull. Soc. Anthropol.* 6: 377–393.

Clarke E. (1963). Apoplexy in the Hippocratic writings. *Bull. Hist. Med.* 37: 301–314.

Clarke E. and O'Malley C. D. (1968). *The Human Brain and Spinal Cord*. Berkeley: University of California Press.

Creutz W. (1934). *Die Neurologie des 1.–7.* Jahrhunderts n. Chr. Leipzig: Thieme.

Critchley M. (1930). The anterior cerebral artery, and its clinical syndromes. *Brain* 55: 120–165.

Critchton A. (1798). *An Inquiry into the Nature and Origin of Mental Derangement*. London: T. Cadell Jr. & W. Davies.

Damasio A. (1983). Pure alexia. *Trends Neurosci.* 6: 93–96.

Damasio A. R. (1985). The frontal lobes. In Heilman K. S. and Valenstein E. (eds.), *Clinical Neuropsychology*. New York: Oxford University Press, pp. 339–402.

Damasio A., Damasio H., and Van Hoesen G. W. (1982). Prosopagnosia: anatomic basis and behavioral mechanisms. *Neurology* 32: 331–341.

Damasio A. R. and Kassel N. F. (1978). Transcortical motor aphasia in relation to lesions of the supplementary motor area. *Neurology* 28: 396.

Damasio A. R. and Van Hoesen G. W. (1983). Emotional disturbances associated with lesions of the limbic frontal lobe. In Heilman K. M. and Satz P. (eds.), *Neuropsychology of Human Emotion*. New York: Guilford Press, pp. 85–110.

Damasio A., Yamada T., Damasio H., Corbett J., and McKee J. (1980). Central achromatopsia: behavioral, anatomic and physiologic aspects. *Neurology* 30: 1064–1071.

Damasio H. (1983). A computed tomographic guide to identification of cerebral vascular territories. *Arch. Neurol.* 40: 138–142.

Davidson C., Goodhart S. P., and Needles W. (1934). Cerebral localization in cerebrovascular disease. *Res. Publ. Assoc. Res. Nerv. Ment. Dis.*, 13: 435–465.

Dejerine J. (1892). Contribution à la l'étude anatomopathologique et clinique des differentes varietés de cécité verbale. *Mem. Soc. Biol.* 4: 61–90.

Donley J. E. (1909). John James Wepfer, a renaissance student of apoplexy. *Bull. Johns Hopkins Hosp.* 20: 1–8.

Duret H. (1874). Recherches anatomiques sur la circulation de l'encéphale. *Arch. Physiol. Norm. Pathol.* 1: 60–91, 316–353, 664–693, 919–957.

Foix C. (1926). Sur l'anatomie pathologique de l'aphasie. *Ann. Anat. Pathol.* 3: 787–814.

Foix C., and Hillemand P. (1925). Les syndromes de l'artére cérébrale antérieure. *Encephale* 20: 209–232.

Foix C. and Levy M. (1927). Les ramollissements sylviens. *Rev. Neurol. (Paris)* 2: 1–51.

Gall F. J. and Spurzheim G. (1809). *Recherches sur le Systeme Nerveux en Général, et Sur Celui du Cerveau en Particulier*. Paris: F. Schoell (reprint, Amsterdam: Bonset, 1967).

Gawel M. (1982). The development of concepts concerning cerebral circulation. In Rose. F. C. (ed.), *Historical Aspects of the Neural Sciences*. New York: Raven Press, pp. 171–178.

Geschwind N. (1965). Disconnection syndromes in animals and man. *Brain* 88: 237–295. 585–644.

Geschwind N. (1970). Language disturbances in cerebrovascular disease. In Benton A. L. (ed.), *Behavioral Change in Cerebrovascular Disease*. New York: Harper & Row, pp. 29–36.

Geschwind N., and Fusillo M. (1966). Color naming defects in association with alexia. *Arch. Neurol.* 15: 137–146.

Gesner J. A. P. (1770). *Samlung von Beobachtungen aus der Arzneigelahrtheit und Naturkunde*. Nördlingen: C. G. Beck.

Greenblatt S. (1973). Alexia without agraphia or hemianopia; anatomical analysis of an autopsied case. *Brain* 96: 307–318.

Hécaen H. and Angelergues R. (1962). Agnosia for faces (prosopagnosia). *Arch. Neurol.* 7: 92–100.

Heidenhain A. (1927). Beitrag zur Kenntnis der Seelenblindheit. *Monatsschr. Psychiatr. Neurol.* 66: 61–116.

Heubner H. B. O. (1874). *Die luetische Erkrankung der Hirnarterien*. Leipzig: Vogel.

Hoessley G. F. (1965). Intracranial hemorrhage in the seventeenth century. *J. Neurosurg.* 24: 493–496.

Kleist K. (1934). *Gehirnpathologie*. Leipzig: Barth.

Levin H. S. and Rose J. E. (1979). Alexia without agraphia in a musician after transcallosal removal of a left ventricular meningioma. *Neurosurgery*. 4: 168–174.

Liepmann H. and Maas O. (1907). Fall von linkseitiger Agraphie und Apraxie bei rechtseitiger Lahmung. *J. Psychol. Neurol.*, 10: 214–227.

Mackay G. and Dunlop J. C. (1899). The cerebral lesions in a case of complete acquired colour-blindness. *Scott. Med. Surg. J.*, 5: 503–512.

Major R. H. (1945). *Classic Descriptions of Disease*, 3rd ed. Springfield, IL: Charles C. Thomas.

McHenry L. C. (1969). *Garrison's History of Neurology*: Springfield, IL: Charles C. Thomas.

Meadows J. C. (1974a). Disturbed perception of colours associated with localized cerebral lesions. *Brain* 97: 615–632.

Meadows J. C. (1974b). The anatomical basis of prosopagnosia. *J. Neurol. Neurosurg. Psychiatry* 37: 489–501.

Meyer A. (1971). *Historical Aspects of Cerebral Anatomy*. London: Oxford University Press.

Meyer A., and Hierons R. (1962). Observations on the history of the "circle of Willis." *Med. Hist.* 6: 119–130.

Morgagni G. B. (1769). *The Seats and Causes of Disease, Investigated by Anatomy*. Translated by B. Alexander. London: A. Millar & T. Cadell.

Pfeiffer R. A. (1928). *Die Angioarchitektonik der Grosshirnrinde*. Berlin: Springer.

Quaglino A. and Borelli G. (1867). Emiplegia sinistra con amaurosi; guaragione; perdita totale della percezione dei colori and della memoria della configurazione degli oggetti. *G. Oftalmol. Ital.* 10: 106–117.

Rubens A. B. (1975). Aphasia with infarction in the territory of the anterior cerebral artery. *Cortex* 11: 239–250.

Rubens A. B. (1976). Transcortical motor aphasia. In Whitaker H. and Whitaker H. A. (eds.), *Studies in Neurolinguistics*. Vol. 1. New York: Academic Press, pp. 293–303.

Shellshear J. L. (1920). The basal arteries of the forebrain and their functional significance. *J. Anat.* 15: 27–35.

Siegel R. E. (1968). *Galen's System of Physiology and Medicine*. Basel: Karger.

Soury, J. (1899). *Le Système Nerveux Central*. Paris: Carre & Naud.

Stuss D. T. and Benson, D. F. (1986). *The Frontal Lobes*. New York: Raven Press.

Verrey D. (1888). Hémiachromatopsie droite absolute. *Arch. Ophthalmol.* 8: 289–300.

Vincent F. M., Sadowsky C. H. Saunders R. L., and Reeves A. G. (1977). Alexia without agraphia, hemianopia or color naming defect: a disconnection syndrome. *Neurology* 27: 689–691.

Wilbrand H. (1892). Ein Fall von Seelenblindheit und Hemianopsie mit Sectionsbefund. *Dtsch. L. Nervenheilk.* 2: 361–387.

Willis T. (1664). *Cerebral Anatomy*. London: J. Flesher.

6

Spatial Thinking in Neurological Patients: Historical Aspects

This chapter sketches the development of knowledge and ideas about diverse defects of spatial thinking in patients with brain disease. It covers the period beginning with the inception of these ideas somewhat over 100 years ago to the 1960s. The review is necessarily selective and incomplete since the literature on the topic is enormous. However, it should provide a historical background for discussion of the current status of the field.

Hughlings Jackson

The idea that a lesion in the brain could produce a specific defect in thinking, orientation, or action with respect to space arose within the context of the broader concept of agnosia. The origins of the latter concept can be traced in the evolving thought of Hughlings Jackson. As early as 1864, Jackson raised the question of whether perception, particularly visual perception, might not have its seat in the right cerebral hemisphere. Ten years later, in his famous paper on the nature of the duality of the brain, he discussed the possibility in greater detail, expressing the opinion that the posterior part of the right hemisphere served the function of visual recognition and memory (Jackson, 1874). As he phrased it, "the hinder part of the brain on the right side is the chief seat of the revival of images in the *recognition* of object, places, etc. [p. 101]." As an example of a defect in this capacity caused by disease, he cited the case of a

---

Reprinted with permission from M. Potegal (Ed.), *Spatial Abilities: Developmental and Physiological Foundations*. New York: Academic Press. © 1982. Academic Press, Inc.

The personal investigations cited in this chapter were supported by Research Grant NS-00616 from the National Institute of Neurological and Communicative Disorders and Stroke.

patient who exhibited what is now called disorientation for place. Although she was in the London Hospital, she asserted that she was in a place in Holborn where she had worked for some years. But Jackson admitted that the evidence for locating "perception" in the right hemisphere was not strong, remarking that "as will be seen, my facts are very few [p. 103]."

Two years later, Jackson's ideas took more definite form when he described a patient who proved to have a tumor in the posterior right hemisphere and whose "first symptoms were those of what I call imperception. She often did not know objects, persons and places." The first indication that something was amiss with this 59-year-old woman was when she lost her way going from her home to a nearby park, a route she had been taking for 30 years. Over the course of the next few weeks, she showed odd lapses of behavior. For example, she made mistakes in dressing herself, a type of disability that later was given the name of "dressing dyspraxia." After admission to the hospital, she was not able to identify the different nurses attending her. Collectively these deficits in recognition, orientation, and action constituted what Jackson called *imperception*, "a defect as special as aphasia." However, his term was not adopted by other clinicans who later described the same constellation of deficits under the rubric of *mindblindness* or *visual agnosia*.

The next major contribution to this topic came from the physiological laboratory. Having shown that extensive destruction of the occipital lobes produced blindness in dogs and monkeys, Hermann Munk (1878) then described the effects of a more limited lesion in the same area. The animal (in this case, the dog) obviously could see since he ambulated freely and avoided obstacles. Yet he seemed to have lost the capacity to grasp the meaning of many visual stimuli that he appeared to perceive clearly. For example, he showed no signs of special recognition of his master, nor did he react appropriately to a threatening gesture or to the sight of a piece of meat. Munk called this disturbance in visual behavior *mindblindness* and he ascribed it to a loss of visual memory images that prevented the animal from relating current visual experience to past experience.

Munk's idea of a higher order disturbance in which visual associational or memory processes are impaired against a background of intact visuosensory capacity received a skeptical reception from his fellow physiologists, who were inclined to interpret mindblindness as an expression of defects in visual discrimination. Some clinicans also doubted the reality of mindblindness, feeling that the condition was essentially a reflection of defective visual acuity, and their position was supported by Munk's own contention that mindblindness resulted from a lesion in the same areas as served foveal vision. However, other clinical observers readily accepted the concept since they were convinced that they had seen patients with the same impairment Munk had described in dogs. Case reports, such as those by Wilbrand (1887) and Lissauer (1890), established that mindblindness or visual object agnosia did exist in human subjects. The primary deficit shown by these patients was an inability to recognize objects or persons despite apparently adequate visual acuity. In addition, some showed spatial disorientation, as reflected in losing one's way along familiar routes both indoors and outdoors, not being able to describe the location of familiar streets and buildings or to describe the disposition of the furniture in one's living room or bedroom. Since not all patients with visual object agnosia showed these spatial disabilities, the designation of *visuospatial agnosia* was given to them to indicate their essential independence from disorders of object recognition.

Badal and Spatial Thinking

Another trend in clinical investigation emphasized impairment in spatial thinking independently of sensory modality. The pioneer study of this type was that of a Bordeaux ophthalmologist, Jules Badal (1888), who entitled his paper "Contribution to the Study of Psychic Blindness; Alexia; Agraphia; Inferior Hemianopsia; Disorder of the Sense of Space" (cf. Benton, 1969; Benton & Meyers, 1956). His patient showed a large number of diverse deficits but her chief complaint was spatial disorientation. She could not find her way in her apartment or in the immediate neighborhood and she would not leave home without a guide. She could not answer simple questions about the spatial relations of the main streets of Bordeaux although she had long been thoroughly familiar with them. Like Jackson's patient, she showed dyspraxia for dressing. "She could not dress herself alone without putting on her clothes in reverse, taking the left sleeve for the right. It took her an infinite time to determine the order in which the different articles of clothing should be put on." She showed faulty visual guidance of hand movements in reaching (cf. Damasio & Benton, 1979). "She also had great difficulty in finding objects which she needed, even when they were in front of her. She would reach for it and her hand would constantly pass over it as if influenced by a false projection due to paralysis of the eye muscles. However, there was no diplopia, no strabismus and the eye movements were executed in a normal manner [p. 101]." Her central visual acuity was excellent. If her attention could be directed to them—for she had great difficulty in maintaining and shifting ocular fixation—she could name the smallest letters on the eye chart and she showed no difficulty in recognizing or naming the smallest objects.

But, as suggested by the title of his paper, Badal's main point was that the patient suffered from an impairment in spatial perception that transcended the visual modality. Although her auditory acuity appeared to be intact, she made errors in identifying the direction of the source of sounds. Impairment of spatial perception in the somesthetic modalities was manifested in defective body schema performances. She showed gross finger agnosia, not being able to state which of her fingers had been touched, and she could no longer distinguish between the right and left sides of her body. These errors in localization were made whether her eyes were open or closed.

Similar cases with visual disorientation and difficulty in making spatial judgments but with intact visual acuity and visual object recognition were described by Foerster (1890), Dunn (1895), Peters (1896), Meyer (1900), and Lenz (1905). Discussing the fact that one of his patients showed a serious disability in reading, Meyer pointed out that this type of reading failure, which reflected a disturbance in spatial orientation, was not to be confused with true alexia which was of a linguistic character.

In 1909 Balint described a patient with a rather distinctive assemblage of deficits associated with inaccurate visual judgments. The most prominent features of the syndrome, which Balint described as "psychic paralysis of gaze, optic ataxia, and spatial disturbance of attention [p. 51]" and which is now called *Balint's syndrome*, were maintenance of ocular fixation on a point in the visual field with seeming inability to shift fixation, inattention to objects and events in other parts of the visual field, and misreaching for objects. These impairments in oculomotor and visuomotor function were accompanied by a number of perceptual deficits, such as difficulty in estimating distances, in reading long polysyllabic words (although simpler words could be read), and in identifying figures such as a hexagon or an octagon although simpler figures such as a triangle or square were readily identified. Attention was generally fixated on a point in the right visual field with consequent neglect of stimuli in the left field. There were many expressions of impairment in the execution of visually guided movements. Besides misreaching for objects, the patient was unable to draw or copy or to use a knife accurately in cutting. But he could recognize objects and read single letters.

An interesting development of this early period is seen in Rieger's (1909) hypothesis that the brain contains two distinct but interacting apparatuses, one serving verbal–conceptual functions and the other spatial–practical functions. His ideas were developed further by Reichardt (1918) who described visuospatial and visuoconstructional defects in association with lesions of the right hemisphere and contrasted them with the linguistic impairments associated with left-hemisphere disease.

Thus, by 1910, a fairly large number of specific deficits in performance, indicative of imapirment of spatial thinking, had been described. As Table 6–1 shows, these deficits could be perceptual, amnesic, or praxic in nature. Thinking about their neurological basis followed two lines. The dominant point of view was that these disabilities were the product of bilateral disease involving the occipital and posterior parietal and temporal areas, and this position received substantial support from autopsy study. Thus, the brain of Foerster's (1890) patient showed bilateral softening confined to the occipital and parietal lobes (Sachs, 1895) and the brain of one of Meyer's (1900) patients showed bilateral

TABLE 6–1. Performance Deficits Described in the Literature as of 1910

1. Inability to follow routes
2. Defective topographic or geographic memory
3. Difficulty in judging distance
4. Difficulty in reading
5. Inattention in left visual field
6. Misreaching for objects
7. Dyspraxia for dressing
8. Difficulty in locating objects
9. Disturbances in ocular fixation

occipital lobe disease. Autopsy study of Balint's (1909) patient showed bilateral atrophy of the occipital, parietal, and temporal lobes with the most marked changes evident in the posterior parietal and temporal areas. The prevailing view was that this extensive destruction of visual association cortex resulted in a loss of visual memory images.

A second line of thought emphasized the role of the right hemisphere in the mediation of spatial thinking. As has been seen, Jackson considered the posterior part of the right hemisphere to be a center for visual recognition and memory, including spatial memory. In the 1890s, a Philadelphia physician, T. D. Dunn (1895), specifically localized spatial orientation in the right hemisphere. Having described a patient who could not remember the spatial relations of familiar streets or even of the rooms in his house but who could still recognize objects, faces, and simple words, he postulated the existence of a "geographic center" in the right hemisphere for what he called "the sense of location." Since his patient did not have visual object agnosia or facial agnosia, Dunn denied that it was necessary to invoke a generalized loss of visual memory images as the underlying disability, the patient having only loss of "optical images of locality."

Further support for a specific association between spatial disorientation and disease of the right hemisphere came from the observations of Peters (1896) and Lenz (1905), each of whom called attention to the relatively high frequency of spatial disorientation in patients with left homonymous hemianopia. However, in contrast to Dunn, both authors were extremely cautious in making inferences from their observations. Peters declined to draw a conclusion and Lenz only raised the question of whether "the right occipital lobe is perhaps more strongly related to orientation than the left."

The Contribution of Walther Poppelreuter

Study of patients with traumatic head wounds during and directly after World War 1 added further knowledge about the visuospatial defects associated with brain injury. The most comprehensive and detailed investigation was that of Poppelreuter (1917), who was the first to apply experimental–psychological methods such as tachistoscopy and the instrumental measurement of depth perception in the evaluation of these patients. As a consequence, he was able to show that defective depth perception was extraordinarily frequent in patients with occipital wounds. About one-third of them (with or without visual-field defects) proved to have some degree of impairment when acuity of depth perception was quantitatively assessed. Poppelreuter further pointed out that most of these patients did not complain of having difficulties in depth perception in everyday life.

He also studied accuracy in reaching for objects and found that misreaching could occur with different degrees of severity, that it might be present in the whole visual field or only in the periphery, and that patients with intact fields, as well as hemianopics, showed the defect. He emphasized the motor or behavioral aspects of misreaching and believed that the traditional explanation of it in terms of a disturbed "sense of locality" was incorrect. Rather it was a disturbance of coordination between sensory and motor processes, that is, an apraxia and not a disturbance in perception. Visuosensory capacity and distance judgment can be completely intact in a patient who misreaches. Thus, misreaching or defective visual guidance of hand movements reflects "not an alteration in the content of perception but a disturbance of the mechanism of localization."

Poppelreuter studied the exploration of visual space in his patients by means of his "field of search" test in which 57 diverse visual stimuli (numbers, letters, geometric figures) were presented in an irregular array and the subject was required to point to stimuli named or shown by the examiner. Relying on quantitative measures of performance, Poppelreuter was able to demonstrate that visual exploration was significantly prolonged in many patients, particularly those with occipital or bilateral wounds. Hemianopic defect per se did not appear to have an important influence on performance. Decades later Teuber, Battersby, and Bender (1949; Teuber, 1964) utilized this procedure to investigate the exploration of visual space in both adults and children with brain damage and found prolongation in searching time not only in those with parieto-occipital lesions but also in those with frontal damage. In some patients with unilateral injury the deficit was particularly severe in the contralateral visual field.

Misreaching for objects or inaccurate pointing to them was only one form of what Poppelreuter called *visual apraxia*. Other forms of the disability were awkwardness in manipulating objects (e.g., cutting with scissors), defective visually guided locomotion (e.g., rail-walking), and visuoconstructional defects such as poor copying of designs, failure in block designs tasks, and inaccurate construction of block models. In discussing these performances he noted once again that visual-field defects were not closely related to them and he emphasized that these visuomotor deficits were independent of both disturbances in form perception, as disclosed by tachistoscopic or "mixed figures" tests, and impairment in distance judgment.

Karl Kleist and Constructional Apraxia

One of Poppelreuter's more important contributions was his emphasis on visuoconstructive disabilities as a distinctive type of disturbance that could be shown by patients with brain disease. This theme was then taken up by Karl Kleist (1922/1934), who earlier had made similar observations (Kleist, 1912) and who now coined the term *constructional apraxia* for the disability he defined as a disturbance "in formative activities such as assembling, building, and drawing, in which the spatial form of the product proves to be unsuccessful, without there being an apraxia of single movements."

As a neurologist, Kleist was particularly interested in the site of the lesions that led to constructional apraxia. He agreed with Poppelreuter that, at least in its pure form, constructional apraxia represented a failure in integration between perceptual and motor processes rather than a perceptual defect per se. Thus it was, in modern terminology, a "disconnection symptom" (Geschwind, 1965). At the same time, Kleist was aware that impaired visuoperceptual capacity could also be expressed in defective visuoconstructive performances and he conceded that it was often difficult to decide whether an observed visuoconstructive disability was a "true" constructional apraxia or the direct reflection of visuoperceptive impairment. In any case, what *he* meant by *constructional apraxia* was the disconnection symptom, not the motoric expression of a perceptual deficit. Indeed, that is why he called it an *apraxia*, that is, a disturbance in purposeful motor activity within a setting on intact sensory and motor capacity. With respect to the neurological basis for the disability, Kleist placed the crucial lesion in the parieto-occipital territory of the left or dominant hemisphere, the functional effect of such a lesion being to disconnect the visual association areas (Areas 18, 19, 39) from anterior motor and preomotor regions and hence to prevent visual information from reaching executive motor centers.

Kleist's description and particularly that of his student Hans Strauss (1924) established constructional apraxia as a form of motoric visuospatial disorder associated with brain disease. However, his insistence that it was purely a praxic or "executive" disability was for the most part ignored and sometimes actively challenged. For example, Kroll (1929), Kroll and Stollbun (1933), Lange (1936), and Schlesinger (1928) pointed out that disturbances in spatial orientation and visual perception were almost always part of the clinical picture of "constructional apraxia." Consequently, the term was generally applied to any visuoconstructional failure, whether or not it occurred within a setting of perceptual and orientational disability.

On the neurological side, Kleist's localization of the crucial lesion underlying constructional apraxia was also challenged by subsequent by subsequent clinical study which indicated that in fact the deficit was more frequently shown by patients with right-hemisphere disease than by those with left-hemisphere damage (Benton, 1962; Benton and Fogel, 1962; Dide, 1938; Hécaen, Ajuriaguerra, and Massonet, 1951; Lange, 1936; McFie, Piercy, and Zangwill, 1950; Paterson and Zangwill, 1944; Piercy, Hécaen, and Ajuriaguerra, 1960; Piercy and Smyth, 1962). As has been mentioned, this point had already been made by Reichardt (1918), who contrasted visuospatial and visuoconstructive defects associated with right-hemisphere disease with the linguistic defects produced by lesions of the left hemisphere. Kleist took account of Reichardt's observations but questioned their validity on the grounds that his cases may have had left-hemisphere lesions that were not evident on macroscopic examination and also that some of his patients may have been left-handed.

Despite the accumulating evidence in its favor, the idea that there is a close association between constructional apraxia and disease of the right hemisphere was not readily accepted by neurologists. Admittedly, the early contributions to the topic, consisting of single case studies or global clinical impressions, could easily be discounted. Only after the more systematic studies of Zangwill, Hécaen, and their co-workers (1944–1951) were published was it necessary to consider the reported correlation seriously. However, even when the correlation was accepted, its neuropsychological meaning was not clear. It was not possible to consider the right hemisphere to be "dominant" for visuoconstructive or visuospatial activity in the same sense that the left hemisphere was considered to be dominant for language functions, for the two situations were not at all comparable. Aphasic disorder resulting from disease of the nondominant right hemisphere in a right-handed patient (i.e., so-called crossed aphasia), was recognized as a highly unusual phenomenon, occurring in not more than 1 or 2% of cases (Russell and Espir, 1961; Zangwill, 1960). But, of course, constructional apraxia resulting from disease of the left hemisphere in right-handed patients was not at all unusual. It was only a matter of a bias toward a somewhat higher frequency in patients with lesions of the right hemisphere (Benton, 1962; Benton and Fogel, 1962).

This empirical finding that, although it is more frequent and more severe in patients with right-hemisphere disease, constructional apraxia is also shown by a substantial proportion of patients with disease of the left hemisphere posed a problem of interpretation. One proffered explanation more or less reflected the observed facts. It hypothesized a partial "dominance" of the right hemisphere for visuoconstructive functions in the form of their "bilateral but unequal representation" in the two cerebral hemispheres (Piercy and Smyth, 1962). Another explanation, first advanced by Duensing (1953), held that there are two distinctive types of visuoconstructive disability, of fundamentally different character.

One type, equivalent to the "true" constructional apraxia of Kleist, is of an executive or motor nature and is related to the disruption of mechanisms in the left hemisphere. The other type results from a basic impairment in visuospatial thinking and is related to disruption of mechanisms in the right hemisphere.

Piercy and Smyth (1962) undertook to evaluate the cogency of the two competing explanations by investigating the relationship between constructional performance and the status of visuoperceptive ability in patients with right- and left-hemisphere disease. A number of tests requiring the copying of designs and the construction of block and matchstick models were employed to assess constructional ability and Raven's Progressive Matrices provided the measure of visuoperceptive capacity. It was reasoned that if the hypothesis of two distinctive types of visuoconstructive disability in relation to side of lesion is correct, then a close association between defective constructional performance and visuoperceptual impairment should be seen in patients with right-hemisphere lesions but not in those with disease of the left hemisphere, at least some of whom should show constructional apraxia within a context of intact visuoperceptive capacity. The results were unequivocal. Constructional performances and score on the Raven test were very closely associated in both hemispheric groups. The two groups differed only in respect to level of performance, the patients with right-hemisphere damage showing more severe impairment on both the constructional and perceptual tasks. Piercy and Smyth concluded that the theory of two distinctive types of visuoconstructive disability could not be supported and that the concept of "bilateral but unequal representation" in the two hemisphere was the more likely possibility.

However, a study the same year by Costa and Vaughn (1962) generated different results. Giving the WAIS block designs and the Raven matrices to patients with unilateral lesions, they found a close correlation (r = 0.83) between the two performances in those with right-hemisphere disease but only a minimal positive association (r = 0.33) in those with left-hemisphere disease. Although the authors did not draw a specific conclusion, their findings were consonant with the existence of discrete visuoperceptual and executive types of constructional impairment.

Qualitative analysis of the constructional performances provided another approach to the question of whether there existed distinctive types of disabilities that were differentially related to side of lesion. It was argued that impaired visuospatial functions should be reflected in productions characterized by distortion of the spatial relations among the elements of the construction. Construction from a model should be as defective as construction to verbal command because of the pervasive visuoperceptual disability. In contrast, executive or psychomotor impairment with attendant awkwardness in manipulation of the pencil or blocks should be reflected in constructions that are coherent and spatially correct but simplified and lacking in elaboration. Constructions from a model should be superior to those from verbal command since the model could facilitate slavish copying and the making of corrections when indicated. Fragmentary evidence in favor of this distinction was adduced by a number of investigators, among them Hécaen et al. (1951), Duensing (1953), McFie and Zangwill (1960), Piercy et al. (1960), and Arrigoni and De Renzi (1964). However, the detailed comparative study by Warrington, James, and Kinsbourne (1966) of drawing performance in relation to side of lesion failed to confirm most of the hypothesized qualitative differences in the productions.

Thus, by the late 1960s there were a number of unresolved questions about constructional apraxia, the primary ones being whether it represented one or more than one disability and what was the exact nature of its relationship to side of lesion in patients with unilateral brain disease. In addition, the question of whether or not constructional apraxia was merely a reflection of general mental impairment was raised (Benton, 1967, 1969).

Types of Impairment

The casualties of World War I provided an abundance of case material for detailed study and this led to the development of classifications of types of visual disorientation. Gordon Holmes (1918; Holmes and Horrax, 1919) divided into two categories the disorders of visual orientation and attention that he observed: *(1)* disturbances in localization, orientation and distance perception, as reflected in misreaching for objects, inability to learn routes, and difficulty in reading connected text; *(2)* oculomotor defects, such as the inability to shift fixation on verbal command and absence of the blink reflex.

On his part, Kleist (1922/1934) distinguished between disturbances of visuospatial *perception* (as reflected in defective bisection of lines, pointing to objects, or distance judgments) and visuospatial *agnosia* or *amnesia* (as reflected in the forgetting of geographic and topographic relationships). The neurological significance of the distinction was that the perceptual disorders were related to lesions in the calcarine region and its immediate vicinity (Areas 17 and 18). These lesions might be unilateral (producing, for example, mislocalization in one visual half-field) or bilateral (producing, for example, defective depth perception). In contrast, the agnosic or amnesic disorders were related to lesions of the outlying Area 19 primarily involving the left hemisphere.

Russell Brain (1941) made still another distinction between defective localization of stimuli within grasping distance (as in misreaching for objects) and defective localization of stimuli beyond arm's reach (as in poor distance judgments). Some of his patients showed impairment in one form of localization and not in the other, dissociations that he attributed to differences in the site of the causative lesions. He suggested that lesions involving the connections between visual cortex and the hand and arm area of the parietal somatosensory cortex produced mislocalizations within arm's reach whereas those affecting the connections between the visual cortex and the leg area resulted in impaired localization of more distant stimuli within "walking distance," as he phrased it. Later Birkmayer (1951) made a similar distinction.

Brain also offered a classification of forms of visual disorientation. The first form was defective localization of objects in space and this could be subdivided into three types, depending on whether it resulted from impaired visual acuity, hemianopia, or impairment of cerebral integrative processes. This last type was true agnosia for spatial relationships and could be exhibited in either one half-field, as Riddoch (1935) had shown, or in the entire field. Patients with visuospatial agnosia, particularly if it is present throughout the visual field, "cannot find their own way round objects when they run into them, set out in the wrong direction to get to others which they clearly see, and have difficulty in finding their way about and learning the topography of a room [p. 268]."

A second type of disorientation was loss of stereoscopic vision, an uncommon disorder previously described by Riddoch (1917) and Holmes and Horrax (1919). Another rare disorder was visual allesthesia, that is, the referral of visual stimuli to the opposite half-field, comparable to the more extensively described tactile allesthesia in which stimuli applied to one side of the body are referred to the opposite side (cf. Benton, 1959). Brain had not seen such a case and mentioned it only for the sake of completeness in listing.

A more important type of disorientation was neglect or unawareness of the left half of visual space shown by patients with extensive lesions of the parieto-occipital territory of the right hemisphere. Comparable to the neglect of the left side of the body seen in patients with right parietal lesions, this unawareness of the left half of space produces an inability to follow routes because of a tendency to avoid making turns to the left when indicated.

Finally, Brain listed loss of topographical memory as an independent form of visual disorientation, pointing out that a patient may have serious visuospatial problems on the perceptual level and yet be able to describe routes and spatial interrelationships accurately. Although most of the cases of this type described in the literature had proven to have bilateral disease, Brain expressed the opinion that the crucial lesion was in the left occipital area.

Disturbances of the Body Schema

As has been noted, Badal included his patient's inability to discriminate the left and right sides of her body and to identify her fingers as expressions of a "disorder of the sense of space." Many clinical investigators followed his example in viewing these and other disturbances of the body schema as reflecting a basic impairment in spatial thinking. After Gerstmann (1924, 1927) described finger agnosia as "a circumscribed disturbance of orientation towards one's body," Lange (1930, 1933) and Stengel (1944) suggested that this rather peculiar deficit as well as the other elements of the Gerstmann syndrome (right–left disorientation, agraphia, acalculia) should be considered as part of a more comprehensive syndrome of spatial disorientation involving external space and constructional praxis as well as the body schema.

There were, however, competing explanations. Head (1926) interpreted impairment in right–left discrimination to be a specific expression of the same disturbance in "symbolic formulation and expression" that defined aphasia. Consequently, he included tests of right–left orientation in his battery for the assessment of aphasic patients. Moreover, these "hand, eye and ear" tests, as he called them, included nonverbal imitation tasks as well as tasks requiring naming or understanding the names of body parts. Supporting Head's interpretation, Benton (1959) cited the extraordinarily high frequency with which aphasic patients showed disturbed left–right awareness and finger recognition as evidence that the occurrence of these deficits in patients with unilateral brain disease reflects a disturbance of language or symbolic thinking.

Ajuriaguerra and Hécaen (1949) and Benton (1959) pointed out that disorientation with respect to external space did not necessarily imply disorientation toward one's own body and, conversely, that disturbances in the body schema did not necessarily imply the occurrence of conventional visual disorientation as described by Poppelreuter and Kleist. However, the frequent concurrence of the two types of orientational disability, particularly in the form of neglect of the left half of space *and* of one's body, was noted by Pinéas (1931), Brain (1941), Critchley (1953), and other observers. Brain believed that visuospatial orientation and body awareness were intimately related and that the posterior parietal region connecting the visual cortex with the somatosensory area in the postcentral gyrus provided an anatomical basis for this association.

Auditory–Spatial Discrimination

Apart from single case reports, such as those of Badal (1888), Penfield and Evans (1934), Ross and Fountain (1948), and Wortis and Pfeffer (1948), the spatial aspects of audition in patients with brain disease were not investigated until the 1950s when Sanchez–Longo and Forster (1958; Sanchez–Longo, Forster, and Auth, 1957) reported their studies of auditory localization. In the first study the performance of five patients with unilateral temporal lobe lesions were compared to a group of control patients with the finding that four of the five patients were grossly inaccurate, their mean error of localization being larger than the poorest of the 20 control subjects. Moreover, in analogy with visual localization, every patient showed a larger error of localization in the auditory field contralateral to the side of lesion. The results were confirmed in a second study of a larger number of patients. In addition, a group of patients with lesions not involving the temporal lobe were assessed with the finding that their overall performance level was within the normal range. The observation that patients with unilateral temporal lobe injury often show particularly severe impairment in localization in the contralateral field was consonant with the earlier case reports of Penfield and Evans (1934) and Wortis and Pfeffer (1948).

However, Walsh (1957), presenting click stimuli through earphones and manipulating time and intensity differences between the clicks as cues to localization of the apparent direction of the source of sound, reported that patients with temporal lobe lesions performed quite adequately. A second study, in which sounds were transmitted through air to assess "real" rather than "apparent" localization, produced the same results. The three patients with temporal lobe lesions were able to localize the source of the sound. Walsh's treatment of his data was rather impressionistic (in contrast to the quantitative analyses of Sanchez–Longo and Forster) and it is not clear that patients performed on a normal level of accuracy. In any case, his results were in accord with those earlier reported by Ross and Fountain (1948).

The study of Shankweiler (1961) introduced some new elements into an already rather confused picture. Two of his basic findings were negative. There was no evidence for particularly severe impairment of localization in the contralateral auditory field in patients with unilateral lesions nor did those with temporal lobe disease show more severe defects than those with parieto-occipital or frontal lesions. However, he did find that the patients with right-hemisphere lesions were poorer in performance than those with left-hemisphere lesions, significantly on one auditory localization task (pointing to the source of a sound) and nonsignificantly on a second task (discrimination of angular differences). Pointing out that auditory localization takes place in a visually organized space, Shankweiler considered that the observed between-hemispheres difference in accuracy of localization was not unexpected in view of the established association between visuospatial deficits and disease of the right hemisphere. Another finding, which perhaps explains some of the discordant results of previous studies, was that for both control subjects and patients the correlation between performances on the two auditory localization tasks (pointing versus verbal judgment) was not significant.

Teuber (1962), employing dichotic clicks with manipulation of time and intensity differences to assess auditory localization, reported results that were in accord with those of Shankweiler. Patients with right-hemisphere lesions performed more poorly than those with left-hemisphere disease. In addition, performance level tended to be specific to the task. A patient might perform adequately on the intensity difference task but not on the time difference task or vice versa. Teuber concluded that "brain injury can impair binaural localization based on time and intensity differences, but the effects are dissociable, suggesting at least partial separation of neural mechanisms underlying these two forms of localication [p. 154]."

Tactile-Spatial Performances

The concept that the tactile and kinesthetic senses have a spatial component as well as methods for measuring that component arose from the inspired work of Ernst Heinrich Weber (see Ross and Murray, 1978), two of whose studies have recently appeared in English translation (Weber, 1978). He devised the tactile compass to measure the accuracy of discrimination of two points on the skin and later developed the procedure of having a subject indicate a point on the skin that had been touched in order to measure the accuracy of tactile localization. The two-point threshold is primarily a measure of tactile acuity, analogous to visual acuity. Nevertheless, that there is a spatial component in the task of discriminating two points on the skin surface is indicated by the significant correlation between this performance and the error of tactile localization (Boring, 1930). However, it was generally agreed that the task of localizing a stimulated point on the skin was the more direct measure of the "sense of space."

Beginning in the 1870s, two-point discrimination and single point localization were intensively studied both in patients with lesions of the central nervous system and in those with peripheral nerve injuries. It was readily established that impaired performance could occur as a consequence of disease of the somatosensory system at any level from the peripheral nerve to the cerebral cortex. Thereafter attention was focused on a number of questions. One of these was whether these tactile "spatial" deficits could occur independently of more basic defects in tactile sensitivity or were merely expressions of these defects. A second question concerned the neurological basis of impaired tactile—spatial performances.

With regard to the question of the relationships of tactile–spatial defects to impaired sensitivity, there was a gradual accumulation of evidence that defective two-point discrimination and point localization could be shown in the absence of defects in tactile sensitivity and, conversely, that patients with severely impaired tactile sensitivity (i.e., raised thresholds to pressure, pain, and temperature) could show intact localizing capacity. In 1901 Otfrid Foerster reviewed the pertinent literature and described the findings in a large sample of his own patients to establish these facts. However, at the same time he pointed to the close association between defects in tactile localization and disturbances in kinesthetic sensitivity, as reflected in raised thresholds for the detection of passive movements of the fingers, hands and arms.

Recalling the longstanding controversy between proponents of nativist and empiricist theories of the genesis of space perception, Foerster adduced clinical evidence to support the proposition that the apprehension of spatial characteristics and relations is not an inherent attribute of sensory experience but instead gradually develops as associations between different sensory experiences are formed. Thus, the tactile sense of space is the resultant of the establishment of connections between tactile, visual, and kinesthetic experience. If kinesthetic experience is impoverished, as in cases of congenital paralysis, or is impaired as a consequence of acquired disease of the nervous system, then tactile experience is deprived of its spatial component and this is reflected in defective performance on spatial tasks such as point localization.

At the same time, other somatosensory tests of a spatial character were developed and applied for clinical and investigative purposes. Position sense, that is, a patient's awareness of the position in which his arm, finger, or toe has been placed, was assessed by his verbal report or his imitation of the position. Recognition of the direction of lines drawn on the skin surface was another procedure used to assess the spatial aspects of tactile perception. A more complicated maneuver was to draw numerals or letters on the forearm, palm, or finger tips and determine whether or not the patient could identify them. His failure to do so was labeled *agraphesthesia*.

Over the decades there was much discussion about the meaning of failing performance on these spatial tasks. Broadly speaking, there were two schools of thought on the subject. One group saw these deficits as expressions of a primary disorder of spatial thinking in which the patient is unable to organize sensory information into a coherent spatial framework. Head (1920), for example, ascribed inaccurate point localization and position sense to the impairment of spatially organized "schemata" relating to the body surface and to posture. The other group insisted that failing performance was merely the result of more basic disorders in sensitivity such as raised or unstable sensory thresholds, disturbances in sensory processes over time, and fatigability, so that in fact the patient did not receive the sensory information required to localize accurately or discriminate between two stimulated points. The controversy is still not resolved.

However, all neurologists agreed that failure on these somatosensory spatial tasks was a sensitive indicator of the presence of brain disease and, specifically, of disease of the parietal lobes. The detailed investigation of sensory disturbances from cerebral lesions carried out by Head and Holmes (1911; Head, 1920; Holmes, 1927) showed this clearly and later work only confirmed their findings. The study of Shy and Haase (1957), in which 25 patients with verified focal lesions in the parietal lobe were given a battery of 12 sensory tests, found that four of the five most frequently encountered defects were of a spatial character, namely, impaired position sense, inaccurate point localization, raised thresholds for two-point discrimination and inability to identify numerals drawn on the skin. The one nonspatial deficit in this set of five was a raised threshold for the perception of passive movement which, as Foerster (1901) had shown decades earlier, was closely correlated with tactile–spatial defects. In contrast, sensory thresholds for pressure, pain, and temperature were altered in relatively few patients and all of these showed one or more spatial deficits. Shy and Haase suggested that somatosensory deficits could be arranged in a hierarchical order in relation to overall severity of impairment, as shown in Table 6–2. They conceded, however, that there were cases whose pattern of deficits did not conform to the schema.

With respect to the neurological basis of these somatosensory deficits, clinical investigators such as Foerster (1901) and Head (1920) demonstrated that impairment could be produced by lesions at any level of the nervous system. Head and Sherren (1905), for example, found that defective two-point discrimination was closely associated with impaired sensitivity to tactile pressure in patients with peripheral nerve injuries and indeed was a remarkably persisting deficit that might be present after all other sensory capacities had returned to normal. Head and Thompson (1906) found that defective two-point discrimination was a frequent consequence of spinal cord disease but in this instance it could appear independently of any important disturbances of tactile sensitivity. Nevertheless, Head believed that lesions below the level of the cortex were more likely to result in basic sensory impairment (i.e., raised or unstable thresholds to light pressure, pain, and temperature) than were cortical lesions, which primarily impaired the discriminative aspects of sensory experience.

Clinical study during the last 2 decades of the nineteenth century established that the cortical mechanisms medating somatosensory responses were primarily located in the parietal lobe. However, the precentral gyrus, which today is usu-

TABLE 6–2. Levels of Severity of Defect in Parietal Lobe Disease*

LEVEL	DEFICITS
I	Impaired position sense
II	I plus slowed perception of passive movement (normal threshold)
III	II plus raised threshold for passive movement and defective point localization
IV	III plus raised two-point threshold and agraphesthesia
V	IV plus astereognosis, defective roughness discrimination and temperature sense
VI	V plus raised threshold for pressure and pain

*Adapted from Shy and Haase (1957).

ally designated as a motor area, was often included in the somatosensory region, the combined precentral and postcentral gyri constituting a sensorimotor region. Moreover, it was found that lesions in the posterior part of the parietal lobe, as well as in the postcentral gyrus, could produce various forms of impairment. Thus, Head (1920) concluded that "loss of sensation of the cortical type may be produced by a lesion of the pre- and post-central convolutions, the anterior part of the superior parietal lobule, and the angular gyri. These portions of the hemisphere contain the sensory centres [p. 759]." However, it was not possible to relate different forms of impairment to lesions in specific loci within this extended somatosensory cortical region.

It was understood that, in consonance with the facts of contralateral innervation, unilateral parietal disease would produce tactile impairment on the opposite side of the body. However, beginning in 1906 and extending through the 1930s, a number of clinicians reported instances of bilateral impairment in patients with apparently unilateral lesions. The earliest papers described bilateral defects in tactile object identification in association with unilateral lesions but later studies, such as those of Bychowsky and Eidinow (1934) and Koerner (1938), reported bilateral disturbances of sensitivity to pressure, pain, and vibration. Little attention was paid to these scattered papers until the publication of the large-scale study of Semmes et al. (1960) who demonstrated that bilateral impairment in pressure sensitivity, two-point discrimination, point localization, and the detection of passive movement was not a rare finding in patients with unilateral lesions. Subsequent studies generally confirmed their finding. A second observation that these bilateral defects were encountered with particularly high frequency in patients with left-hemisphere disease was not consistently supported. Subsequently, Carmon and Benton (1969) found bilateral impairment in the perception of the direction of punctate stimuli applied to the skin in patients with right-hemisphere disease but not in those with left-hemisphere lesions. They interpreted their findings as indicating that the right hemisphere plays a particularly important role in the mediation of behavior requiring the appreciation of spatial relations in the tactile as well as the visual modality. The significance of a supramodal spatial factor in the mediation of tactile form discrimination was emphasized in studies by Semmes (1965), De Renzi and Scotti (1969), and Dee and Benton (1970) which found a close relationship between defect on the tactile task and corresponding defect in visuospatial performances.

Concluding Comments

Disorders in spatial thinking associated with disease of the nervous system were recognized by clinicians as early as the 1880s. These disorders were typically studied within a single sensory modality. Vision was investigated in great detail and types of visuospatial disorder were formulated by Kleist, Brain, and other neurologists. The occurrence of specific disorders, which were often defined in terms of level (e.g., sensory, integrative, mnesic), was then related to the locus and extent of the causative lesion. Spatial deficits in the somatosensory modality, such as inaccurate tactile localization and impaired position sense, were also investigated, mainly in relation to their value in diagnosis but also as a vehicle for studying integrative processes in the central nervous system. In contrast, the spatial aspects of audition received relatively little attention. The concept that brain disease can produce a generalized impairment in spatial thinking that affects performance in all sensory modalities was advanced. Over the decades there was a slow accumulation of evidence pointing to the paramount importance of the right hemisphere in mediating spatial performances.

The exact nature of the interrelations among the diverse performance deficits that are regarded as indicative of "spatial disorientation" remains to be determined. Clinical observation attests that patients may show dissociated deficits, that is, failure on one spatial task but not the other. For example, although perceptumotor spatial disability, as reflected in failing visuoconstructional performance, is usually associated with visuoperceptual spatial disability, as reflected in failing performance on discrimination tasks, some patients show one type of deficit but not the other (Costa and Vaughn, 1962; Dee, 1970). There is also evidence that the neuropathological bases for distinctive types of disabilities may differ. Defective three-dimensional block construction, a perceptuomotor spatial disability, is shown by a substantial proportion of aphasic patients with left-hemisphere disease but impaired appreciation of the direction of lines, a visuoperceptual-spatial disability, is not characteristic of these patients (Benton, 1973; Benton, 1975; Benton et al., 1978). Moreover, despite theorizing about the dependence of orientation in external space on the integrity of the body schema, clinical observation discloses numerous instances of dissociated impairment, as documented in the section on disturbances of the body schema in this chapter.

The intriguing concept of a supramodal spatial disability deserves further exploration. An association of visuospatial (and visuoconstructive) performance deficits with tactile—spatial deficits has been described by a number of investigators (Corkin, 1965; Dee & Benton, 1970; DeRenzi & Scotti, 1969; Milner, 1965). It seems likely that the basis for the relationship is that in sighted persons all spatial performances—visual, auditory, somesthetic—take place within a visually organized spatial matrix. However, the observed occurrence of dissociated visual and tactile spatial deficits raises the question of whether the determining factors may not be neuropathological rather than behavioral in nature.

References

Ajuriaguerra J. de. and Hécaen H. (1949). *Le Cortex Cérébral*. Paris: Masson et Cie.

Arrigoni G. and De Renzi E. (1964). Constructional apraxia and hemispheric locus of lesion. *Cortex* 1: 170–197.

Badal J. (1888). Contribution a l'étude des cécités psychiques: Alexie, agraphie, hémianopsie inférieure, trouble du sens de l'espace. *Archives d'Ophtalmologie* 8: 97–117.

Balint R. (1909). Seelenlähmung des Schauens, optische Ataxie, räumliche Störung der Aufmerksamkeit. *Monatsschrift fuer Psychiatrie und Neurologie* 25: 51–81.

Benton A. L. (1959). *Right-Left Discrimination and Finger Localization: Development and Pathology*. New York: Hoeber-Harper.

Benton A. L. (1962). The visual retention test as a constructional praxis task. *Confinia Neurologica* 22: 141–155.

Benton A. L. (1967). Constructional apraxia and the minor hemisphere. *Confinia Neurologica* 29: 1–16.

Benton A. L. (1969). Disorders of spatial orientation. In Vinken P. L., and Bruyn G. W. (eds.), *Handbook of Clinical Neurology*, Vol. 3, Ch. 13. Amsterdam: North Holland.

Benton A. L. (1973). Visuoconstructive disability in patients with cerebral disease: Its relationship to side of lesion and aphasic disorder. *Doc. Ophthalmol.*, 34: 67–76.

Benton A. L. & Fogel M. L. (1962). Three-dimensional constructional praxis. *Arch. Neurol.* 7: 347–354.

Benton A. L., Hannay H. J., and Varney N. R. (1975). Visual perception of line direction in patients with unilateral brain disease. *Neurology* 25: 907–910.

Benton A. L. and Meyers R. (1956). An early description of the Gerstmann syndrome. *Neurology* 6: 838–842.

Benton A. L., Varney N. R., and Hamsher K. (1978). Visuospatial judgment: A clinical test. *Arch. Neurol.* 35: 364–367.

Birkmayer W. (1951). *Hirnverletzungen: Mechanismus, Spaetkomplikationen, Funktionswandel*. Wien: Springer-Verlag.

Boring E. G. (1930). The two-point limen and the error of localization. *Am. J. Psychol.* 42: 446–449.

Brain W. R. (1941). Visual disorientation with special reference to lesions of the right cerebral hemisphere. *Brain* 64: 244–272.

Bychowsky G. and Eidinow M. (1934). Doppelseitige Sensibilitaetstoerungen bei einseitigen Gehirnherden. *Nervenarzt* 7: 498–506.

Carmon A. and Benton A. L. (1969). Tactile perception of direction and number in patients with unilateral cerebral disease. *Neurology* 19: 525–532.

Corkin S. (1965). Tactually-guided maze learning in man: Effects of unilateral cortical excisions and bilateral hippocampal lesions. *Neuropsychologia* 3: 339–351.

Costa L. D. and Vaughan H. G. (1962). Performances of patients with lateralized cerebral lesions: Verbal and perceptual tests. *J. Nerv. Ment. Dis.* 134: 162–168.

Critchley M. (1953). *The Parietal Lobes*. London: Edward Arnold.

Damasio A. R. and Benton A. L. (1979). Impairment of hand movements under visual guidance. *Neurology* 29: 170–178.

Dee H. L. (1970). Visuoconstructive and visuoperceptive deficit in patients with unilateral cerebral lesions. *Neuropsychologia* 8: 305–314.

Dee H. L. and Benton A. L. (1970). A cross-modal investigation of spatial performances in patients with unilateral cerebral disease. *Cortex* 6: 261–272.

De Renzi E. and Scotti G. (1969). The influence of spatial disorders in impairing tactual discrimination of shapes. *Cortex* 5: 53–62.

Dide M. (1938). Les désorientations temporo-spatiales et la préponderance de l'hémisphère droit dans les agnoso-akinésies proprioceptives. *Encéphale* 33: 276–294.

Duensing F. (1953). Raumagnostische und ideatorisch-apraktische Stoerung des gestaltenden Handelns. *Deutsche Zeitschrift fuer Nervenheilkunde* 170: 72–94.

Dunn T. D. (1895). Double hemiplegia with double hemianopsia loss of geographic centre. *Transactions, College of Physicians of Philadelphia* 17: 45–56.

Foerster O. (1901). Untersuchungen ueber das Localisationsvermoegen bei Sensibilitaetsstoerungen: Ein Beitrag zur Psychophysiologie der Raumvorstellung. *Monatsschrift fuer Psychiatrie und Neurologie* 9: 31–42.

Foerster R. (1890). Ueber Rindenblindheit. *Graefes Archiv fuer Ophthalmologie* 36: 94–108.

Gerstmann J. (1924). Fingeragnosie: Eine umschriebene Stoerung der Orientierung am eigenen Koerper. *Wiener Klinische Wochenschrift* 37: 1010–1012.

Gerstmann J. (1927). Fingeragnosie und isolierte Agraphie-ein neues Syndrom. *Zeitschrift fuer die gesamte Neurologie und Psychiatrie* 108: 152–177.

Geschwind N. (1965). Disconnexion syndromes in animals and man. *Brain* 88: 237–294, 586–644.

Head H. (1920). *Studies in Neurology*. London: Oxford University Press.

Head H. (1926). *Aphasia and Kindred Disorders of Speech*. Cambridge: The University Press.

Head H. and Holmes G. (1911). Sensory disturbances from cerebral lesions. *Brain* 34: 102–254.

Head H. and Sherren J. (1905). The consequences of injury to the peripheral nerves in man. *Brain* 28: 116–338.

Head H. and Thompson T. (1906). The grouping of afferent impulses within the spinal cord. *Brain* 29: 537–741.

Hécaen H., Ajuriaguerra J. de, and Massonet J. (1951). Les troubles visuoconstructifs par lésion pariéto-occipitale droite. *Encéphale* 40: 122–179.

Holmes G. (1918) Disturbances of visual orientation. *B. J. Ophthalmol.* 2: 449–468, 506–516.

Holmes G. (1927). Disorders of sensation produced by cortical lesions. *Brain* 50: 413–427.

Holmes G. and Horrax G. (1919). Disturbances of spatial orientation and visual inattention, with loss of stereoscopic vision. *Arch. Neurol. Psychiatry* 1: 385–407.

Jackson J. H. (1864) Clinical remarks on defects of expression (by words, writing, signs, etc.) in diseases of the nervous system. *Lancet* 1: 604–605.

Jackson J. H. (1874). On the nature of the duality of the brain. *Medical Press and Circular* 17: 19. (Reprinted in *Brain*, 1915, 38, 80–103.)

Jackson J. H. (1876). Case of large cerebral tumour without optic neuritis and with left hemiplegia and imperception. *Royal Ophthalmic Hospital Reports* 8: 434–444.

Kleist K. (1912). Der Gang und der gegenwaertige Stand der Apraxieforschung. *Ergebnisse der Neurologie und Psychiatrie* 1: 342–452.

Kleist K. Kriegsverletzungen des Gehirns in ihrer Bedeutung fuer die Hirnlokalisation und Hirnpathologie. In von Schjerning O. (ed.), *Handbuch der Aerztlichen Erfahrung im Weltkriege*, Bd. 4. Leipzig: Barth, 1922/1934.

Koerner S. C. (1938). Die Beeinflusskeit der Sensibilitaet an symmetrischen Hautgebieten bei einseitiger Hirnschaedigung und bei Gesunden. *Deutsche Zeitschrift fuer Nervenheilkunde* 145: 116–130.

Kroll M. (1929). *Die neurologischen Symptomenkomplexe*. Berlin: Springer.

Kroll M. and Stollbun D. (1933). Was ist konstruktive Apraxie? *Zeitschrift fuer die gesamte Neurologie und Psychiatrie* 148: 142–158.

Lange J. (1930). Fingernosie und Agraphie. *Monatsschrift fuer Psychiatrie und Neurologie* 76: 129–188.

Lange J. (1933). Probleme der Fingeragnosie. *Zeitschrift fuer die gesamte Neurologie und Psychiatrie* 147: 594–620.

Lange J. (1936). Agnosien und Apraxien. In Bumke O. and Foerster O. (eds.), *Handbuch der Neurologie*, Bd. 6. Berlin: Springer-Verlag.

Lenz G. (1905). *Beitraege zur Hemianopsie*. Stuttgart.

Lissauer H. (1890). Ein Fall von Seelenblindheit nebst einem Beitrag zur Theorie derselben. *Archiv fuer Psychiatrie und Nervenkrankheiten* 21: 222–270.

McFie J., Piercy M. F., and Zangwill O. L. (1950). Visual-spatial agnosia associated with lesions of the right cerebral hemisphere. *Brain* 67: 167–190.

McFie J., and Zangwill O. (1960). Visual-constructive disabilities associated with lesions of the left hemisphere. *Brain* 83: 243–260.

Meyer O. (1900). Ein-und doppelseitige homonyme Hemianopsie mit Orientierungstoerungen. *Monatsschrift fuer Psychiatrie und Neurologie* 8: 440–456.

Milner B. (1965). Visually-guided maze learning in man: Effects of bilateral hippocampal, bilateral frontal, and unilateral cerebral lesions. *Neuropsychologia* 3: 317–338.

Munk H. (1878). Weitere Mittheilungen zur Physiologie der Grosshirnrinde. *Archiv fuer Anatomie und Physiologie* 2: 162–178.

Paterson A. and Zangwill O. L. (1944). Disorders of visual space perception associated with lesions of the right cerebral hemisphere. *Brain* 67: 331–358.

Penfield W. and Evans J. P. (1934). Functional defects produced by cerebral lobectomies. *Res. Publ. Assoc. Res. Nerv. Ment. Dis.* 13: 352–377.

Peters A. (1896). Ueber die Beziehungen zwischen Orientierungsstoerungen und ein-und doppelseitige Hemianopsie. *Archiv fuer Augenheilkunde* 32: 175–187.

Piercy M. F., Hécaen H., and Ajuriaguerra J. de. (1960). Constructional apraxia associated with unilateral cerebral lesions—left and right sided cases compared. *Brain* 83: 225–242.

Piercy M. F. and Smyth V. (1962). Right hemisphere dominance for certain nonverbal intellectual skills. *Brain* 85: 775–790.

Pinéas H. (1931). Ein Fall von raeumliche Orientierungsstoerung mit Dyschirie. *Zeitschrift fuer die gesamte Neurologie und Psychiatrie* 133: 180–195.

Poppelreuter W. (1917). *Die psychischen Schaedigungen durch Kopfschuss im Kriege 1914–1916: die Stoerungen der niederen und hoeheren Sehleistungen durch Verletzungen des Okzipitalhirns*. Lepizig: Voss.

Reichardt M. (1918). *Allgemeine und spezielle Psychiatrie: ein Lehrbuch fuer Studierende und Aerzte*, II Aufl., Jena, Germany: G. Fischer.

Riddoch G. (1917). Dissociation of visual perceptions due to occipital injuries, with special reference to appreciation of movement. *Brain* 40: 15–57.

Riddoch G. (1935). Visual disorientation in homonymous half-fields. *Brain* 58: 376–382.

Rieger C. (1909). Ueber Apparate in dem Hirn. *Arbeiten aus der Psychiatrischen Klinik Wuerzburg* 5: 176–197.

Ross H. E. and Murray D. J. (1978). Introduction. In E. H. Weber, *The Sense of Touch*. London: Academic Press.

Ross S. J. and Fountain G. (1948). Phenomenon of cutaneous sensory extinction. *Arch. Neurol. Psychiatry* 59: 107–113.

Russell W. R. and Espir M. L. E. (1961). *Traumatic Aphasia*. London: Oxford University Press.

Sachs H. (1895). Das Gehirn des Foerster'schen Rindenblinden. *Arbeiten aus der Psychiatrischen und Nervenklinik Breslau* 2: 55–122.

Sanchez-Longo L. P. and Forster F. M. (1958). Clinical significance of impairment of sound localization. *Neurology* 8: 119–125.

Sanchez-Longo L. P., Forster F., and Auth T. L. (1957). A clinical test for sound localization and its applications. *Neurology* 7: 655–663.

Schlesinger B. (1928). Zur Auffassung der optischen und konstruktiven Apraxie. *Zeitschrift fuer die gesamte Neurologie und Psychiatrie* 117: 649–697.

Semmes J. (1965). A non-tactual factor in stereognosis. *Neuropsychologia* 3: 295–315.

Semmes J., Weinstein S., Ghent L., and Teuber H. L. (1960). *Somatosensory Changes after Penetrating Brain Wounds in Man*. Cambridge: Harvard University Press.

Shankweiler D. (1961). Performance of brain-damaged patients on two tests of sound localization. *J. Comp. Physiolog. Psychol.* 54: 375–381.

Shy G. M. and Haase G. R. (1957). Sensorische Stoerungen bei Scheitellappenlaesionen. *Deutsche Zeitschrift fuer Nervenheilkunde* 176: 519–542.

Stengel E. (1944). Loss of spatial orientation, constructional apraxia and Gerstmann's syndrome. *J. Ment. Sci.* 90: 753–760.

Strauss H. (1924). Ueber Konstruktive Apraxie. *Monatsschrift fuer Psychiatrie und Neurologie* 63: 739–748.

Teuber H. L. (1962). Effects of brain wounds implicating right or left hemisphere in man: Hemisphere differences and hemisphere interaction in vision, audition and somesthesis. In V. B. Mountcastle (ed.), *Interhemispheric Relations and Cerebral Dominance*. Baltimore: Johns Hopkins Press.

Teuber H. L. (1964). The riddle of frontal lobe function in man. In Warren J. M. and Akert K. (eds.), *The Frontal Granular Cortex and Behavior*. New York: McGraw-Hill.

Teuber H. L., Battersby W., and Bender M. B. (1949). Changes in visual searching performance following cerebral lesions. *Am. J. Physiol.* 159, 592.

Walsh E. G. (1957). An investigation of sound localization in patients with neurological abnormalities. *Brain* 80: 222–250.

Warrington E. K., James M., and Kinsbourne M. (1966). Drawing disability in relation to laterality of cerebral lesion. *Brain* 89: 53–82.

Weber E. H. (1978). *The Sense of Touch: De Tactu*, translated by H. E. Ross; *Der Tastsinn* translated by D. J. Murray. London: Academic Press.

Wilbrand H. (1887). *Dei Seelenblindheit als Herderscheinung und ihre Beziehungen zur homonymen Hemianopsie*. Wiesbaden: J. F. Bergmann.

Wortis S. B. and Pfeffer A. Z. (1948). Unilateral auditory-spatial agnosia. *J. Nerv. Ment. Dis.* 108: 181–186.

Zangwill O. L. 1960. *Cerebral Dominance and Its Relation to Psychological Function*. Edinburgh: Oliver & Boyd.

Part II

THE APHASIC DISORDERS

7

Early Descriptions of Aphasia

ARTHUR L. BENTON and ROBERT J. JOYNT

One of the features of the spirited and prolonged discussion that followed Paul Broca's famous pathological demonstrations before the Académie de Médecine of Paris in 1861 was the "exhumation," to use the caustic term of Desiré Bernard, of ancient and long-forgotten descriptions of aphasia. Thus, Jules Falret (1864) in his analysis of the various clinical forms of aphasia, mentioned case reports by Johann Gesner (1770) and Alexander Crichton (1798) as being among the earliest in the field. Trousseau (1931) went farther back, citing the anecdotes of the elder Pliny as evidence that aphasia was known as early as the first century A.D., and quoting the comments of Schenck von Grafenberg (1585) to the effect that he had observed patients who were unable to speak because of loss of memory.

The discovery of "prehistoric" case reports and references dealing with aphasia continued through the latter decades of the century and into the present century. Coupland (1874), Jastrowitz (1875), and Ebstein (1913), called attention to Goethe's description in *Wilhelm Meisters Lehrjahre* (1795), and Ogle (1874), to the still earlier self-description of Samuel Johnson. Külz (1875) presented a German translation of Linné's (1745) brief but most interesting account of expressive aphasia; later. Hultgren (1916) discussed it at some length. Bernard (1889) pointed out that Johann Schmidt's description of alexia in 1676 compared quite favorably with later reports. Soury (1899) cited the very early references to traumatic aphasia by Nicolò Massa (1558) and Francisco Arceo (1588). Gans (1914) presented a German translation of the description by Rommel (1683) of a case of what he regarded as "transcortical" motor aphasia.

Reprinted with permission from the *A. M. A. Archives of Neurology* August 1960, Vol. 3 pp. 205–221.

That the early history of aphasia continues to be of considerable interest to neurologists is evidenced by the recent contributions to it by a number of authors. In 1943, Viets possibly unaware of the German translation of Külz, published an English translation of the case report of Linné. More recently, Antoni (1957) apparently unaware of the contributions of both Külz and Viets, again called attention to it and indicated his feeling that it has been unjustly neglected in historical surveys of the field. Some years ago, Riese (1947) cited Goethe's account as being the "first description containing basic features of aphasia," an opinion with which many students would not agree. In 1950, Eliasberg (1950) called attention to the descriptions of Spalding (1983) and Herz (1791) which appeared in the *Magazin für Erfahrungsseelenkunde*. Most recently, Hoff et al. (1958) have provided an account of the self-description in 1787 by the French scientist Grandjean de Fouchy of his transitory aphasia.

Since the early history of aphasia has claimed our own interest, we believe that it would be of value to assemble in systematic fashion all the older allusions and case reports which have been cited by various authors at various times and places. In making this collation, we have depended almost completely upon references in the literature to guide us to the original writings and have not undertaken an independent examination of original sources which might contain hitherto undiscovered material. The survey is not altogether nonevaluative in nature. Some descriptions are obviously more adequate than others and deserve to be recognized as such. At the same time, there is no doubt that some students have read into certain writings a much greater import than they actually possess, and these misinterpretations warrant correction. On the whole, the facts are clear enough and speak for themselves. The period covered in this survey extends from the possible references to aphasia in the Hippocratic Corpus to the end of the eighteenth century.

Ancient Descriptions

Hippocratic Corpus (ca. 400 B.C.)—There are many references to "aphonia" in the Hippocratic writings, usually in the adjectival form *aphōnos* (Aphorisms, Epidemics, Sacred Disease, Coan Prognosis). The term is used to designate one of the features of apoplexy or epilepsy and also occurs in descriptions of the course of protracted, usually fatal, illnesses. It is rendered in the English translations of Adams (1939) and Jones (1923–31) as "speechless," "loss of speech," or "loss of power of speech." However, the new translation by Chadwick and Mann (1950) usually gives it as "aphonia" or "loss of voice," although in some places it is rendered as "speechless" or "aphasia."

It is sometimes remarked that Hippocrates "must" have appreciated the distinction between aphasia and aphonia, since in one case description (Epidemics

III, Case 3) it is noted that the patient was *anaudos* ("without voice or utterance, speechless"), as well as *aphōnos* as "aphonia." Adams and Jones, since they have consistently translated *aphōnos* as "speechless" or the equivalent, are obliged to break the rule in the translation of this passage. Both now render *anaudos* as "speechless" and utilize another term for *aphōnos*. Adams gives it as "loss of articulation"; Jones, as "voiceless."

There is no doubt that the physicians of the Hippocratic School observed aphasic or aphasia-like manifestations in patients with cerebral disease or dysfunction. So must have generations of physicians before them. The distinction of the School in this respect lies in the very frequent specific references to these conditions. However, it is usually impossible to judge exactly what was meant by the terms *aphonos* and *anaudos*. That they were distinguished from one another is suggested by the use of both terms in the case description cited above. On the other hand, the varying contexts in which the descriptive term *aphonos* appears suggest that sometimes it meant aphasia, sometimes anarthria, sometimes loss of voice. In one passage (Coan Prognosis, No. 315 in the Chadwick-Mann translation), the term *hypaphōnon* ("partial loss of speech or dumbness") is used. It is probable that, as in our own day, the same term was used by different writers to mean different things.

There is a passage in the Coan Prognosis (No. 353 in the Chadwick-Mann translation) which associates temporary speechlessness (*anaudiē*) following convulsions "with paralysis of the tongue, or of the arm and right side of the body." When this is combined with the observation that "an incised wound in one temple produces a spasm in the opposite side of the body" (Coan Prognosis, No. 448 in the Chadwick-Mann translation), it is seen that the essential ingredients for relating aphasia to a lesion of the left hemisphere were present in the Hippocratic writings. But, of course, there is no evidence that the correlation was actually made.

Valerius Maximus (ca. A.D. 30) (Kempf, 1888)—This Latin author and commentator notes that a learned man of Athens, after being struck in the head by a stone, lost his memory of letters, to which he had been particularly devoted, but retained his memory of everything else. This is perhaps the earliest reference to a traumatic alexia to be found in Western literature.

Pliny (A.D. 23–79) (Holland, 1601)—In his *Clinique Médicale*, Trousseau (1931) quoted Pliny to illustrate the thesis that "the physiological conditions of aphasia" were not unknown in antiquity. The relevant lines, which come after an account of some wonderous feats of memory, are as follows:

> And yet there is not a thing in man so fraile and brittle againe as it, whether it be occasioned by disease, by casual injuries and occurrents, or by feare, through which it faileth sometime in part, and otherwhiles decaieth generally, and is cleane lost. One with the stroke of a stone, fell presently to forget his letters onely, and could read no more; otherwise his memory served him well ynough. Another, with

> a fall from the roufe of a very high house, lost the remembrance of his own mother, his next kinsfolke, friends, and neighbours. Another, in a sicknesse of his forgot his owne servants about him: and *Messala Corvinus* the great Oratour, upon the like occasion, forgot his owne proper name.

From a perusal of this charming passage, the reader may decide for himself the extent to which Pliny understood "the physiological conditions of aphasia." In any event, the passage does make clear reference to a case of traumatic alexia, quite possibly the same "very learned man of Athens" mentioned by Valerius Maximus.

Soranus of Ephesus (A.D. 98–135)—The treatises on acute and chronic diseases by Soranus, chief exponent of the Methodist sect, are known to us through the writings of Caelius Aurelianus, who flourished about A.D. 450 (Drabkin, 1950). In his discussion of "paralysis" ("On Chronic Diseases," Book II), in which he distinguished between sensory and motor impairment and between flaccid and spastic paralysis, Caelius points out that while paralysis of the tongue leads to faulty articulation of speech, such paralysis "may be distinguished from cases of loss of speech resulting from some other disease. For in these latter cases, the tongue does not change color or the condition of its surface, or lose sensation or mobility, or change position." According to Creutz (1934), most of the medical writers of this period made the same distinction between impairment of speech or of the voice due to paralysis of the tongue and that due to other causes. The nature of the speech impairments which were referable to other factors remains an open question. No doubt it included aphasia but it may also have had reference to loss of voice from localized peripheral affections. In this respect, it is noteworthy that, directly after making the distinction between loss of speech due to paralysis of the tongue and that due to other causes, Soranus makes an apparently analogous distinction between "paralytic" anosmia and other types. "When the organ of smell is paralyzed, it can no longer detect odors. But this paralysis is to be distinguished from the disease of the nostrils called 'ozaena.' "

Sextus Empiricus (ca. A.D. 200) (Patrick, 1899)—The great skeptic philosopher finds a place in this review because he is commonly supposed to be among the first to use the term *aphasia*. It need only be pointed out that Sextus had in mind a particular philosophic position of the Skeptics, namely, "nonassertion," which referred not at all to the clinical condition of aphasia.

> We explain Aphasia as follows: The word *phasis* is used in two ways, having a general and a special signification. According to the general signification, it expresses affirmation or negation, as "It is day" or "It is not day"; according to the special signification, it expresses an affirmation only. . . . Now Aphasia is the opposite of *phasis* in its general signification, which, as we said, comprises both affirmation and negation. It follows that Aphasia is a condition of mind, according to which we say that we neither affirm nor deny anything.

One cannot help but remark that Hughlings Jackson's conception of aphasia as "a loss of power to propositionise" approaches this use of the term by the Greek Skeptics. From such a point of view, Trousseau's choice of it acquires an aura of prescience. However, whatever may be the relations in a deeper sense between modern concepts of aphasia and its technical meaning in ancient philosophy, it must be conceded that Sextus Empiricus has no real place in the early history of aphasia.

Renaissance Descriptions

Antonio Guainerio (?–1440) (Guainerio, 1481)—Guainerio's references to aphasia are perhaps the earliest of the Renaissance descriptions. Pointing out that when too much phlegm accumulates in the posterior ventricle "the organ of memory can retain little or nothing," he mentions: "I had under my care two old men, one of whom did not know more than three words . . . The other . . . rarely or never recalled the right name of anyone. When he summoned someone, he did not call him by name." From this brief description and Guainerio's interpretation of the disorder as being essentially one of memory, it might be guessed that the first patient suffered from a motor aphasia, the second from an amnestic aphasia.

Baverius de Baveriis (ca. 1480) (Baverius de Baveriis, 1543)—Among the *Consilia* of Baverius of Imola is one (No. 65) dealing with a patient, "an excellent young man," who suffered from "inability to move one side of the body with inability to speak, much sleeping, and weakness of nerves." The inability to speak, which is not further described, is ascribed to "weakness of the seventh pair of nerves, by which the tongue is moved." The side of the body affected is not specified. Whether the patient was dysphasic or dysarthric can hardly be determined from these few lines. In another *Consilium* (No. 2), a pregnant woman is described as "having a cramp in the vertebrae of the neck, so that she cannot raise herself up, and also having a cramp in tongue so that it impedes her speech."

Paracelsus (1493–1541)—Ebstein (1915) has called attention to the fact that this formidable figure of Renaissance medicine, who apparently was well aware of the relationship of paralysis and speech disturbances to disease of the brain, also pointed out that centrally determined deficits of speech, as well as of hearing and vision, could occur in the absence of paralysis. The relevant passage in *Der grossen Wundartzney* . . . (cited by Ebstein) runs as follows:

> Wounds of the head which cause sudden death or epilepsy. . . . It should be recognized that when the chambers of vision, hearing or speech are affected; this is not stroke or paralysis; these are wounds in and of themselves which do not heal completely unless they be very slight.

Ebstein infers from this passage that Paracelsus recognized that focal symptoms, particularly speech disturbances, could occur as a consequence of head injuries.

Nicolo Massa (?–1569)—Massa (1558), one of the great anatomists and syphiologists of his day, describes a case of traumatic aphasia or anarthria which he cured by surgical intervention.

> Also restored to health by my efforts was a handsome young man, Marcus Goro, who was wounded by the sharp point of a spear having on one side an axe and on the other a sword, which they call a halberd. There was a fracture not only of the cranial bone but also of the meninges and the brain substance extending to the basal bone. Because this was protruding, a silver tube, which extended to the basal bone and exerted pressure on it, was placed in the wound. In addition to all his other misfortunes, the young man was speechless for eight days. Asked by many distinguished officials, I came there and noted that . . . the fracture of the bone was about the length of the external ear, a half-finger deep and equally wide. . . . Since the doctors declared that they had seen no bone, I concluded that the reason for the loss of voice was that part of the bone was lodged in the brain. I took an instrument from a certain surgeon who was in attendance and extracted the bone from the wound, whereupon the patient began to speak at once, saying, "Praise God, I am cured." This drew much applause from the doctors, nobles, and attendants who were present.*

Francisco Arceo (1493–1573?) (Arceo, 1588)—In citing Massa's case report, Soury (1899) mentions that a similar experience was also related by the Spanish surgeon Arceo, who describes quite briefly the condition of a workman who was struck on the head by a falling stone. Parts of the skull were depressed into the brain, and for several days after the accident the patient was "not onely speechles, but lay without moving." Arceo reflected the bone fragments back into place and, in doing this, observed that the meninges were inflamed. Three days later, "he spake, yet unperfecklie, and as men of troubled minde are wonte to doe." In due time, the patient recovered completely and "married a wife. For he was then a young man."

Johann Schenck von Grafenberg (1530–1598)—As we have mentioned, Trousseau (1931) cited Schenck von Grafenberg as being one of the early physicians who appreciated the essential nature of aphasia. In his lectures, the following passage from Schenck's *Observationes* (1585) is quoted:

> I have observed in many cases of apoplexy, lethargy, and similar major diseases of the brain that, although the tongue was not paralyzed, the patient could not speak because, the faculty of memory being abolished, the words were not produced.

* Translated by Mrs. Lillian C. Nelson.

Seventeenth-Century Descriptions

In the seventeenth century there appeared two case reports, one by Schmidt, the other by Rommel, which attained a level of description that was significantly above anything which had hitherto appeared. Both cases are described in sufficient detail so that not only is there no doubt that the patients were truly aphasic but also the type of language disability which was manifested is made clearly evident. Since, to our knowledge, English versions of these reports are not available, full translations of them will be presented.

Johann Schmidt (1624–1690)—In 1673, Schmidt (Schmidt, 1676) made observations on a case of aphasia which were published three years later in the *Miscellanea* of the Academia Naturae Curiosorum of Leipzig. They concerned a patient who suffered from a motor aphasia following a stroke. In due time, the aphasia receded but the patient remained completely alexic.

On Loss of Reading Ability Following Apoplexy with Preservation of Writing*

A leading citizen among us, Nicholas Cambier, an old man of 65 years, was seized with a very severe attack of apoplexy which all his attendants feared would lead to his death. Many remedies were applied, including copious venesection, irritating enemas to stimulate the sleeping faculties, cupping with deep incisions of the scapular and nuchal regions, together with inunction of the neck, forehead and nose and, from time to time, essences and spirits for the head to the degree that his condition would permit.

Upon his return home, it was evident that his right side was paralyzed and that he had difficulty in speaking. He muttered a good deal but was incapable of expressing the feelings of his mind; he substituted one word for another so that his attendants had difficulty in determining what he wanted. He then developed epilepsy with severe convulsions; this disappeared and he returned to his former state. Thus was the wretched man tortured. Finally, by the goodness of God, these terrible enemies were overcome. At no time had they carried the threat of immediate death.

A final evil remained to be overcome. He could not read written characters, much less combine them in any way. He did not know a single letter nor could he distinguish one from another. But it is remarkable that, if some name were given to him to be written, he could write it readily, spelling it correctly. However, he could not read what he had written even though it was in his own hand. Nor could he distinguish or identify the characters. For if he were asked what letter this or that was or how the letters had been combined, he could answer only by chance or through his habit of writing. It appeared that he wrote without deliberation. No teaching or guidance was successful in inculcating recognition of letters in him.

It was otherwise with a certain stone cutter in our country. Wilhelm Richter came to see me after his apoplexy receded because he was not able to read at all

* Translated by Mrs. Lillian C. Nelson.

> or to recognize letters. However, he learned the alphabetic elements of the language again in a short time. He then combined them and attained perfection in his reading.

This case report of Schmidt, dating back almost three centuries, is indeed a remarkable one. It provides, so far as we are aware, the first unmistakable descriptions of paraphasia and alexia. Moreover, as Desiré Bernard (1889) pointed out, Schmidt took pains, by a comparison of his two cases, to show that the course of an acquired impairment in reading could vary. In his brief discussion following the case reports, Schmidt mentions the patient's inability to read script which he himself had just written as being the most "memorable" feature of his first case. This phenomenon has been repeatedly observed since his time and its significance is still a subject of lively interest.

Peter Rommel (1643–1708)—Rommel (1683), who designated his case a "rare aphonia," described a patient with motor aphasia and incapacity for repetition but with consideration retention of capacity for serial speech and for understanding of oral and written language. A translation of his report reads as follows:

On a Rare Aphonia*

> The wife of Senator H., of the imperial city of Laufen, a highly respected lady 52 years of age, fell ill seven years ago, after which she was bled without medical consultation, as unfortunately is so often the case. After a fairly strenuous walk which she took after dinner, she suffered a mild delirium and apoplexy with paralysis of the right side. At the same time, she lost all speech with the exception of the words, "yes" and "and." She could say no other word, not even a syllable, with these exceptions: the Lord's Prayer, the Apostles' Creed, some Biblical verses and other prayers, which she could recite verbatim and without hesitation but somewhat precipitously. But it is to be noted that they were said in the order in which she was accustomed to saying them for many years and, if this regular sequence were interrupted and she were asked to recite a prayer or Biblical verse not in its accustomed place, she either could not do it at all or only after a long interval and with great difficulty. I tried this test myself and was astonished to hear her reciting some prayers. However, when I requested her to repeat a prayer that she had already recited she could not do it even after great effort, until her maid, who had long been familiar with the order of the prayers, would recite it. Then she would recite the requested prayer, although with some difficulty. Similarly, I asked her to repeat some words in the order in which I said them, e.g., "God will help." Stimulated to effort, she tried several times, but was unsuccessful. Overcome with misery, she burst into tears. Then we tried to determine whether she could repeat very short sentences consisting of the same words found in her prayers. However, she was also unsuccessful in this.
>
> Nevertheless, her memory was excellent. She grasped and understood everything that she saw and heard and she answered questions, even about events in the remote past, by affirmative or negative nods of the head. In her own way, she

* Translated by Mrs. Lillian C. Nelson.

> showed censure or approval of things done badly or well in her household. She attended church, listened to the sermons and claimed that she received great comfort from them. At home she even read the Holy Writ and other theological books but complained that what she read impressed her less and was forgotten more readily than what she heard. The fingers of her right hand were contracted and the whole arm was deprived of movement and warmth, but not, however, of feeling.
>
> Otherwise, she has been in excellent health, has a very good appetite, sleeps well and, in spite of her age, menses are regular. Indeed she states that in general she is healthier than she was before. She has given up all medication, since she took a variety of drugs prescribed by the most eminent physicians with her condition remaining the same. She now lives content with her lot.

This case report must be considered to be outstanding. The defects and preserved capacities of the patient are clearly delineated; indeed, the description of her language disorder compares favorably with that to be found in most contemporary clinical reports. In referring to his case as one of "rare aphonia," Rommel had in mind, of course, what he considered to be the striking feature of the clinical picture, namely, the discrepancy between the patient's impairment in spontaneous verbal expression and in repetition and her retained capacity for serial speech. Thus he must be given credit for presenting the first descriptive analysis of this commonly encountered aphasic profile.

Eighteenth-Century Descriptions

As might be expected, many descriptions of aphasia or allusions to it appeared during the eighteenth century. A number of them are outlined below. No doubt systematic examination of the medical literature of the period would disclose additional instances.

Duc de Saint-Simon (1675–1755)—A note by Cullerre (1906) called attention to a brief description of an aphasic, in the memoirs of the Duc de Saint Simon (1958), which possesses a feature of special interest. Among the entries for the year 1718 the following statement about the diplomatist and military leader, the Duc d'Harcourt, appears:

> Marshall d'Harcourt finally died on 19 October, at the age of only 55 years. Having been reduced by several apoplectic attacks to the point where he could not utter a single syllable, he would indicate with a pointer the letters of a large alphabet which was set before him and which an ever watchful secretary would accordingly write and form into words. He would do this with all the impatience and despair imaginable.

Cullerre points out that this visual use of the letters of the alphabet to form words is, in a sense, a precursor of the diagnostic test of movable letters employed by Trousseau and other clinicians to determine the status of "internal language" in their aphasic patients. He also remarks that the brief allusion to the intense affective state of the Duc as he coped with the difficulties of expressing his thoughts foreshadows the more detailed observations of Trousseau on this aspect of aphasic behavior.

Gerard van Swieten (1700–1772)—Van Swieten's oft-quoted reference (Van Swieten 1742–46) to aphasia reads as follows:

> I have seen many patients whose cerebral functions were quite sound after recovery from apoplexy, except for this one deficit: In designating objects, they could not find the correct names for them. These unfortunate people would try with their hands and feet and an effort of their whole body to explain what they wanted and yet could not. This disability often remained incurable for many years.

Brief as this description is, it points clearly to the type of aphasic deficit shown by these patients, and one seems to be on safe ground in considering it to be an unmistakable allusion to amnestic aphasia.

Carl Linné (1707–1778)—In 1745, Linné published a case report (Linnaeus, 1745) describing the condition of an educated man who, in conjunction with a "sleeping sickness" (cataphora), showed markedly disordered speech. Initially he showed paraphasic disturbances, speaking "as it were, a foreign language, having his own names for all words, e.g., to drink *To Ti,* etc." After this, it was found that he was incapable of writing any name, even his own or those of his wife and children. If a name which he was apparently trying to say was spoken to him, he would say "yes," but he could not repeat the word, saying "cannot." Yet he seemed to be able to read names with understanding, and "when he wanted to mention the names of any of his colleagues, he pointed to the *Catalogum Lectionum* in which the name was found." The aphasia receded shortly before his death. Linné remarks that the patient had thus lost "first, the memory of all nouns and, second, the ability to express nouns."

An English translation of Linné's report has been published by Viets (1943) and a German translation by Külz (1875). As Nils Antoni (1957) has pointed out, Linné presents a fairly clear, if brief, description of a paraphasia followed by severe expressive aphasia, including loss of capacity for repetitive speech. The patient retained some capacity for reading. The exact extent to which he could understand oral speech remains questionable; apparently considerable understanding of spoken language was retained. According to Hultgren (1916), the learned patient was Arvid Arrhenius, Professor at the University of Uppsala.

Olof Dalin (1708–1763)—In their papers, both Hultgren and Antoni called attention to the fact that, directly preceding Linné's communication in the proceedings of the Royal Swedish Academy of Science, there is another description of aphasia by the historian and litterateur Olof Dalin (1745). It reads as follows:

On a Mute Who Can Sing*

Jon Persson, a farmer's son from Ofvankihl, in the parish of Juleta in Sörmanland, born in 1703, brought up in the usual simple way to know his Christianity and to read; in 1736, after he had been married for three years, he had an attack of a violent illness which resulted in a paralysis of the entire right side of the body and complete loss of speech. After almost half a year in bed, he began to move to some degree but he limped and carried his right arm in a sling.

For two years he went to a mineral spring at Juleta parsonage which many people had found to be helpful. However, he did not note any improvement except that he was able to walk more steadily and to pronounce correctly the small but often important word, "yes." However, he gained one advantage, which was later observed and which is the occasion for his present notoriety. He can sing certain hymns, which he had learned before he became ill, as clearly and distinctly as any healthy person. However, it should be noted that at the beginning of the hymn he has to be helped a little by some other person singing with him. Similarly, with the same type of help, he can recite certain prayers without singing, but with a certain rhythm and in a high-pitched, shouting tone. Yet this man is dumb, cannot say a single word except "yes" and has to communicate by making signs with his hands.

To be sure, he has always been somewhat simple-minded and naïve. Yet now, as in the past, he is quite normal in his own way, in his ability to hear and understand, and he is God-fearing, quiet and well behaved.

The vicar of Juleta parish, Joh. Ihering, whose personal and signed statement is the source of my information, has kept him in the vicarage for eight years and has made every effort to determine whether this is a deception or illusion on the part of the man for the purpose of providing himself with food more easily. However, the vicar has found the case to be completely genuine. Parishioners of higher and lower rank offer the same testimony. I have also personally seen this man and have heard him sing.

The strange and varied effects that accompany a stroke are only too familiar. I wish to add nothing to this account other than to make the comment that people who stammer are able to sing without impediment and quite distinctly although they cannot utter ten whole words in succession when they speak.

Why Dalin, who was primarily an important literary figure, should have concerned himself with this case and taken the trouble to report it to the Academy becomes understandable when one considers his background. Hultgren points out that he intended to become a physician and actually studied medicine for a time. Exactly why he abandoned his medical studies is not known. The attitude of therapeutic nihilism expressed by his teacher, Stobaeus, may have operated to reduce his interest. His esthetic and emotional sensitivity may have been a determining factor. In all probability, the change was dictated more by an intense love for literature than by any animus against medicine, for Dalin maintained his interest in science and medicine throughout his life. He was

* Translated by Prof. Arthur A. Wald.

elected a member of the Academy of Science in 1742 and served as its president in 1749.

Dalin's description is of interest in demonstrating, as did the earlier case report of Rommel, that the capacity for serial speech may be retained by a patient with motor aphasia even when he has lost all other aspects of expressive language. It is of particular interest because of the specific reference to singing, which is, in essence, melodic serial speech. Apparently the patient retained understanding of spoken language to a considerable degree, but here, as in so many case reports, it is impossible to judge whether there was a significant loss in this area as well. Dalin's remarks about the ability of stammerers to sing with fluency suggests that this phenomenon had been observed before and that he was merely calling it to the attention of the reader.

Giovanni Battista Morgagni (1682–1771)—Morgagni's great *De Sedibus* . . . , published in 1762, includes numerous brief descriptions of cases of speechlessness associated with apoplexy, head injury, and cerebral disease in which autopsy study disclosed injury or disease of the brain. They posses three noteworthy features. The first is the frequency with which Morgagni took pains to point out that, although the patient could not talk, he was able to understand spoken language.

> But before the thirtieth day, the fever came on again with a coldness: and to this was added, about the thirty fourth day, an apoplectic affection, with a loss of speech, and a privation of motion in the whole right side of the body, though the sense remained at the same time. However, she show'd by nods and signs that she understood what was said.
>
> . . . .
>
> But many errors in diet being committed, and some febrile accessions having already preceeded, about the eleventh day a very violent epileptic convulsion attack'd him: and when this remitted, the patient did not speak: although he signified that he understood what others said.
>
> . . . .
>
> . . . he scarcely spoke at all, and when he did, he stammer'd; but he answered in such a manner, by nods and signs, to those who ask'd him questions, that you might perceive his internal senses to be strong and perfect.

The second noteworthy feature of Morgagni's work is that, as would be expected in the *De Sedibus*, his clinical descriptions are supplemented by the findings of autopsy. These examinations showed that various types of cerebral lesion—trauma, vascular accident, and tumor—could be associated with paralysis and motor speech impairment.

The third characteristic of his observations which deserves mention is the frequency with which motor speech disorders are described in concurrence with right hemiplegia and subsequent autopsy evidence of disease or injury of the left cerebral hemisphere. Morgagni amassed considerable clinicopathologic evidence in support of the association between paralysis of one side of the body and the presence of disease in the opposite cerebral hemisphere, and he discussed the matter at some length. On the basis of this, Ebstein (1915) concluded that Morgagni (and his master, Valsalva) had established the relationship between aphasia, right hemiplegia and disease of the left cerebral hemisphere. He writes: "These extracts are quite sufficient to indicate that not only does clinical and autopsy observation of contralateral innervation originate with Valsalva and Morgagni but also the association of right hemiplegia with speech disorders. In the future we can speak frankly of the Valsalva-Morgagni doctrine or law."

There seems to be little doubt that Ebstein overstates the case for Morgagni. Incidental description without interpretation does not amount to discovery. Despite the frequency with which motor speech disorder and right hemiplegia appear together in his descriptions and his clear appreciation of crossed innervation, there is no evidence whatever that Morgagni actually correlated aphasia with right hemiplegia or with lesions in the left cerebral hemisphere. Possibly the best evidence that he drew no conclusions about the relationship between aphasia and right hemipiegia (or left hemisphere disease) is the fact that, although the *De Sedibus* was one of the most widely used medical works for several decades after its publication, not only in the original Latin but also in English, French, and German translations, it does not seem to have suggested this relationship to its many readers.

Morgagni's descriptions are typically brief, and the exact nature of the expressive speech disorders which he mentions is never quite clear. In our search, we have encountered no description of a deficit in the understanding of speech which is sufficiently specific to suggest sensory aphasia.

Johann Gesner (1738–1801)—Gesner devoted a section of about 75 pages to the subject of "Die Sprachamnesie" in the second volume (1770) of his *Samlung von Beobachtungen aus der Arzneygelahrtheit*. In it he presents a number of descriptions of aphasic patients, based on either his personal observations or those of older writers, as well as a discussion of the psychopathology of these conditions.

The first case (later cited by Crichton, 1798, and Falret, 1864) is one of jargon aphasia. A 73-year-old man had a seizure in which he experienced a cramp in the muscles of the mouth and at the same time "an itch like the crawling of ants which he tried to eliminate by rubbing." About two weeks later there was a sudden onset of a confusional state which was accompanied by "a very peculiar impairment of speech." He articulated fluently but uttered incomprehensible neologisms. He had no paralysis but did show a slight unsteadiness in gait. He also wrote jargon and his written words corresponded phonetically to the words as pronounced. He could not write his name nor could he read. Nevertheless, it was evident that he was not grossly demented and retained his understanding of objects in the environment. He was aware of the fact that he was speaking jargon.

The second case report summarizes a description by Wepfer of a middle-aged man, who showed a pronounced impairment in memory immediately following a sleeping sickness of nine days' duration. He seemed to have forgotten past events and for a period of some weeks failed to recognize his wife and children. He could not read, although his vision was unimpaired. In due time, however, he recognized his family, was able to recite the Lord's Prayer and the Psalms and to read some words, being more successful in Latin than in German. He would often write whole lines and paragraphs in an elegant hand, but what he wrote made no sense. By means of gestures and isolated words he was able to convey that he recognized his friends, but he could not call them by name. He was concerned about household affairs and would offer "advice" to his wife in the form of many meaningless words. Often he would start a conversation, speaking reasonably and clearly, and then falter in the middle of it. All other abilities were found to be unimpaired.

The third case report describes the condition of an abbot who, just as he was about to give some instructions to a peasant, found himself unable to do so. The impairment lasted for three days. He could recognize objects but could not read. There were no sensory or motor deficits. He improved gradually, but as late as the eighth day it was noted that he would still use inappropriate words in conversation. He could recite the Lord's Prayer fluently but faltered when he attempted longer psalms or songs. In due time, he partially regained the ability to read, the degree of recovery being greater for Latin than for German. He himself felt that he had suffered some decline in judgment, in the ability to calculate, and in the capacity for understanding the speech of others.

The next case is one taken from the writings of Friedrich Hoffmann. A man found himself afflicted with a sudden loss of memory. He could not speak, read, or write but was able to understand what others said to him. He retained his memory for past events and was able to indicate that a physician should be sent for.

There follows a description of an elderly patient whose tongue became paralyzed. After a day of treatment (Spanish flies and venesection) he began to speak again, "but he used the same words to name various objects words that seemed to come from a foreign language." During the course of the next few weeks he improved to the point that he could read newspapers with understanding. However, he could not read aloud.

The final case report concerns a patient who was personally observed by Gesner. After a severe stroke, a teacher found that, although he recognized letters and words, he invariably misspoke when he read them aloud. He was aware of the deficit, remarking: "I know this letter and realize that I have seen and spoken it countless times; yet when I want to say it aloud, I say something else. This has made me so disturbed and bitter that I do not like to attempt it any more." Nevertheless, his understanding of what was said or read aloud to him seemed to be completely intact.

Gesner's discussion of the psychopathology of these conditions is quite lengthy, has many interesting features, and deserves more detailed consideration than can be given it here. Very briefly stated, he attributes the language deficits not to general intellectual decline or to a loss of memory "in general," as was the habit of some older writers, but to a specific impairment in verbal memory. This impairment in memory consists in the inability to associate images or abstract ideas with their expressive verbal symbols. Paraphasic substitutions occur when the idea which the patient has in mind is a vivid one and he has a strong need to express it. Thus, when a patient utters a neologism or an inappropriate word, he is manifesting a forgetting of speech and not a disorder in thinking or understanding. The basic cause of these language deficits is disease of the brain which reflects itself in a weakness or inertia of the relationships between the different parts of that organ.

It is evident that Gesner's contribution to the clinical and theoretical aspects of aphasia was a major one. His case descriptions indicated clearly that expressive aphasia could not be interpreted as merely a paralysis of the tongue or any other organ. He showed that jargon aphasia was typically accompanied by jargon agraphia and that there could be a phonetic correspondence between the two modalities of expression. As in the previous case reports of Rommel and Dalin, it is noted that the capacity for serial speech may be retained by a patient who shows gross impairment in the other aspects of expressive language. That one deals here with distinctive language deficits, and not with a generalized disorder in thinking, is repeatedly emphasized.

Gesner's theoretical analysis also represented a major advance in thinking about aphasia. He was the first to advance the idea that the basic psychopathology of these disorders consists in a failure to associate image or idea with linguistic sign. This concept was destined to become the basic idea underlying the views of most 19th century clinicians concerning aphasia.

Jean Paul Grandjean de Fouchy (1707–1788)—Hoff et al. (1958) have called attention to this early self-observation of a transitory paraphasia. At the time of the incident (1783), de Fouchy, a man of broad interests and many talents, was 76 years old. The directly pertinent lines in his account, which is translated in full by Hoff et al., read as follows:

> Toward the end of dinner, I felt a little increase of pain above the left eye, and in that very instant I became unable to pronounce the words that I wanted. I heard what was said, and I thought of what I ought to reply, but I spoke other words than those which would express my thoughts, or if I began them I did not complete them, and I substituted other words for them. I had nevertheless all movements as freely as usual. . . . I saw all objects clearly, I heard distinctly what was being said; and the organs of thought were, it seemed to me, in a natural state. This sort of paroxysm lasted about a minute.

Johann Joachim Spalding (1714–1804)—This description, by an eminent German theologian, of his experiences during an episode of paraphasia and dysgraphia was reported in 1783. A translation of it appeared in Alexander Crichton's "Inquiry into the Nature and Origin of Mental Derangement" (1798) and was reprinted in Forbes Winslow's "On the Obscure Diseases of the Brain and Disorders of the Mind" (1868). In 1950, Eliasberg (1950) presented a fresh English translation in a paper on the "prehistory" of aphasia.

Spalding relates how, after a rather busy morning, he had begun to write a receipt for some monies received and discovered that he could not continue after having written the first two words, "for I could not recollect the words which belonged to the ideas I had in mind." Exerting every effort, he started to write again slowly and deliberately, only to find that he was writing words other than those intended. Turning to the person who was waiting for the receipt, he could not express himself clearly but managed by a combination of monosyllables and gestures to get him to understand that he was not to wait for the receipt. There followed "a tumultuous disorder in my senses, in which I was incapable of remarking anything in particular, except that one series of ideas forced themselves involuntarily on my mind. . . . I endeavoured to speak, in order to discover whether I was capable of saying anything that was connected, but although I made the greatest efforts of attention, and proceeded with the utmost caution, I perceived that I uniformly spoke other words than those I intended. My mind was as little master of the organs of speech, as it had been before of my hand in writing."

According to Spalding's estimate, this state of affairs lasted about half an hour and was followed by a period of about the same duration during which he felt constrained to speak slowly and deliberately. By afternoon he was sufficiently recovered to be able to write the description which was subsequently published.

Spalding's self-description is an extremely interesting one but did not add anything that was essentially new to the fund of existing knowledge. As Eliasberg has pointed out, a theoretical explanation of the deficits was attempted by the philosopher, Moses Mendelssohn (1783).

Samuel Johnson (1707–1784)—Ogle (1874) was probably the first medical writer to call attention to Dr. Johnson's description of the aphasic and agraphic disturbances accompanying his stroke, which occurred about 3 o'clock in the morning of June 17, 1783. In a letter (June 19, 1783) to Mrs. Thrale, he wrote:

> On Monday the 16. I sat for my picture and walked a considerable way without inconvenience. In the afternoon and evening I felt myself light and easy, and began to plan schemes of life. Thus I went to bed, and in a short time waked and sat up as has long been my custom, when I felt a confusion and indistinctness in my head which lasted, I suppose about half a minute; I was alarmed and prayed God, that however he might afflict my body he would spare my understanding. This prayer, that I might try the integrity of my faculties I made in Latin verse. The

> lines were not very good, but I knew them not to be very good, I made them easily, and concluded myself to be unimpaired in my faculties. [Chapman, 1952].
>
> Soon after I perceived that I had suffered a paralytick stroke, and that my Speech had been taken from me. I had no pain, and so little dejection in this dreadful state that I wondered at my own apathy, and considered that perhaps death itself when it should come, would excite less horror than seems now to attend it.
>
> . . . .
>
> I then wrote a card to Mr. Allen, that I might have a discreet friend at hand to act as occasion should require. In penning this note I had some difficulty, my hand, I knew not how nor why, made wrong letters. . . . I have so far recovered my vocal powers, as to repeat the Lord's Prayer with no very imperfect articulation. My memory, I hope, yet remains as it was.

Johnson seems to have recovered quickly from these impairments in speech and writing. However, examination of printed versions of the letters which he wrote after the stroke shows occasional repetition of words, suggesting that recovery from the dysgraphia may not have been complete. That his ability to write varied from time to time may be inferred from a letter written (in a clear hand) on May 10, 1784, to June Langton, which begins: "I am sorry that your pretty Letter has been so long without being answered; but when I am not pretty well, I do not write plain enough for young ladies." Critchley's detailed analysis of Johnson's writing, which is based on photocopies of his letters written before and after the stroke, should clarify this question.

Ryklof Michel van Goens (1748–1810)—Van Goens, a philologist and classical scholar, contributed a description of a case of paraphasia to Volume VII (1789) of the *Magazin für Erfahrungsseelenkunde*. The report was subsequently summarized by Crichton (1798) and Forbes Winslow (1868). The patient, who was the wife of the professor of mathematics at the University of Utrecht, was herself a mathematician and astronomer. The pertinent passages in van Goens' report (1789) are as follows:

> After an illness, she suddenly was afflicted with a forgetting, or, rather, an incapacity or confusion of speech. . . . If she desired a chair, she would ask for a table; if she wished to have a book, she would ask for a glass. If one said to her the desired word, for which she had substituted another, she could not repeat it.
>
> Sometimes she herself perceived that she misnamed objects; at other times, she was annoyed when a *fan*, which she had asked for, was brought to her, instead of the *bonnet*, which she thought she had requested. This unusual disorder persisted for several months.
>
> Her speech was generally confused and rather clumsy, but her amnesia applied only to certain words. Otherwise, her memory was sufficiently intact that she continued to manage the household. She was able to even show her husband the position of the stars on a chart as correctly as when she had been completely well. She recovered gradually and has enjoyed the full use of her mental powers for several years.

Marcus Herz (1747–1803)—This case report by Herz, a prominent physician and intellectual figure of his time in Berlin, was published in 1791 and was quoted by Crichton (1798) and Forbes Winslow (1868). It was summarized by Eliasberg (1950), who interpreted the patient's disorders as being due to a "combination of subcortical aphasia with conduction aphasia." The English version in Crichton's book (which we have compared with the original and found to be essentially accurate) runs as follows.

> In August 1785, I was called to an officer of the artillery, a man about 40 years old, who, as I was informed, was seized with a palsy in consequence of cold and violent anger. His tongue, hands, and feet were lamed by the attack. He was under the care of one of our first physicians, at whose desire I was consulted concerning the propriety of using electricity. From the time that this remedy was first employed until the following year, I never saw him; but then he sent for me again, as his own physician, he said, had deserted him.
>
> I found him so much recovered as to have the complete use of his feet; his hands were also much stronger; but in regard to his speech, the following very remarkable circumstance was to be observed. He was unable to articulate distinctly any words which either occurred to him spontaneously, or when they were slowly and loudly repeated to him. He strenuously exerted himself to speak, but an unintelligible kind of murmur was all that could be heard. The effort he made was violent and terminated in a deep sigh. On the other hand, he could read aloud with facility. If a book, or any written paper, was held before his eyes, he read so quickly and distinctly, that it was impossible to observe that there was the slightest fault in his organs of speech. But if the book or paper was withdrawn, he was then totally incapable of pronouncing one of the words which he had read the instant before. I tried this experiment repeatedly, not only in the presence of his wife, but of many other people. The effect was uniformly the same.

It is difficult to see how this patient's condition can be accounted for by postulating a "combination of subcortical motor aphasia with conduction aphasia." We doubt the justification of considering him a case of aphasia at all. Taking all the recorded facts into consideration—the bilateral paralysis and "paralysis of the tongue" which followed some kind of emotional upset, which lasted for a year, and which was apparently cured in large part by "electricity," together with the peculiar combination of absolute incapacity for spontaneous or repetitive speech, and complete fluency in reading aloud—we think that the weight of evidence favors a diagnosis of hysteria.

Johann Wolfgang von Goethe (1749–1832)—Goethe's description of motor aphasia, which appears in "*Wilhelm Meisters Lehrjahre*" has been cited and quoted many times (cf. Coupland (1874), Jastrowitz (1875), Ebstein (1913), Riese (1947). The novel was first published in 1795, and it is surmised that Goethe's experience with aphasia was based on the fact that his maternal grandfather, Johann Wolfgang Textor, had a stroke with right hemiplegia and aphasia as residuals. The relevant passage reads in one English translation (1871) as follows:

> But, unfortunately, this happiness was but of short duration; my father was suddenly seized with palsy, which attacked his right side, and deprived him of the power of speech. We were obliged to guess at everything he wanted, for he never expressed the words which he intended to utter. Oftentimes this was to me fearfully distressing, particularly upon occasions when he insisted upon being left alone with me—he would signify, by violent gestures, that every other person should retire; but when we were left together, he found himself unable to express his thoughts. His impatience then became extreme, and his distress was deeply afflicting. This much seemed certain—that there was something which he was anxious to confide to me of the utmost importance to myself. I cannot express the anxiety which I felt to know it. Formerly I could see his wishes in his eyes—but this was no longer the case. His eyes no longer spoke.

This brief description of a motor aphasia is sufficiently specific to identify the disorder as such. The incapacity of the patient to express himself, his emotional reaction to his ability, and his use of gesture to communicate are presented clearly enough. However, in the light of what we know about earlier descriptions of aphasia, it seems obvious that Goethe's account is no way outstanding and hardly worthy of being singled out for special mention. It is certainly incorrect to claim any priority for it as the first adequate or near-adequate description of aphasia or to suggest that Goethe might be "actually considered the discoverer of the speech center" (Bryk, 1909)

Alexander Crichton (1763–1856)—In his book, Crichton (1798) discusses what he calls "a very singular defect of memory," which "ought rather to be considered as a defect of that principle, by which ideas, and their proper expressions, are associated, than of memory; for it consists in this, that the person, although he has a distinct notion of what he means to say, cannot pronounce the words which ought to characterize his thoughts." In addition to citing Gesner's first case as an illustration of the deficit, Crichton also reports a personally observed case of paraphasia.

> The first case of this kind which occurred to me in practice was that of an attorney, much respected for his integrity and talents, but who had many sad failings, to which our physical nature too often subjects us. Although nearly in his 70th year, and married to an amiable lady much younger than himself, he kept a mistress whom he was in the habit of visiting every evening. The arms of Venus are not wielded with impunity at the age of 70. He was suddenly seized with a great prostration of strength, giddiness, forgetfulness, insensibility to all concerns of life, and every symptom of approaching fatuity. His forgetfulness was of the kind alluded to. When he wished to ask for any thing, he would constantly make use of some inappropriate term. Instead of asking for a piece of bread, he would probably ask for his boots; but if these were brought, he knew they did not correspond with idea he had of the thing he wished to have, and was therefore angry; yet he would still demand his boots or shoes, meaning bread. If he wanted a tumbler to drink out of, it was a thousand to one he did not call for a certain chamber utensil; and if it was the said utensil he wanted, he would call it a tumbler

> or a dish. He evidently was conscious that he pronounced wrong words for when the proper expressions were spoken by another person, and he was asked if it was not such a thing he wanted, he always seemed aware of his mistake, and corrected himself by adopting the appropriate expression. This gentleman was cured of his complaint by large doses of valerian, and other proper medicines.

Crichton's description of paraphasia is clear enough but added little to the knowledge already gained from older case reports. However, it is noteworthy that, like Gesner (with whose work he was familiar), Crichton characterized the deficit as being one not merely of memory but, rather, of the associative bonds between ideas and their linguistic expression.

Comment

In the elucidation of clinical phenomena, accurate recognition and adequate description usually precede formulations about causation and pathogenesis. Aphasia is no exception to this rule. As this historical survey shows, the published literature on aphasia before 1800 was primarily, but not exclusively, descriptive. Taken in its totality, this literature constitutes what was "known" about aphasia in 1800, i.e., what a well-informed student *would* know about aphasia. This body of knowledge may be analyzed from three standpoints—the clinical manifestations of aphasia, conceptions of its essential psychopathology, and ideas about its neuropathologic basis.

Clinical Manifestations—As we have seen, the oldest descriptions referred merely to "speechlessness," usually complete, sometimes partial. From a reading of these descriptions, it is usually not possible for one to be confident that the described conditions represented forms of motor aphasia rather than of anarthria. Perhaps the first clear (but extremely brief) reference to aphasic disorders is that of Guainerius (1481), with his citation of one patient who knew only three words, and of another, who rarely could recall the names of people, although presumably he could talk. The first unmistakable description of a motor aphasia (in the form of paraphasia) seems to be that of Schmidt (1673). This was soon followed by Rommel's (1683) superb account of a patient who was incapable of spontaneous or repetitive speech but who could recite prayers and verses. The earliest unmistakable allusion to amnestic aphasia is that of van Swieten (1742). The coincidence of aphasia and agraphia was observed by Linné (1745). Gesner (1770) contributed the first adequate descriptions of jargon aphasia, showed that it could be accompanied by jargon agraphia, and described differential impairment in reading in patients who knew Latin as well as their native language. Alexia was mentioned by Valerius Maximum and Pliny, but was first adequately described by Schmidt. The case reports of Dalin (1745), van Goens (1789), and Crichton (1798) provided descriptions of various clinical features of aphasia, such as unawareness of the disability and the intense affective reactions to frustration which are so often observed. A number of interesting self-descriptions, most notably that of Spalding (1783), had been published.

In brief, almost all the clinical forms of aphasia—complete motor aphasia, paraphasia, jargon aphasia, agraphia, and alexia—had been described before 1800. The unawareness of defect which may accompany paraphasia and jargon aphasia had been noted, as well as the coincidence of aphasia and agraphia. Retention of capacity for serial speech (in the form of recital of prayers and of signing) when spontaneous, conversational, and repetitive speech was gravely impaired had been remarked. Differential impairment in reading one language as compared with another and characteristic frustration reactions had been described.

The one major form of aphasia which seems to have been missed is sensory aphasia in the form of impairment in comprehension of oral speech. To be sure, Gesner mentioned the self-evaluation of one of his patients to the effect that he had suffered some impairment in understanding the speech of others. However, beyond this, there is no mention of specific impairment in speech comprehension in the early literature. Indeed, quite often emphasis was placed on the patient's retained capacity for understanding spoken language within the setting of defective expression of speech (cf. Rommel, Morgagni, Dalin, Gesner).

A number of possible reasons may be suggested for this failure to identify sensory aphasia as such. Gross lack of comprehension of oral language was probably interpreted either as a manifestation of dementia or as a loss of hearing. Less severe impairment in comprehension possibly went unrecognized because of the patient's retained capacity to respond appropriately to simple questions and requests. On the basis of our current understanding of jargon aphasia, it must be assumed that the patients of Gesner and Crichton did in fact have receptive deficits which escaped attention. It may be noted that sensory aphasia remained virtually unrecognized as a specific language deficit for another three-quarters of a century, until the appearance of Wernicke's monograph, in 1874.

The milder forms of agrammatism or syntactic aphasia, as manifested in telegraphic speech, alterations of intonation, and syntactical poverty, are also not mentioned in the early literature.

Psychopathologic Conceptions—The earliest interpretation of severe motor aphasia was that it was due to paralysis of the tongue. In cases of expressive language deficit, in which it was obvious that the action of the tongue and the other peripheral speech organs was unimpaired, recourse was had to a global explanation of "loss of memory." Alexia was interpreted as a partial loss of memory, one that was restricted to letters. Linné characterized his patient's paraphasia and subsequent Broca-type aphasia as a loss of memory for nouns and an inability to express them.

Gesner's (1770) more specific conception that paraphasia and jargon aphasia were due to an interruption in the connections between an image or an idea and its expressive linguistic sign constituted a notable advance in theorizing about expressive aphasic disorders. The same idea was presented by Crichton (1798). Developed in greater detail, this conception formed the basis for the classical theory of aphasia which was developed in the 19th century and which, it must be said, still guides the thinking of many clinicians, despite the cogent criticisms of such men as Jackson, Head, Pick, and Goldstein.

Neuropathology—From the earliest times it was recognized that aphasic disorders were due to disease or injury of the brain or, at least, of the ventricles. The differentiation of such centrally determined speech deficits from those caused by peripheral factors seems to have been made quite early (e.g., by Soranus), although one cannot be absolutely certain on this point. At any rate, the distinction was clearly made by Renaissance physicians. In due time it was observed that aphasic disturbances were often associated with stroke or convulsions and that they could occur as a consequence of trauma, fever, vascular accident, or tumor. The clinicopathologic correlations of Morgagni provided incontrovertible evidence of these relationships.

The association of aphasia with right hemiplegia was not remarked, despite the repeated incidental observation of the clinical combination of aphasia and dextral paralysis. This relationship escaped the notice of even so keen and careful a student as Morgagni, who had had the opportunity of observing so many instances of this concurrence. The failure to make this correlation was not, of course, peculiarly distinctive of medical observation before 1800. Scores of aphasic patients with dextral paralysis must have been observed during the first 60 years of the nineteenth century. Yet, with the exception of Marc Dax, no clinician noted the association until Broca's demonstrations in 1861 forced recognition of it.

When one asks why this relationship, which now seems so obvious to us, escaped the attention of earlier observers, a reasonable answer would appear to be that such a correlation did not make "sense." Nor does it make "sense" even today. In spite of the theoretical speculations which have been advanced to explain the association, it remains a "low-order" relationship, established by empirical observation and admittedly of tremendous clinical importance. Yet its basic psychoneurologic significance still eludes us.

Nor, with one exception, did the early workers attempt neuropathologic localization of aphasia along the anterior-posterior dimension of the brain—a question which only a short time later Gall and Bouillaud were to raise so forcefully. The exception is represented by the few remarks of Guainerius (1481), who ascribed the aphasia of his elderly patients to an excessive accumulation of phlegm in the posterior ventricle, deducing this from the premise that the "organ of memory" was in this region.

In conclusion, this analysis of the literature on aphasia from the Hippocratic writings to 1800 shows that the early contributions to the subject were not quite as few as is often assumed to be the case. A substantial amount of clinical knowledge had been gained by the beginning of the nineteenth century. This body of knowledge, which was created for the most part by contributions in the seventeenth and eighteenth centuries, was elaborated and augmented in the first half of the nineteenth century, as clinical information accumulated and an interest in the problem of localization developed. However, it does not appear that the *basic* character of this body of knowledge was altered by the contributions of the first half of the nineteenth century. Instead, there seems to have been a continuous and gradual development of the field until the latter half of the nineteenth century, when the intense interest in aphasic disorders which followed Broca's discovery introduced new conceptions and created an incomparably richer corpus of knowledge.

Summary

This survey of the literature on aphasia from the Hippocratic writings to 1800 indicates that:

1. Most of the clinical forms of aphasia (e.g., motor aphasia, jargon aphasia, amnestic aphasia, alexia, agraphia) had been described and certain common features of aphasic disorders (e.g., retention of capacity for serial speech, concurrence of jargon aphasia and jargon agraphia, unawareness of disability) had been noted. However, sensory aphasia had not been recognized as a specific entity.
2. It was known that aphasia could occur as a consequence of various diseases of the brain, but no important ideas about localization had been advanced.
3. The thesis that the basic psychopathology of aphasic disorders was an interruption in the connections between images or ideas and their linguistic signs had been advanced.
4. The outstanding early contributions appear to be those of Johann Schmidt (1673) on alexia, of Peter Rommel (1683) on motor aphasia, and of Johann Gesner (1770) on jargon aphasia and the theory of aphasic disorders.

Acknowledgments

We are greatly indebted to Dr. Dorothy M. Schullian, History of Medicine Division, National Library of Medicine, and to Miss Ada M. Stoflet, Reference Division, State University of Iowa Libraries, for their generous aid in locating source material and securing biographical information on the early contributors. We are also grateful to Prof. Gustav Bergmann for many valuable suggestions and criticisms during the course of this study, and to Mrs. Gladys Bartholow, State University of Iowa Medical Library, for help in obtaining source material.

References

Adams F. (1939). *The Genuine Works of Hippocrates*. Baltimore: Williams & Wilkins.

Antoni N. (1957). "En lärd man i Upsala." *Opuscu. Med.* 2: 153–160.

Arceo F. (1588). *A Most Excellent and Compendious Method of Curing Woundes in the Head*. London: Thomas East for Thomas Cadman.

Baverius de Baveriis (1543). *Consiliorum de Re Medica Sive Morborum Curationibus Liber*. Argentinae: Libraria Balthasari Pistoris.

Bernard D. (1889). *De l'aphasie et de ses Diverses Formes*. Paris: Lecrosnier et Babé.

Bryk, O. (1909). *Entwicklungsgeschichte der reinen und angewandten Naturwissenschaft im XIX Jahrhundert*. Leipzig: J. A. Barth.

Chadwick J. and Mann W. N. (1950). *The Medical Works of Hippocrates*. Oxford: Blackwell Scientific Publications.

Chapman R. W. (1952). *The Letters of Samuel Johnson, with Mrs. Thrale's Genuine Letters to Him*. Oxford: Clarendon Press.

Coupland S. (1874). Description of aphasia by Goethe, *Brt. Med. J.* 1: 19.

Creutz W. (1934). *Die Neurologie des 1.–7. Jahr-hunderts nach Chr.* Leipzig: Georg Thieme.

Crichton A. (1798). *An Inquiry into the Nature and Origin of Mental Derangement, Comprehending a Concise System of the Physiology and Pathology of the Human Mind and a History of the Passions and Their Effects*. London: T. Cadell, Jr., and W. Davies.

Critchley M. *Dr. Johnson's Aphasia* (in press).

Cullerre A. (1906). Un Aphasique au XVIIIe siècle. *Chronique Médicale* 13: 300, 1906.

Dalin O. (1745). Berättelse om en dumbe, som kan siunga. *K. Swenska Wetensk. Acad. Handlingar* 6: 114–115.

Drabkin I. E. (1950). *Caelius Aurelianus: On Acute Diseases and on Chronic Diseases*. Chicago: University of Chicago Press.

Ebstein E. (1913). Goethes Anteil an der Lehre von der Aphasie. *Ztschr. ges. Neurol. u. Psychiat.* 17: 58–64.

Ebstein E. (1915). Das Valsalva-Morgagnische Gesetz: ein Beitrag zur Vorgeschichte der Aphasie. *Deutsche Ztschr. Nervenh.* 53: 130–136, 1915.

Eliasberg W. (1950). A contribution to the pre-history of aphasia. *J. Hist. Med.* 5: 96–101.

Falret J. (1864). Des troubles du langage et la mémoire des mots dans les affections cérébrales, *Arch. Gén. Med.* 3: 336–354, 591–609.

Gans A. (1914). Über einen im Anfang des 18. Jahrhunderts von Dr. Peter Rommel klassisch beschriebenen Fall von transcorticaler motorischer Aphasie. *Ztschr. ges. Neurol. u. Psychiat.* 24: 480–482.

Gesner J. A. P. (1769–76). *Samlung von Beobachtungen aus der Arzneygelahrtheit und Naturkunde*. Nördlingen: C. G. Beck.

Goethe J. W. (1871). *Wilhelm Meister's Apprenticeship*. Translated by R. Dillon Boylan. London; Bell and Daldy.

Grandjean de Fouchy J. P. (1784). Observation anatomique. *Histoire de l'Académie Royale des Sciences, Mémoires*, 399–401.

Guainerio A. (1481). *Opera Medica*. Pavia: Antonius de Carcano.

Herz M. (1791). Wirkung des Denkvermögens auf die Sprachwerkzeuge. *Magazin für Erfahrungsseelenkunde* 8 (Pt. 2): 1–6.

Hoff H. E., Guillemin R., and Geddes L. A. (1958). An 18th century scientist's observation of his own aphasia, *Bull. Hist. Med.* 32: 446–450.

Holland P. (1601). *The Historie of the World, Commonly Called the Natural Historie of C. Plinius Secundus.* London.

Hultgren E. O. (1916). Historiska Notiser i Afasiläran. *Svenska läk.-sällsk. förhandl.* 42: 1022–1037.

Jastrowitz M. (1875). Historische Notiz über Aphasie. *Berl. klin. Wchnschr.* 12: 323.

Jones W. H. S. (1923–31). *Hipprocrates.* New York: G. P. Putnam's Sons.

Kempf K. (1888). *Valerii Maximi Factorum et Dictorum Memorabilium Libri Novem.* Leipzig: B. G. Teubner.

Külz E. (1875). Zur Geschichte der Aphasie. *Berl. klin. Wchnschr.* 12: 699.

Linnaeus C. (1745). Glömska of alla substantiva och isynnerhet namn. *K. Swenska Wetensk. Acad. Handlungen* 6: 116–117.

Massa N. (1558). *Epistolarum Medicinalium Tomus primus.* Venetiis, ex Officina Stellæ Iordani Zilleti.

Mendelssohn M. (1783). Psychologische Betrachtungen auf Veranlassung einer von dem Herrn Oberkonsistorialrat Spalding an sich selbst gemachten Erfahrung. *Magazin für Erfahrungs-seelenkunde* 1 (Pt. 3): 46–75.

Morgagni G. B. (1769). *The Seats and Causes of Disease Investigated by Anatomy.* Translated by Benjamin Alexander, M.D. London.

Ogle, J. W. (1874). Part of a clinical lecture on aphasia, *Brt. Med. J.* 1: 163–165.

Patrick M. M. (1899). *Sextus Empiricus and Greek Scepticism.* Cambridge: Deighton Bell & Co.

Riese W. (1947). The early history of aphasia. *Bull. Hist. Med.* 21: 322–334.

Rommelius P. (1683). De Aphoniâ Rarâ. *Miscellanea Curiosa Medico-Physica Academiae Naturae Curiosorum* 2 (Ser. 2): 222–227.

Saint-Simon L. (1958). *Mémoires.* Paris: Gallimard.

Schenck a Grafenberg J. (1585). *Observationes Medicæ de Capite Humano.* Lugduni.

Schmidt J. (1676). De oblivione lectionis ex apoplexia salva scriptione. *Miscellanea curiosa medicophysica Academiae naturae curiosorum* 4: 195–197.

Soury J. (1899). *Le Systeme Nerveux Central: Structure et Fonctions: Histoire Critique des Théories et des Doctrines.* Paris: Carré et Naud.

Spalding J. J. (1783). Ein Brief an Sulzern über eine an sich selbst gemachte Erfahrung. *Magazin für Erfahrungsseelenkunde* 1 (Pt. 1): 38–43.

Trousseau A. (1931). *Clinique Médicale de l'Hôtel Dieu de Paris,* Ed. XII. Paris: J.-B. Baillière et Fils.

van Goens R. M. (1789). Einige Beispiele von Geistes-oder Gedächtnissabwesenheit. *Magazin für Erfahrungsseelenkunde* 7 (Pt. 3): 77–80.

Van Swieten G. (1742–46). *Commentaria in Hermanni Boerhaave Aphorismos, de cognoscendis et curandis morbis.* Lugduni: J. & H. Verbeek.

Viets H. R. (1943). Aphasia as described by Linnaeus and as painted by Ribera, *Bull. Hist. Med.* 13: 328–329.

Winslow F. (1868). *On the Obscure Diseases of the Brain, and Disorders of the Mind,* Ed. 4. London: John Churchill & Sons.

8

Aphasia (1800–1860)

It seems to me quite appropriate that the first meeting of this new society devoted to the study of aphasia should begin with a series of historical papers, all the more so since surprising misconceptions about the history of aphasia are held by otherwise well-informed workers in the field.

The period I will discuss as my contribution to this symposium on the history of aphasia is the first 60 years of the nineteenth century—i.e., from 1800 to the fateful case report of Paul Broca in which he described his aphasic patient who was found to have a lesion confined to the left frontal lobe. To assess developments during this period we must consider what the actual state of knowledge was in 1800—i.e., just before Franz Joseph Gall appeared on the scene.

As the detailed account of Benton and Joynt (1960) has demonstrated, that knowledge was remarkably impressive. Almost all the clinical forms of aphasia—for example, complete motor aphasia, paraphasia, jargon aphasia, agraphia, and alexia—had been described. The unawareness of defect that may accompany paraphasia and jargon aphasia had been noted, and the coincidence of aphasia and agraphia had been remarked. Retention of capacity for serial speech, when spontaneous, conversational, and repetitive speech was gravely impaired, had been described. Differential impairment in reading one language as compared with another had also been described.

The one major form of aphasia that had not been clearly recognized was sensory aphasia. Indeed, emphasis was often placed on the patient's retained capacity for understanding spoken language within the setting of defective speech expression. The milder forms of syntactic aphasia also had not been described.

The associationist conception that aphasia was due to an interruption in the

An adaptation of a lecture given at the first meeting of the Academy of Aphasia, Chicago, November 1, 1963. The material dealing with the pre-1800 history of aphasia has been deleted, and some stylistic changes to conform with the deletion have been made.

connections between image or idea and expressive linguistic sign had been advanced.

However, beyond the recognition that aphasia was a manifestation of disease of the brain, there was little interest or knowledge in the neuropathological basis of the disorder. Interest in this aspect of the problem of aphasia came to the fore only at the beginning of the nineteenth century.

The work done during the first 60 years of the nineteenth century may be considered under three rubrics: clinical contributions, theoretical formulations, and contributions to the neuropathology and physiopathology of aphasia.

Clinical Contributions

With regard to clinical study, there were many papers devoted to the phenomenology of aphasia. Most of these did not include new observations, although sometimes their authors seemed to feel that they did. This holds, for example, for the descriptions of Heberden (1801), of Pinel (1809), and of Larrey (ca. 1810), the last two being cited by Gall in his great work.

However, there were a number of studies that were real contributions to knowledge of the clinical phenomology of aphasia. One is the description by Osborne in 1833 of a highly educated patient with severe jargon aphasia who, nevertheless, understood spoken speech quite well and could read with understanding. He was even able to read French and to translate from Latin into English. His writing was only mildly affected, showing no jargon features and only an occasional transposition.

A second is Lordat's case report in 1843 of a priest who became aphasic after a stroke. At first he showed an almost complete motor aphasia but steadily improved until he reached a static condition in which he could say hardly a word in French but could express himself fluently in his native provincial dialect of Languedoc. This is, as far as I know, the first explicit description of a clear dissociation of language loss in a polyglot, although Bouillaud in 1825 had already made reference to a patient who retained some words of patois within the setting of complete inability to speak French.

Bouillaud himself made a number of interesting clinical observations. He cited cases who showed echolalia, automatically repeating the last words of any statement made to them. He also noted the verbosity of some aphasic patients in contrast to those who were virtually speechless.

There is also Marcé's paper in 1856 dealing specifically with impairment in writing. Marcé described a number of cases of agraphia within the setting of oral language disturbances of varying severity and different types, and he postulated the existence of a cerebral center for writing that is related to, but nevertheless distinct from, the coordinating center for oral speech.

Finally, there is an important reference to receptive aphasia in the 1843 monograph of Lordat, which was almost completely ignored or rejected by his contemporaries and indeed for some decades afterward. It is included in his description of his own aphasia. Having discussed his expressive speech difficulties, he notes that he also suffered from impairment in speech comprehension. "I was no longer in a position to absorb the ideas of others because the amnesia which prevented my speaking rendered me incapable of understanding the sounds which I heard quickly enough so that I could grasp their meaning. It required time for the effort to recall each sound and the conversation was too fluent to permit me to understand a sufficient number of words."

Thanks to these clinical contributions, the well-informed physician of 1860 was incomparably more aware of the complexities of the aphasic disorders than his counterpart of 1800. Whatever might be its true cause, aphasia, he knew, was *not* the consequence of partial or complete paralysis of the tongue. He also knew that aphasia could present in diverse forms, that these diverse forms could appear together or be dissociated, and that they could be partial or complete.

Theoretical Formulations

This enriched clinical knowledge led to more sophisticated formulations of the nature of aphasia. A major theoretical advance was made by Bouillaud, whose contribution in this regard was really more important than his better known efforts in the area of the cerebral localization of aphasic disorders. Bouillaud utilized his own observations as well as some that were personally communicated to him as the basis for classifying aphasia disorders into two types that he explicated at some length. In 1825 he wrote:

> [I]t is quite necessary to distinguish two different phenomena in the act of speech, namely, the power of creating words as signs of our ideas and that of articulating these same words. There is, so to speak, an internal speech and an external speech; the latter is only the expression of the former. The nervous system which directs the formation of signs is not identical with that which produces the movements of the organs of speech, for it is not uncommon to observe suspension of speech sometimes solely because the tongue and its congenerous organs refuse the pronunciation of words and sometimes because the memory of these words escape us.
>
> It is important to distinguish clearly between these two causes which can lead to loss of speech, each in its own way; one by destroying the organ of memory of words, the other by an impairment in the nervous principle which directs the movements of speech.

Thus Bouillaud made a fundamental distinction between pure expressive aphasia—the "aphemia" of Broca, the "apraxia of speech" of Liepmann—and amnestic aphasia. It is a distinction that remains valid today.

The other major theoretician of the period was Lordat. Like Bouillaud, he distinguished between verbal amnesia, or loss of memory for words, and what he called "verbal asynergy," or loss of the ability to pronounce words that the patient has clearly in mind. He classified verbal amnesia into various types corresponding to what we would now call paraphasia, deformation of words, and pure word-finding disturbance. His concept of "verbal asynergy" was based on observation of cases of aphasia "in which the patient has a clear idea of the words he should utter and in which the muscles of speech are completely free from paralysis." Lordat also discussed the relationship between intelligence and language and concluded that, contrary to the position of one philosophic school, they were essentially independent. Thus aphasia was neither a sign nor a cause of dementia.

Neuropathological Conceptions

The theoretical psychological analyses naturally had some effect on the problem of the anatomical and physiological basis of the aphasic disorders. Bouillaud, as is well-known, was an ardent champion of the conception of Gall that the seat of language was to be found in the frontal lobes and that aphasia was a consequence of lesions in this area. He marshaled clinical as well as pathological evidence to support this contention. Having pointed out that there were different types of language disorder, he argued that this favored the view that different parts of the brain had different functions.

Bouillaud's ideas were not accepted but neither were they ignored, as some historical accounts would have it. It is true that his localizationist position was rejected in some quarters on a priori grounds. Obviously, a man like Flourens who believed in the mass action of the cerebral hemispheres and denied that they had any direct control of movement, could hardly accept it. However, the more important opposition was on an empirical basis.

In the first place, the neuropathological evidence that Bouillaud himself brought forth to support his thesis was not very good. Reviewing his own autopsied cases as well as those in the literature, he typically presented just a few words on the loci of the lesions and sometimes these few words were very imprecise indeed. In some cases, the flat statement that the lesion was in one or the other anterior lobes (or both) is made. However, in other cases, the locus of the lesion is described as being in the "anterior part of the hemispheres." In still other cases, the locus of the lesions is stated as being "towards the anterior part" of the right or left hemisphere. Yet Bouillaud could be quite critical of the reports of others.

In the second place, empirical testing by others did not confirm the Gall-Bouillaud thesis. For example, Andral (1834) reported the clinical status of 37 patients in whom lesions of the anterior lobes had been found on autopsy. Twenty-one of these patients had shown disturbances of speech while 16 had been free of any speech disorder. On the other hand, Andral stated that he had seen 14 cases of aphasia with lesions of the middle or posterior lobe and without lesions of the anterior lobes. This was a biased approach that did not take into account the number of cases with lesions of the middle or posterior lobes that had not been aphasic; nevertheless, Andral was justified in concluding that "loss of speech is not a necessary result of lesions of the anterior lobes and furthermore it can occur in cases in which anatomical investigation shows no changes in these lobes."

Throughout the history of aphasia the clinical combination of the disorder with the right hemiplegia had been repeatedly observed and reported. Yet the idea of a relationship between the two phenomena was never grasped, even by so astute an observer as Morgagni who described numerous cases of motor speech disorder and right hemiplegia with subsequent autopsy evidence of disease of the left hemisphere. With the exception of Marc Dax, no one in the first half of the nineteenth century noted the association despite the fact that they must have observed the coincidence again and again. For example, Bouillaud in 1825 presented 29 cases with and without aphasia and with and without lesions of the anterior, middle and posterior lobes in his *Traité*. Twenty-five of these cases had lesions confined to a single hemisphere, 11 to the left hemisphere and 14 to the right. Eight (73%) of the 11 left hemisphere cases were aphasic, while only 4 (29%) of the 14 right hemisphere cases were aphasic. A similar bias can be seen in the case material of Andral. But, preoccupied as they were with the question of the anterior–posterior dimension in localization, neither Bouillaud nor Andral gave thought to the hemispheric locus of the lesions. However, the association between lesions of the left hemisphere and aphasia did not escape the attention of Marc Dax, who wrote what was essentially a private memoir or sealed communication on the subject in 1836. From an historical standpoint, this piece of work belongs to the period of Broca for it was not published until 1865. Hence it is more appropriate for Dr. Joynt to consider it in his discussion of the significance of Broca's discovery.

The controversy about the role of the frontal lobes in aphasia, which began in 1825 with the publication of Bouillaud's classic paper and his book, and continued with increasing sharpness through a number of decades, has received a fair amount of attention from medical historians. Sober evaluation suggests that it generates more noise and heat than light and that its intrinsic importance, as compared with other developments during the same period, has been overrated. It is true, that the bitter struggle between the camp of Bouillaud and the opposition led directly to Broca's autopsy studies, which in their turn initiated a new era in the study of aphasia.

References

Andral G. (1834). *Clinique Médicale*. Paris: Fortin, Masson.

Benton A. L., and Joynt R. J. (1960). Early description of aphasia. *Arch. Neurol.* 3: 205–222.

Bouillaud J.-B. (1825). Recherches cliniques propres à démontrer que la perte de la parole correspond à la lésion des lobules anterieurs du cerveau. *Arch. Gén. Méd.* 8: 25–45.

Bouillaud J.-B. (1825). *Traité Clinique et Physiologique de l'Encéphalite*. Paris: J. B. Baillière.

Lordat, J. (1843). *Analyse de la Parole pour Servir à la Theorie de Divers cas d'Alalie et de Paralalie*. Paris: J. B. Baillière.

Marcé L. V. (1856). Sur quelques observations de physiologie pathologique tendant à démontrer l'existence d'un principe coordinateur de l'écriture. *Mémoires de la Société de Biologie* 3: 93–115.

Osborne J. (1833). On the loss of the faculty of speech depending on forgetfulness of the art of using the vocal organs. *Dublin J. Med. Chem. Sci.* 4: 157–170.

9

The Memoir of Marc Dax on Aphasia

ROBERT J. JOYNT and ARTHUR L. BENTON

The association of aphasia with right hemiplegia is now regarded as one of the verities of clinical medicine. There are well-known but infrequent exceptions, almost all of them occurring in left-handed patients. It is remarkable that the almost constant relationship of aphasia and right hemiplegia was not recognized generally until the last half of the nineteenth century. Perhaps, as has been suggested by Benton and Joynt, (1960), this correlation was not made because it made little "sense." Even today, its basic psychoneurological significance eludes us, although there has been much theoretical speculation.

The discovery of this association is usually ascribed to Broca (1861, 1863), but this distinction is often dimmed by an accompanying mention of Marc Dax's earlier contribution in 1836, a quarter of a century before Broca's first observation. Dax's memoir is not only interesting in that it is the first mention of the role of the left hemisphere in the function of speech but also because it raises once again the problem of "priority" in scientific observation.

Marc Dax was born in 1770 and died in 1837. He studied medicine in Montpellier, his graduate thesis being an interesting survey of the incidence and nature of the diseases occurring over a 5-year period in the small town of Aigues-Mortes. As Gibson (1962) has recently pointed out, in this thesis Dax called attention to the occasional occurrence of post-seizure focal paralysis in some children he observed. This observation preceded by many years those of

Reprinted with permission from *Neurology, Minneapolis,* September 1964, Vol. 14, No. 9. © 1964, from Lancet Publications, Inc.

Bravais and Todd who are usually credited with the first descriptions of the phenomenon.

Dax had a keen interest in the study of language, and this may account for the special attention which he paid to language disturbances. In 1836, 1 year before his death, he wrote a paper (Dax, 1836) on the association between aphasic disorders and lesions of the left hemisphere for presentation at a regional medical congress at Montpellier. The paper was not published and, as will be seen, there is no evidence that Marc Dax actually presented it at the congress. When it was belatedly submitted for publication in 1865 by his physician-son, Gustav Dax, 4 years after Broca's initial observation (Broca 1865), it initiated a controversy about priority which has persisted up to the present day. At the same time, together with his father's memoir, Gustav Dax (Dax 1865) published a summary of his own observations and views on aphasia.

Since an English version of the memoir by Marc Dax is not available, a full translation of it is presented below:

LESIONS OF THE LEFT HALF OF THE BRAIN COINCIDENT WITH THE FORGETTING OF THE SIGNS OF THOUGHT

In September, 1800, I made the acquaintance of a former cavalry captain who, having been wounded in the head by a sabre blow during a battle, later suffered a major impairment in his memory for words, while his memory for things was preserved in all its integrity. Such a clear-cut distinction between the two forms of memory made me keenly interested in knowing the cause for it.

After two or three years of fruitless inquiry, I finally hoped to find the key to the enigma in the system of Dr. Gall, which was beginning to spread throughout France. This writer indeed assigns a different place in the brain for each of these two forms of memory; on the cranium, the one corresponds, according to him, to the interior of the orbits and the other to the base of the forehead.

I then inquired of the relatives of the cavalry officer, who had recently died, about the part of the cranium which had been wounded. They informed me that it was at the center of the left parietal bone. This reply, which was not at all in accord with the doctrine of the German physiologist was, at the moment, useless for the solution of my problem.

In 1806, the famous naturalist Broussonnet lost his memory for words after an attack of apoplexy. He lived for about a year after this attack, but his residence in a city far from where I live deprived me for a long time of some ideas which would have provided me with the history of his illness and the details of the autopsy. In 1809, I made a third observation on the forgetting of words in a man suffering from a cancer of the face, from which he died a few months after my visit.

These three examples were without connection for me and taught me nothing until I had occasion to read Cuvier's eulogy of Broussonnet in 1811. Here I noted, among other things, that a large ulcer on the left side of the brain had been found. Immediately, my thinking went back to the subject of my first observation, who had been wounded on the left side; and, as for the third, I recalled very clearly that the cancerous tumor was on the left half of the face.

I was struck by this identity of site in the only three examples which I had been able to observe over a period of eleven years. On the other hand, I found them to be too small in number to persuade me that there was a general law here, without taking into account the unlikelihood that the functions of one half of the brain could differ in this respect from the functions of the other half. Nevertheless, at the end of 1812 a fourth observation, and a fifth at the beginning of 1813, gave me hope of being able to convert my first observations into a general rule. This hope was conspicuously confirmed by a sixth example in 1814, which I owe to the kindness of Dr. Pariset, now permanent secretary of the Royal Academy of Medicine, and who at that time had already made a distinguished name for himself in important medical literature.

Since then I have continued to collect similar observations, more than forty in number at the present time, without encountering a single exception during this long period of time. Even if some exceptions should appear in the future, they would not invalidate the rule inasmuch as they would be small in number. In the same way, decussation continues to be considered as a general law of the organism even when, in an incalculable number of cerebral lesions, observers have noted eight or ten which were on the same side as the hemiplegia. I would not even regard as an exception a disease of the left hemisphere without alteration of speech, particularly if the disease were slight or if it had developed slowly. A true exception, which I have not seen as yet, would be impairment of memory from words resulting from a disease that was confined to the right hemisphere.

To the observations gathered in my practice, I could add from my reading some that are approximately the same. I have taken them from the writings of Morgagni, the Mémoires de l'Académie Royale de Chirurgie, the works of Mauduyt on medical electricity, medical journals, the periodical collection of the Société de Médecine de Paris, and the Révue Médicale. From all the preceding I believe it possible to conclude not that all diseases of the left hemisphere necessarily impair verbal memory but that, when this form of memory is impaired by disease of the brain, it is necessary to look for the cause of the disorder in the left hemisphere, and to look for it there even if both hemispheres are diseased.

Diverse interpretations have been made of loss of memory for words. Gall and his school attribute it to a lesion of the anterior lobes of the brain; however, several cases have been observed in which the anterior lobes were destroyed by a disease without impairment of this form of memory.[1] Bouillaud seems to attribute the cause to a paralysis of the tongue in a dissertation entitled *Recherches Pathologiques et Cliniques sur l'Influence du Cerveau dans les Mouvements Musculaires, et Spécialement sur ceux des Organes de la Parole.*[2] However, among the patients who are under consideration here, the majority continue to speak, saying one word for another; their tongues are not at all paralyzed. I have observed one, among others, who was completely deprived of his speech; however, when I asked him to move his tongue, he moved it with great fluency. If he were given a drink disagreeable to the taste, he showed from his grimace that he distinguished flavors very well. Therefore, there was no impairment either of the sensitivity or of the movement of the tongue.

This absence of speech without paralysis of its principal organ had been noted

1. *Revue médicale,* septembre 1826, p. 365 et suivantes.
2. *Ibid.*, avril 1825, p. 143.

as early as the 16th century. The following passage written by a German physician named Atheus is found in the collection of Schenkius: "I have observed in many cases of apoplexy, lethargy and similar major diseases of the brain that, although the tongue was not paralyzed, the patient could not speak because the faculty of memory being abolished, the words were not produced."[3]

I prefer the explanation of Professor Lordat, who attributes this phenomenon not to paralysis of the tongue, but to impairment in the synergies of the muscles which cooperate in the execution of speech, synergies of simultaneous muscular movements which are formed by habit and which are linked together so that finally they respond to one another without the intervention of the will.[4] These synergies cannot only be disturbed abruptly by disease but also by old age, as Castel pointed out so well at a meeting of the Académie Royale de Médecine de Paris.[5]

There now remains a very interesting problem to resolve: why does it happen that alterations of the left cerebral hemisphere are followed by loss of memory for words? While we await a satisfactory answer to this question, I hope that my work will not be useless for the diagnosis and treatment of diseases of this type. When the cerebral disorder is not accompanied by hemiplegia or when the latter is slow in developing, it is possible to fail to recognize the nature of the disease, or, at least, the site which it occupies, and this knowledge would be indispensable for the correct application of topical and derivative remedies. In this case, suspension or aberration of speech would eliminate all uncertainty.

I could report several cases in which this circumstance enlightened me usefully for the welfare of patients, but I will limit myself to a single example. A lady fainted and fell from the chair in which she had been sitting. Although I left promptly to see her, when I appeared, she had already recovered. Had she suffered a fainting spell or a syncope? Did the short duration of the attack permit one to suspect an apoplectic affection? I did not think so at first but the patient, in describing to me what she had experienced, said: "After regaining consciousness, I was unable to speak for a moment." These words were a ray of light to me, and, two days later, called in great haste to the same patient (who had just suffered a similar accident, but one much more intense than the first, because I found her completely mute this time) I had no need for reflection to know the nature, the site or the treatment of this illness. I promptly applied a large number of leeches to the left temple and in a few minutes, as the blood flowed, her speech was gradually restored. A half hour later, the patient had recovered and, taking some precautions, she has continued to enjoy good health for several years.

I hope that the new point of view which I propose here not only will be useful for the treatment of the disorders under consideration, but also that it will be helpful in clarifying medicolegal issues. A patient of this type can draw up a will and can direct his business affairs, because his intelligence is ordinarily very well conserved, and it would be unjust and cruel to declare him incompetent and to regard him as suffering from insanity. I hope also that it will lead to research which will not be useless to the progress of science.

3. Joann. Schenkii, *Obs. med. libri* VII, in folio, p. 180, edit. de Lyon. (Atheus sent his observations to Schenkius in 1585.)

4. *Recueil périodique de la Sociéte de médecine de Paris*, décembre 1820, p. 317, and *Revue médicale*, septembre 1821, p. 25.

5. *Revue médicale*, juin 1831, p. 491.

Discussion

From a scientific standpoint, Marc Dax's generalization on the role of the left hemisphere in speech was hardly derived from well-documented observations. The clinical descriptions were scanty, and the pathological confirmation was entirely lacking. Dax made no mention of handedness nor did he, in any way, link hand preference to hemispheric localization of speech function. Moreover, Dax's references to Bouillaud were quite inexact as Bouillaud had not ascribed this form of speech derangement to paralysis of the tongue; even the title of Bouillaud's article (1825) was not cited correctly by Dax. Many years later, after the memoir had become well known, Bouillaud (1869) reproached Marc Dax for these oversights. Nonetheless, Marc Dax did make, and for the first time, a clinical observation of the highest importance.

The question of who should have the credit for this observation is unsettled and raises interesting points of historical priority. In 1861, Broca reported two instances of aphasia with lesions in the left third frontal convolution (Broca, 1861, Joynt, 1961). He made no mention at that time of the significance of both these lesions occurring on the left side. Later, at a meeting of the Anthropological Society of Paris on April 2, 1863, Broca reported on eight autopsies (Broca 1863) of patients with aphasia and noted that they all had lesions in the third frontal convolution. He added, ". . . and, a most remarkable thing, in all of these patients the lesion existed on the left side. I do not dare to draw a conclusion and I await new facts." In 1865, Broca expanded his views of the special role of the left hemisphere in speech and also discussed his priority in making this observation (Broca, 1865). He had read Marc Dax's paper as published by his son in 1865 and, naturally, wished to read the original presentation along with any discussion. He searched in vain throughout the medical literature for the original report or even for a reference to the 1836 paper. He then asked the librarian of the Montpellier faculty of medicine to make personal inquiries regarding the 1836 presentation. The librarian reported that he had interviewed 20 physicians who had attended the 1836 congress at Montpellier, and none could recall such a presentation. Hence Broca was, with good reason, quite skeptical that Marc Dax had actually presented his paper at the congress.

The discussion on priority was reopened by Broca in 1877 (Broca 1877). He stated that he had obtained a manuscript of the Marc Dax paper, purportedly presented in 1836, and compared it with the Gustav Dax manuscript on aphasia. Broca admits that the style, the mode of expression, and the discussion all demonstrated a difference in origin. Therefore, he did not doubt that the paper was written in 1836 by Marc Dax for presentation, but he did not believe that it was ever presented. Broca speculated that Marc Dax probably felt unsure of his ground and did not have the courage to face a discussion as there was no confirmation of his cases by autopsy findings.

There is suggestive evidence that Gustav Dax, the son, did know of the preferential involvement of the left hemisphere in aphasia prior to Broca's 1863 report. Presumably, this knowledge was gained from his father—for Gustav Dax had prepared an extensive treatise of his own on aphasia (Dax, 1877) entitled: "Observations intended to prove the constant coincidence of the derangements of speech with a lesion of the left cerebral hemisphere." In the introduction, Gustav Dax pays respect to his father's memory and mentions his father's views on the localization of lesions responsible for the loss of speech. This work of Gustav Dax was received by the Academy of Medicine of Paris on March 24, 1863. Broca's statement on the eight cases of aphasia with left hemisphere lesions was delivered on April 2, 1863. Unfortunately, the commission appointed by the academy to examine Gustav Dax's essay did not publish a report on it until 2 years later. Additional support for Dax's claim was provided in 1879 by Caizergues, who reported that he had discovered a copy of Marc Dax's memoir when classifying the papers of his grandfather who had been dean of the faculty of medicine at Montpellier (Caizergues, 1879).

There is, therefore, excellent evidence that Marc Dax did make his observation prior to Broca. There is, however, no evidence that Marc Dax made his observations known to the world other than through the distribution of a report of his findings to a few colleagues. In short, Marc Dax had made an observation for which he was unwilling to take public responsibility, and hence he recorded it in the form of an essentially private communication. It would seem that he believed that he had hit upon a fact of great significance, but he was not sure of it. The concurrent desires for recognition if he were right and for protection if he were not right led to conflict about the advisability of making an oral or written public statement. The compromise solution to this conflict was a "sealed" or "private" communication, a maneuver which had been employed by a number of investigators before Dax who found themselves in a similar predicament and which has been resorted to by a few since his time.

References

Benton A. L. and Joynt R. J. (1960). Early descriptions of aphasia. *Arch. Neurol.* (Chic.) 3: 205–221.

Bouillaud J. B. (1825). Recherches cliniques propres à démontrer que la perte de la parole correspond à la lésion des lobules anterieurs du cerveau. Et a confirmer l'opinion de M. Gall sur le siège de l'organe du langage articulé. *Arch Gén. Méd.* 8: 25–45.

Bouillaud J. P., cited by Bayle, M. (1939). Les fondateurs de la doctrine française de l'aphasie. Thése pour le Doctorat en Médecine, Univ. de Bordeaux, p. 54.

Broca P. (1861). Remarques sur le siège de la faculté du langage articulé; suivies d'une observation d'aphemie. *Bull. Soc. Anat.* (Paris) 6: 330–357.

Broca P. (1836) Localisation des fonctions cérébrales. Siége du langage articulé. *Bull. Soc. Anthrop.* (Paris) 4: 200–203.

Broca P. (1865). Sur la siége de la faculté du langage articulé. *Bull. Soc. Anthrop.* (Paris) 6: 377–393.

Broca P. (1877). Rapport sur un mémoir de M. Armand de Fleury intitulé: De l'inégalité dynamique des deux hémispheres cerebraux. *Bull. Acad. Méd.* (Paris) (Series 2) 6: 508–539.

Caizergues R. (1879). Notes pour servir a l'histoire de l'aphasie. *Montpellier Méd.* 42: 178–180.

Dax, M. (1865). Lesions de la moitié gauche de l'encéphale coincident avec l'oublie des signes de la pensée. *Gaz. hbd. Méd. Chir.* (Paris) 2: 259–262.

Dax G. (1865). Notes sur la même sujet. *Gaz. hbd. Méd. Chir.* (Paris) 2: 262.

Dax G. (1877). Observations tendant à prouver la coïncidence constante de dérangements de la parole avec une lesion de l'hémisphere gauche du cerveau. *Montpellier Méd.* 38: 313–340 and 508–529; 39: 112–130, 226–237, and 413–421. (Complete publication of article which was originally submitted to the Paris Academy of Medicine on March 24, 1863, according to Souques, A. (1928). Quelques cas l'anarthrie de Pierre Marie. Rev. neurol. 35: 319–368. The original article also was submitted to the Paris Academy of Science on March 23, 1863. *C.R. Acad. Sci.* [Paris] 61: 534, 1863.)

Gibson W. C. (1962). Pioneers in localization of function in the brain. *JAMA* 180: 944–951.

Joynt R. J. (1961). Centenary of patient "Tan": His contribution to the problem of aphasia. *Arch. Intern. Med.* 108: 953–956.

10

Johann A. P. Gesner on Aphasia

Our present knowledge of aphasic disorders is the product of an evolution which spans millennia. Delineation of these conditions, their differentiation from other types of disorder of speech and language, and ideas about their causation and basic nature developed very gradually. The earliest medical writings (including the Hippocratic Corpus) made reference only to a general "speechlessness" or "loss of voice" which seemingly covered all types of impairment of speech and language, including not only those which today would be called aphasic but also those due to frank paralysis and to disturbed states of consciousness, as well as those of psychogenic origin.

The beginnings of a differentiation between aphasic and nonaphasic disorders of speech can be found in the writings of some post-Hippocratic authors. Thus Caelius Aurelianus distinguished between impairment of speech due to paralysis of the tongue and "cases of loss of speech resulting from some other disease." According to Creutz (1934), the same distinction was made by most medical writers of the late classical period. One can also point to the reference to a case of traumatic alexia by Valerius Maximus (*c.* A.D. 30), and to Galen's assertion that "word memory" could be lost as a consequence of head injury, as further indications that distinctions between various types of speech and language disorder were being made. By this time also the decisive role of abnormalities of the brain or its ventricles in causing some types of speech disorder was clearly recognized.

Renaissance medicine witnessed further developments. First, the distinction between speech impairment due to "paralysis of the tongue" and an amnesic type of speech disorder was clearly drawn. Secondly, an initial speculative step in the topical localization of language function was taken by Antonio Guainerio when he advanced the conception that certain types of aphasia were due to a

Reprinted with permission from *Medical History*, Vol. 9, 1965.

loss of memory caused by excessive accumulation of fluid in the posterior ventricle. Finally, the concept of the cerebral origin of aphasic (or anarthric) disabilities became a practical medical reality when physicians and surgeons, such as Nicolo Massa and Francisco Arceo, inferred from the observation of aphasia following head injury that fragments of the skull might have become lodged in the brain and interfered with its functions. Acting on this inference, they searched for and removed the fragments from the brain, this intervention being followed by restoration of speech in the patients.

Two quite important contributions to knowledge of aphasia appeared in the seventeenth century. In 1676, the Danzig physician Johann Schmidt published the first reasonably clear description of alexia and paraphasia. A few years later, Peter Rommel described a patient with severe expressive aphasia who nevertheless showed preserved capacity for serial speech (an observation which was made again some 60 years later by Olof Dalin). A few further observations on aphasia were made during the first half of the eighteenth century, the most notable perhaps being Van Swieten's brief description of anomia and Linné's account of a patient with paraphasic disturbances.

All these contributions were extremely brief, even though some of them, such as those of Schmidt and Rommel, were remarkably informative in spite of their brevity. Many details, which we would consider today to be of decisive importance, were not mentioned; moreover, all the reports were of an essentially descriptive nature, little attention being paid to the mechanisms underlying the observed clinical phenomena. However, in 1770 there appeared what it is fair to describe as the first major work devoted to the subject of aphasia. This was a chapter by Johann Augustin Philipp Gesner (1738–1801) entitled "Die Sprachamnesie" in the second volume of his *Samlung von Beobachtungen aus der Arzneigelahrheit und Naturkunde*. The chapter, which covers 73 octavo pages, is about 7000 words in length.

Gesner was a prolific medical writer whose interests were quite broad. In addition to his original writing, he translated Latin and French treatises into German and was actively engaged in editorial work. His five-volume *Samlung* (Gesner, 1769–76), published over a span of eight years, was perhaps his major work. He also wrote a series of four "recent advances" volumes entitled *Die Entdeckungen der Neuesten Zeit in der Arzneygelahrheit* (Gesner, 1777–88) which covered contemporary developments in all branches of medicine.

Die Sprachamnesie

The first paragraph of "*Die Sprachamnesie*" reads as follows:

> I relate the history of a disease which appears worthy of attention not only because it is certainly uncommon but also because it belongs among those documents in

the literature on the human mind which are instructive to psychologists and because I am able to report the opinions and prescriptions of some famous and distinguished physicians who were consulted about it.

There follows the history as it was written by the patient's own physician in a letter dated 6 February 1769. Herr K. D. was a 73-year-old man who had seldom been ill and had always enjoyed the fruits of a regular life. His only complaint during recent years had been bouts of catarrh which would last some weeks and were accompanied by the production of an extraordinarily viscous material. In December of the previous year he had once again begun to suffer from catarrh. In the beginning of January he experienced a cramp in the muscles of the mouth and at the same time an itching sensation like the crawling of ants. The cramp was relieved by taking some pinches of cherry brandy. Unexpectedly, on 26 January, he showed a quite distinctive impairment in speech, together with some mental confusion. He spoke fluently but used "extremely unusual and self-made words that nobody could understand." The speech impairment had persisted unchanged until the date of the letter from the patient's physician. The mental confusion appeared to have increased. There was no evidence of paralysis in any part of his body. "These are the main features of a disease which I at least have never encountered in my 30 years of practice."

There follow eight letters which were written by four consulting physicians between 6 February and 16 July 1769 and which include observations, interpretations of the underlying pathology and a variety of prescriptions. The observations indicate that the patient could neither write nor read. One of the consultants (W. A———r), the author of three of these eight letters, concludes that "the incapacity to make himself understood by us through words or other signs is neither in the tongue nor in other members, for the tongue is skilful enough to produce three times as many words as are necessary. I cannot explain this in other than these terms: nothing is wrong in this patient except the higher mental performances." This consultant also pointed out that, if the cause of the difficulty were in the tongue, the patient would not be incapable of writing, as he obviously was.

Gesner's opinion was first sought about a year after the onset of the patient's illness. There is no evidence to indicate that the actually saw the patient. However, having reviewed the observations and opinions of earlier consultants, he also "wanted to know about those phenomena which pertain to the more speculative part of medicine. I therefore requested the answers to some questions, which will be mentioned presently. These answers were provided not by a physician but by a man who personally observed the patient daily and whose eyes had been opened by worldly wisdom." The report of this observer reads in part as follows:

> The words which Herr K. D. pronounces are for the most part meaningless sounds. However, their total number is not very great, in that a meaningless word is often repeated successively and only occasionally replaced by others which are equally

incomprehensible. These sounds sometimes disappear completely and one does not hear them any more; instead, new coinages appear which last a longer or shorter time. For example, the sound "began," without fixed meaning, which occurred constantly at the beginning of the illness is no longer uttered a half-year later. Instead, one hears a newly created word, "Zettejuset" or "Zettennoset," countless times during the course of a day. Numerals, such as 40, 50, 60, 70, 80, 90, which he uses to serve him in the course of speech, are also to be added to this category.

Doubtlessly these sounds are not always associated with the same ideas for him. They express, or at least are intended to express, all those ideas which he wishes to communicate with others. Their total number is scarcely 100. Thus his currently favourite word "Zettejuset" can mean more than 1000 things. It is also used by him indiscriminately and mixed up with other words in such a manner that his speech is incomprehensible.

At the same time there also occur occasional meaningful words which for the most part concern only familiar things and are not always within the power of the speaker. Examples are such expressions as "obedient servant," "most humble servant," "good morning," "I do not wish to," and several other similar expressions which had always characteristically been used by this man of choleric temperament, as well as swear words such as, "Oh God; Oh God" and "Damn Foolishness," whereby he indicates his futile efforts.

For the most part he uses these words in their proper meaning. However, I have also observed that if I drink to his health and he wants to thank me, the word, "Adieu," is brought forth instead of the usual formula. He is likely to say "Good evening" in the morning and "Good morning" in the evening involuntarily. Thus in a quite special sense he seems to have lost complete control of his tongue.

Writing and speaking are equally defective. He cannot write his full name even once. When he tries to write something else (which he seldom does because he is aware of his incapacity) he produces words on paper which are as incomprehensible as those he utters.

Nor can he read. These signs of ideas make no impression on him although other more concrete objects arouse the appropriate concepts in him. It is just this circumstances about which the patient, who always found great pleasure in reading, often complains.

Objects, when they are of an external sensory nature, certainly arouse the correspondingly correct ideas in him. The patient recognizes everyone whom he knew before, asks about the circumstances of people with whom he has associated, makes observations about them in accordance with their status, age, sex, etc., and, as he always been characteristic of him, praises, finds fault, or laughs at them (and with justification).

I cannot actually maintain that I have personally observed a loss of certain concepts in him unless such a loss may be inferred from the fact that he does not like to have excerpts from books presenting general spiritual or moral truths read to him. Nor does he pay any attention to them, which seems to show that many abstract concepts may have been lost and can be aroused only with difficulty, if at all, by the external signs which we call words. Otherwise he understands the speech of those around him completely and often to their admiration, unless it is presented in too diffuse a manner or, as mentioned above, concerns abstract matters. Moreover, he can also make his own ideas recognized through external signs and demonstrations to such a degree that, if one guesses the meaning of the signs, they represent quite correct and coherent ideas.

The patient is also aware that he speaks unintelligently and, when he repeats some of these words, has often laughed and joked about it.

Now after a year his condition is essentially as has been described. However, it can be said that, physically and mentally, he has improved rather than got worse. His mental powers have also become stronger, his ideas being more orderly and more definite. A few comprehensible words have also appeared. In brief, after one has observed and spoken with the patient at some length, nothing seems to be wrong with him except his speech. I do not know that I can better make his condition more intelligible and understandable except by saying that if a person who is not acquainted with the German language and who did not know that the patient was sick should observe him and hear him talk, he would take him for a healthy, ordinary man who is speaking an unfamiliar language.

In his discussion, Gesner first emphasizes that "just as some mental powers become weakened without injury to others, memory also can be specifically impaired to a greater or lesser degree with respect to only certain classes of ideas." Some reports from the literature as well as a personally observed case are cited to illustrate this point.

The first brief case report describes aphasia and alexia in a lawyer following a "sleep" of nine days duration. In due time, he was able to read some words, being more successful in Latin than in German. He would write whole paragraphs in both Latin an German in an elegant hand, but they made no sense nor could he read them. He would often start a conversation, speaking understandably and clearly, and then falter in the middle of it.

A second case report describes a patient, an abbot, who was aphasic and alexic but who retained the capacity to recite familiar prayers. He partially regained his ability to read, the degree of recovery being greater for Latin than for German. The patient himself felt that he had suffered some decline in judgment, in the ability to calculate and even in understanding the speech of others.

A third case report describes a patient who could not speak, read or write but who could understand the speech of others. A fourth and a fifth describe patients who could read silently with understanding but who could not read aloud.

Gesner then points out that memory constitutes voluntary control over ideation or imagination (*Phantasie*). "Speaking and writing are functions of memory while reading and hearing are functions of ideation." The patient suffered essentially from a disturbance of memory which, however, primarily involved language. His poor grasp of the "external signs" of abstract ideas was not due to an impairment in ideation but rather to a weakness of attention which is common enough in old age. This difficulty in appreciating symbolized abstract ideas was apparent only when a whole series of them was presented; the meaning of a single abstract idea presented in isolation was adequately understood. Thus while he was unable to read whole passages, he could identify specific days on the calendar. Moreover, he seemed to be able to read the Bible. Gesner concedes that it is difficult to prove that the patient did indeed read with understanding but he believes this to be likely.

The patient's paraphasic speech is explained as follows:

> The liveliness of an idea and the desire to communicate it quickly to another person often causes us to use inappropriate words, especially when our attention is concentrated on the idea. However, nobody maintains because of this that our ideation or our reason is disturbed. Therefore, I see only a forgetting of speech when Herr K. D. says meaningful words which do not correspond to his ideas or when he utters meaningless sounds that perhaps suggest to us a remote and often incomprehensible similarity to the correct words or give us a false impression of his thought.

Gesner's conceptualization of the anatomic and physiologic correlates of "speech amnesia" is rather vague and at times difficult to follow. Nevertheless, his basic ideas seem reasonably clear. He points out that an actual object or stimulus (even a heard or seen word) has a stronger effect on the mind than does memory. It is therefore understandable why the ability to recognize an object or word could be retained when other performances such as speaking or writing the name of an object, which depend upon memory, are lost. Recognition is subserved by the functioning of the sensory nerves and is essentially a receptive process. Hence it will be impaired only when there is actual injury of the mass of sensory nerves. In contrast, memory can be impaired even in the absence of such injury. The basis for loss of memory can be sought in another type of disease of the brain in which there is a weakness or inertia in the relationship between the different parts of that organ.

> I look for the seat of this amnesia for speech in the interior of the organs, less in their organization as determined by the senses, than in the physical relationships of their parts, and particularly in a sluggishness in these relationships which arises out of dryness or rigidity.

He finds it unlikely that the patient's language disorder should be determined by injury of specific nerve fibres.

> In our case I do not suspect pressure or obstruction of certain vessels because amnesia is practically the only symptom . . . only language is lost. The vessels of the brain are surely not arranged in accordance with categories of physical ideas and therefore it is incomprehensible that these categories should correspond to areas of destruction. The words which have been lost to memory still serve in thinking. The fibre for the idea of a certain word would have to be completely inactive. But it is inactive only for voluntary performances. Moreover, the most common words are still remembered. How could pressure have made this choice?

The chapter concludes with a discussion of the uncertain prognosis in cases of this type and a survey of possible modes of treatment.

Comment

There can be little doubt that this chapter by Gesner on "speech amnesia" was indeed a major contribution and that, from a number of points of view, it represents a landmark in the study of aphasia. The first case report in it was incomparably more comprehensive and detailed than anything that had been published previously. It is a superb description of jargon aphasia and its value was recognized by later writers, such as Alexander Crichton (1798) and Jules Falret, (1864), who cited it in their discussions of disorders of speech and memory. Taken together, this case report and the five additional briefer ones presented in the discussion provide a wealth of information about such diverse clinical features of aphasia as jargon agraphia, differential impairment in reading one language as compared to another, retention of the ability to recite familiar prayers within the setting of grossly defective spontaneous, conversational and imitative speech, and inability to read aloud with at least partial preservation of the ability to read silently with understanding. There is even a suggestion of the existence of a sensory form of aphasia in Gesner's discussion of the first patient's inability to grasp the import of a series of abstract ideas and in his report of the testimony of another patient that the latter experienced difficulty in understanding the speech of other people.

I have mentioned that Gesner's discussion of the physiopathology and psychopathology of aphasia is at times obscure, particularly to a reader without a thorough grasp of the philosophic background of eighteenth-century German medicine. However, the tenor of his thought is clear enough. The jargon speech of his patient does not reflect dementia but rather a type of forgetting. Ideation and memory for words must be distinguished from each other. Ideation is evoked by the perception of physical objects and the action of the sensory nerves. The evocation of words follows ideation, and further neural energy or action is required for it to take place. Hence it is understandable that disease of the brain could impair verbal memory but leave ideation intact, i.e. that a patient might not be able to produce the name of an object but yet be able to recognize the object and know its significance. The material basis for such an impairment in verbal memory is a sluggishness or inactivity (*Trägheit*) in the relationships among the parts of the brain.

I do not think that one reads too much into Gesner's discussion when one sees it as an early statement of an associationist theory of aphasia, i.e. that the disorder consists of a failure to associate the appropriate vocal or graphic linguistic sign (word) with the intended image or idea. Like his predecessors, he spoke of a "forgetting" of words but he went a step further by ascribing this form of amnesia to impairment in what today we would call "associative process." Some 25 years later, Alexander Crichton (1798) stated the idea with greater clarity when he wrote that this "very singular defect of memory . . . ought rather to be considered as a defect of that principle, by which ideas, and their proper expressions, are associated, than of memory."

Gesner does not seem to have made any further original observations on aphasia. After the publication of the *Samlung*, most of his energy was absorbed in the writing of his comprehensive reviews of current developments in the various branches of medicine which appeared over the period of 1777–88. Summaries of his case of jargon aphasia and of another personally observed case (the last case in the chapter on *Die Sprachamnesie*) are included in the first volume of this series, but no other work having clear and specific reference to aphasic disorders, either by himself or other, is cited in any of the four volumes.

References

Creutz W. (1934). *Die Neurologie des 1–7. Jahrhunderts nach Chr.*, Leipzig, Georg Thieme.

Crichton A. (1798). *An Inquiry into the Origin and Nature of Mental Derangement*, London, T. Cadell, Jr., and W. Davies.

Falret J. (1804). Des troubles du langage et la mémoire des mots dans les affections cérébrales, *Arch. Gén. Méd.* 3: 336–54, 591–609.

Gesner J. A. P. (1769–76) *Samlung von Beobachtungen aus der Arzneygelahrheit und Naturkunde*, 5 vols. Nördlingen, C. G. Beck.

Gesner J. A. P. (1777–88). *Die Entdeckungen der neuesten Zeit in der Arzneigelahrheit*, 4 vols. Nördlingen, Karl Gottlieb Becker.

11

Bergson and Freud on Aphasia: A Comparison

In this paper I plan to outline the views that Henri Bergson and Sigmund Freud advanced about the nature of aphasic disorders in the 1890s, to consider how their views differed from prevailing concepts and finally to assess the impact which their positions had on subsequent thinking about aphasia. To begin with, we need to review the status of aphasia theory in 1890, i.e., what was then known about the aphasic disorders and what ideas about their basic nature were generally accepted.

That loss of speech could follow injury to the brain was known at the time of ancient Greek medicine and probably even before then. Through the centuries a fairly substantial literature describing the features of the speech disorders associated with brain disease accumulated (Benton and Joynt, 1960; Benton, 1964, 1981). By 1850 most of the aphasic syndromes familiar to us today had been described, e.g., expressive aphasia with relative preservation of the capacity to understand speech, amnesic aphasia with word-finding disturbance, jargon aphasia and jargon agraphia, and isolated loss of the ability to read. The distinction between a fluent type of aphasic disorder (characterized by disordered speech) and a nonfluent type (characterized by poverty of speech and difficulty in articulation) had been made. The lack of awareness of defect shown by some patients with jargon speech and unequal loss of proficiency in different languages in polyglot patients had been noted. Impairment of speech with preserved ability to sing had been described. Franz Joseph Gall had postulated the existence of centers for speech articulation and word memory in the frontal lobes and his localization was the subject of rather acrimonious debate during the first half of the nineteenth century.

Reprinted with permission from Gordon & Breach Publishers. A. C. Papanicolaou and P.A.Y. Gunter (eds.), *Bergson and Modern Thought*. London: Harcourt Academic Publishers, 1987.

Still, aphasia was scarcely a subject of great interest to either practicing physicians or medical scientists. The disorder had no specific diagnostic significance nor was it possible to correlate it in any meaningful way with brain function. But when, in the early 1860s, Paul Broca established the association between expressive speech disability and focal lesions in and around the third frontal gyrus of the left hemisphere, aphasia became a major topic in neurological medicine (Broca, 1861, 1863, 1865). To physicians Broca's discovery demonstrated that a specific disability could have specific implications about the condition of the brain and hence that it could possess a specific diagnostic significance. To physiologists the association between a behavioral deficit and a limited cerebral lesion suggested that the brain could indeed be divided into defined areas, each with its distinctive functional properties, and this possibility provided a powerful impetus for intensive experimental study of localization of brain function in the 1870s and 1880s.

Broca coined the term "aphemia" to designate the nonfluent expressive speech disorder which he had correlated with left frontal lobe disease. He contrasted it with the fluent speech disorder that was then known as "word amnesia" and that had as its most prominent feature word-finding difficulty and paraphasic utterances, i.e., the incorrect use of words. The aphemic patient understands what is said to him and he is not devoid of ideas. However, because of an impairment in the coordination of the movements of speech, he cannot express his ideas in words. The amnesic patient is also not devoid of ideas but he has lost knowledge of the conventional relations between ideas and words. Because he has lost his appreciation of the symbolic value of words, he cannot understand what is said to him and he uses words inappropriately in his own speech. However, neither form of aphasic disorder involves a disturbance of thinking as such and both should be distinguished from mental deterioration in which condition the patient is speechless because, as Broca phrased it, "of a lack of ideas to express."

Broca himself was not greatly concerned with the neurological mechanisms underlying speech and its disturbance. It was left to a younger physician, Carl Wernicke, to develop a mature theory of the nature of aphasic disorders. In a monograph that appeared in 1874, Wernicke demonstrated that fluent aphasic disorder, characterized by impaired understanding of speech and disordered expressive speech, was specifically associated with disease in the territory of the posterior temporal lobe of the left hemisphere (Wernicke, 1874). Like Broca, he conceived of aphasia as a disorder of the sign function of language. He denied that aphasic patients were necessarily impaired in intellect even though, as a clinician, he knew that many aphasics, perhaps a majority, did in fact show cognitive defects that extended beyond the realm of language. But he insisted that "nothing could be worse for the study of aphasia than to consider the intellectual disturbance associated with aphasia as an essential part of the disease picture."

However, Wernicke went beyond his empirical discovery and his restriction of aphasia to a disorder of the sign function of language to create a model of the neurological mechanisms, derangements of which produced aphasic disorder. His model, and the revisions of it developed by other neurologists, postulated the existence of interconnected cerebral centers of speech in which memory-images of the different modalities of speech were stored. A center for memory-images of the movement patterns of expressive speech was located in Broca's area in the posterior frontal region. A center for auditory memory-images of words was located in Wernicke's area in the posterior temporal lobe. A center for visual memory-images of words was located farther back in the angular gyrus. Whether or not there was a specific center for memory-images of the movement patterns of writing was a subject of debate. Those who believed in the existence of such a center placed it either in the second frontal gyrus above Broca's area or in the supramarginal gyrus close to the center for visual memory-images of words.

The diverse symptom-pictures of aphasia encountered in clinical practice were explained in terms of either a lesion in one or more centers (i.e., the "central" aphasias) or a lesion in the connections between them (i.e., the "conduction" aphasias). A lesion in Broca's area resulted in a loss of motor memory-images and hence produced a primarily expressive aphasia with preservation of the capacity to understand speech. A lesion in Wernicke's area resulted in a loss of auditory-verbal memory-images and hence produced impairment in the understanding of speech. A lesion in the connections between Wernicke's area and Broca's area resulted in a distinctive symptom-picture in which the patient was able to understand speech (since the center for auditory–verbal memory-images was intact) but his speech was disordered and he was unable to repeat what was said to him (since there was defective transmission of information from the auditory–verbal center to the motor speech center). And so on.

This was the dominant theory of the nature of aphasic disorder that was almost universally accepted by neurologists in the 1890s. Aphasia was a disturbance in the utilization of words as signs of ideas with no necessary impairment in intellect. The neurological basis of speech and language consisted of specific cortical areas in which verbal memory images were stored. Aphasia was produced by lesions in these areas or in the connections between them.

In later years these models of the neurological basis of language and its disorders were derided as empty diagram making that bore no relationship to clinical reality. In fact, they were not as unreal or sterile as their critics made them out to be. They achieved some notable successes in deducing the existence of aphasic symptom-pictures that were not known at the time but that were later validated by clinicopathologic study. Moreover, despite their limitations, they exemplified a scientific approach to aphasia that generated empirically testable hypotheses. Thus, Lichtheim (1885), a leading diagram maker, wrote "... whether our interpretations are correct or not will be determined by further observations ... we must not hesitate to draw the consequences deducible from our hypotheses. The more we do so the sooner we will gain information to correct them, or if necessary, abandon them, if this is what the findings indicate. An erroneous view may be of value."

But the models did encounter serious difficulties. Many observations on aphasia and its neurological basis could not be accommodated by them. And they were unacceptable on a more fundamental level. They purported to elucidate the neural mechanisms underlying normal speech and language by postulating the existence of limited cortical areas, the cells of which were the repository of memory-images or representations of word sounds and speech movements. This seemed incomprehensible to at least some thoughtful students of the nervous system who refused to believe that the neural elements comprising these limited cortical areas could be endowed with such extraordinary capacities. It was not that they believed in the functional equipotentiality of all parts of the cerebral hemispheres. Nor did they deny the facts of clinical localization of brain lesions. But they were convinced that the model builders had fallen into the error of confusing a symptom with a function. The British neurologist, Hughlings Jackson, made this point succinctly when he warned that "to locate the lesion which destroys speech and to locate speech are two different things" (Jackson, 1878).

Jackson was one of the few neurologists in the 1870s and 1880s who opposed the assumptions, formulations and conclusions of the "associationist" theory held by the leading neurologists of the time—Wernicke in Germany, Charcot in France, and Bastian in England. First, he denied that aphasia could be defined as a loss of words. Instead, it was an impairment in the utilization of words in thinking. He distinguished between two levels of speech: automatic (or emotional) speech and intellectual speech. The typical aphasic has retained his capacity for automatic speech (as reflected, for example, in oaths and recurring meaningless utterances). At the same time, he has lost the capacity to make meaningful verbal statements ("propositions," as Jackson called them) either to others or to himself. The basic unit of language is not the word, as was assumed by the associationists, but the proposition, the meaningful statement. It is at this level that speech becomes "a part of thought" and it is at this level that aphasic defect manifests itself. Consequently, those forms of thought that require, or are facilitated by, inner verbalization, will of necessity be impaired in the aphasic patient.

Thus Jackson opposed the prevailing associationist theory at every major point. There were no cortical centers of language but only focally situated lesions that impaired language. Aphasia was not a loss of words as signs of thought but a disturbance in verbal thinking itself. The aphasic patient has words at his disposal but he can use them only at a lower level of automatic speech. He cannot use them at a higher level of propositional speech.

For a number of reasons Jackson's views did not attract much attention even in Britain, and Continental neurologists scarcely knew of their existence. However, one person who did read Jackson's papers with interest and appreciation was a youngish Viennese neurologist by the name of Sigmund Freud.

Freud was 35 years old when he wrote his monograph on "The Interpretation of the Aphasias" in 1891 (Freud, 1891). This was 2 years before he and Josef Breuer presented their preliminary communication on hysteria and 4 years before publication of the famous Breuer-Freud monograph on hysteria. With the possible exception of a brief unsigned entry on aphasia in the medical encyclopedia of Villaret (1888), Freud had not written on the topic before. This did not deter him from undertaking to write a major critique of the dominant theory of the nature of aphasia, as reflected in the work of its most authoritative proponents, Carl Wernicke and Leopold Lichtheim. In so doing, he followed the recommendation of Lichtheim. He examined the clinical facts of aphasia and compared them with the deductions emerging from "centrist" theory. Finding that the deductions did not fit the facts, he proposed a different formulation.

Having outlined Wernicke's original model and Lichtheim's more elaborate models, Freud developed his critique. His first point was that, while the models predict aphasic performance patterns in which a specific function is completely lost and other functions are completely intact, in fact the typical clinical picture is one in which all the different speech functions are impaired to a greater or lesser degree. A second weakness of the models is that they fail to account satisfactorily for certain aphasic symptom-pictures that are encountered in clinical practice. Here Freud cited an example that had been offeed by Lichtheim himself, namely the fact that motor aphasics are often alexic, i.e., they show a specific impairment in understanding what they read.

He then went on to deny the validity of the fundamental distinction between central aphasias and conduction aphasias postulated in the models. Influenced by physiological evidence that isolation of a central area from the rest of the brain produces the same effect as excision of that area, he concluded that "the destruction of a so-called center comes about only through simultaneous interruption of several fiber tracts." As had previous authors, he criticized the concept of a center as a specific central area in which memory images were stored and pointed out the confusion engendered by this mixing of anatomic and psychic entities. He concluded that all aphasic disorders were "conduction aphasias," not in the restricted Wernicke-Lichtheim sense, but in the broader sense that they were produced by interruptions in the neural connections within the brain.

Freud did not deny that lesions in the so-called centers, i.e., Broca's area, Wernicke's area and the angular gyrus, produced different aphasic symptom-pictures. But the reason for this specificity was not a peculiar functional endowment of these areas but the circumstance that they were intimately related to specific cortical sensory and motor regions: Broca's area with motor cortex, Wernicke's area with auditory cortex and the angular gyrus with visual cortex. It was thus understandable that lesions in these areas could lead to distinctive aphasic syndromes.

At the same time, Freud laid great stress on a functional, as opposed to a purely morphological, approach to aphasia. He cited Bastian's (1887) schema of three levels of reduced excitability of cortical areas, the least severe being one in which the area responds to direct sensory stimulation as well as stimulation from other areas but not to volitional influences, and the most severe being one in which the area is completely unresponsive. He went on to postulate that the functional state of all areas of the brain entered into the determination of aphasic symptom-pictures and he adopted "as a guiding principle Hughlings Jackson's doctrine that all these modes of reaction represent instances of functional retrogression (disinvolution) of a highly organized apparatus, and therefore correspond to earlier states of its functional development. This means that under all circumstances an arrangement of associations which, having been acquired later, belongs to a higher level of functioning, will be lost, while an earlier and simpler one will be preserved." And he linked Bastian's three levels of excitability to the Jacksonian doctrine.

Thus Freud's basic conception was that the neural mechanism of speech was located in a definite but continuous cortical region that was bounded at one end by the auditory and visual receptive fields and at the other by the frontal motor areas. Disease or injury in this region destroys communication between various parts of it as well as with the rest of the brain. A limited number of aphasic symptom-pictures occur depending on the locus and severity of injury. Above all, aphasic disorders result not from a loss of memory-images but from impairment of the speech apparatus as a whole.

Every point that Freud made already had been made by one or another earlier writer. The concept of centers of speech had been criticized by Hughlings Jackson. The significance of the intimate anatomic relationship of Broca's area, Wernicke's area, and the angular gyrus territory to the primary motor and sensory areas of the cortex had been pointed out as early as 1866 by the British physicians, Moxon (1866), Trousseau (1864, 1877), and Finkelnburg (1889), as well as Jackson, who had insisted that aphasia involved an intellectual change that transcended the mechanisms of speech expression and reception. Freud's real achievement was to organize all these points into a coherent, carefully reasoned critique that could be used to formulate an alternative conception of the basis and nature of aphasic disorder.

Henri Bergson was 37 years old when he addressed the nature of aphasic disorder in his book, *Matière et Mémoire* (Bergson, 1896), which was published in 1896. Thus he was about the same age as Freud was when the latter wrote his monograph on the topic. However, while Freud as a neurologist was interested in aphasia for its own sake, Bergson as a philosopher was interested in the disorder primarily as a source of empirical data that could be used in understanding the relationship between mind and matter or, more specifically, between the mind and the brain. Thus he approached aphasia from the vantage point of his rejection of psychological parallelism in its absolute form, his insistence on the unity of memory, perception and action, and his view that the brain constitutes a mechanism for the initiation of purposeful motor action rather than a storehouse of "pure" or "real" memories.

He mounted an eloquent attack on the concept that the brain is a storehouse of memory images and on the explanation of aphasic "forgetting" in terms of a loss of these memory-images from destruction of the cortical centers in which they are stored. Pointing out that the same word is pronounced differently by different speakers and hence that there must be countless memory-images of it in the brain, he asks the reader whether he can really believe that all these memory-images are stored there. He reminds him that these memories are conceived as fixed entities and thus that it is difficult to imagine how the brain might select a single one for storage and, if it does, how it matches a new perception of a word with its memory-image. Thus, in Bergson's view, the explanation of aphasia as a loss of memory images is quite untenable.

Citing the familiar clinical observation that aphasics have maximal difficulty in producing proper names and least difficulty in producing verbs, with common nouns occupying an intermediate position in this hierarchy of difficulty, he advanced his own concept of the nature of aphasic disorder, namely, that it is a functional disturbance, an impairment in the capacity to actualize memories. In order to be recalled, memories (which are never lost) require a mental attitude in intimate connection with a bodily attitude. Since verbs generally express actions, their recall is facilitated by physical effort and the aphasic patient can engage in such effort in his efforts to produce them. In contrast, proper nouns are fairly remote from bodily activity and physical effort cannot facilitate their recall. The influence of bodily activity is also seen when a patient who is unable to produce the name of an object describes its mode of action.

Above all, verbal understanding is an active, selective process. It is primarily concerned with sentences (i.e., Jackson's "propositions"), which have structure and which carry meaning, and not with isolated words. The failure of an aphasic patient to understand what he hears or sees is a failure in function. It is a failure to achieve a complete perception which by definition includes a coalescence with past experience. Such a complete perception is the product of intellectual effort for it involves reconstructing the continuous flow of speech into a meaningful message. Thus there is an intrinsic intellectual component in the aphasic patient's failure to understand speech. On the expressive side, aphasia is not a mere failure to utilize words as signs of thought but instead a specific arrest in thinking that leads to a verbal deficiency.

Bergson's thought coincides with that of Freud on a number of major points. It is obvious that both writers rejected the notion that the cerebral cortex serves as a repository of memory-images and that aphasia results from a destruction of these memory-images by organic disease. Both maintained that the clinical facts of the localization of the lesions causing aphasia do not justify localizing normal language processes in limited cortical areas. Both viewed aphasia from a functional standpoint as reflecting a breakdown in the efficient operation of a complicated neural mechanism. Both insisted that perception and memory ("association" in Freud's terminology) form a single process.

There is, however, a fundamental difference in the conceptions of the nature of aphasia held by the two men. Freud did not lay great stress on the role of intellectual factors in the disorder except that, by definition, aphasia had to be considered a specific cognitive disability. To Bergson, aphasia was above all an expression of a basic impairment in intellectual activity, of an incapacity to engage the body in the realization of intentions.

It is clear that Bergson's concepts had a significant influence on subsequent thought about aphasia in France. In 1906, that is, 10 years after the publication of *Matière et Mémoire*, the French neurologist Pierre Marie wrote a series of papers under the title "Revision of the Question of Aphasia" (Marie, 1906 a, b, c). In these papers he attacked the prevailing notions about the lesional localization of aphasic disorders, as well as the pluralistic concept of discrete types of aphasia. Maintaining that in fact there was only one basic aphasic disorder, he insisted that it always involved an impairment of intelligence. Marie was not very specific about the characteristics of the aphasic patient's defect in intelligence but apparently what he had in mind was an inability to cope with diverse tasks that were outside the sphere of language, an intellectual passivity and a lack of initiative.

Marie's papers created a furor in French neurological circles and over the next few years a series of spirited, at times rancorous, debates took place. In the end Marie's views won a large following and the idea that at least the major forms of aphasic disorder involved some degree of impairment of intelligence was generally accepted. This was scarcely Bergsonism but it was an important fragment of it. Jules Dejerine, the other major figure in French neurology at the time, also came to accept the proposition that aphasia involves a defect in intelligence. So far as I am aware, neither Marie nor Dejerine mentioned Bergson in their writing. But *Matière et Mémoire* was widely read and some commentators have classified Marie as "the neurological disciple" of Bergson (cf. Hécaen and Angelergues [1965], and Ombredane [1950]. Aspects of Bergson's thought were later reflected in the writing of a number of neurologists such as Van Woerkom (1921, 1923), Mourgue (1921), and Goldstein (1924), all of whom emphasized impairment in intellectual functions, particularly spatial thinking and abstract reasoning, as a cardinal feature of the symptom-picture of aphasia.

The influence of Freud's 1891 monograph (Freud, 1891) is problematic. It is stated that only 257 copies were sold over a 10-year period and that the book was totally neglected (cf. Jones, 1953). If this is so, there is an odd fact associated with the monograph that calls for explanation. In discussing the necessity for distinguishing between failure to name an object and failure to recognize it, Freud coined the tem "agnosia" to denote the failure in recognition and proposed its use. Not many years passed before his suggestion was generally adopted and "agnosia" replaced older terms, such as "mindblindness," "psychic blindness" and "psychic deafness" to designate the disability. Thus Freud's monograph could not have been completely overlooked. In any case, the views which he expressed are certainly found in later writing on aphasia.

Henri Bergson was scarcely a specialist in the field of aphasia. He was not a physician, he had no first hand experience with aphasic patients and his knowledge of the field came entirely from his analysis of the literature. Surprisingly, to a considerable degree, the same can be said of Sigmund Freud. Although he was a neurologist, it does not appear that he had had much actual experience with aphasic patients, his monograph contains no descriptions of patients whom he had personally examined and cared for. Thus, like Bergson, he based his formulation entirely on his analysis of the literature. Would firsthand experience with aphasic patients have caused either to modify his conclusions? The chances are that it would not. What a clinician sees, or at least deems worthy of note, in his assessment of aphasic patients is determined in large part by his own preconceptions. In any case, despite whatever possible handicap may have been imposed by their lack of clinical experience, their superb intellectual gifts enabled Bergson and Freud to make contributions that have a secure place in the history of clinical neuropsychology.

References

Bastian H. C. (1887). On different kinds of aphasia. *Br. Med. J.* 2: 931–936, 985–990.

Benton A. L., and Joynt R. J. (1960). Early descriptions of aphasia. *Arch. Neurol.* 3: 205–222.

Benton A. L. (1981). Contributions to aphasia before Broca. *Cortex* 1: 314–327.

Benton A. L. (1981). Aphasia: historical perspectives. In Sarno M. T. (ed.). *Acquired Aphasia*, New York: Academic Press.

Bergson H. (1896). *Matière et Mémoire*. Paris: Alcan.

Broca P. (1861). Remarques sur le siège de la faculté du langage articulé suivies d'une observation d'aphémie. *Bull. Soc. Anatomique* 6: 330–357.

Broca P. (1863). Localisation des fonctions cérébrales: siège du langage articulé. *Bull. Soc. Anthropologie* 4: 200–203.

Broca P. (1865). Du siège de la faculté du langage articulé. *Bull. Soc. Anthropologie* 6: 337–393.

Finkelnburg F. C. (1870). Niederrheinische Gesellschaft: Sitzung von 21 März in Bonn. (Also published as Finkelnburg's 1870 lecture on aphasia with commentary. Trans. R. J. Duffy and B. Z. Liles. *J. Speech Hearing Dis.* 44: 156–168, 1889.)

Freud S. (1891). *Zur Auffasung der Aphasien*. Leipzig and Wien: Deuticke. (Also published as *On Aphasia*. Trans. E. Stengel. New York: International Universities Press.)

Goldstein K. (1924). Das Wesen der amnestischen Aphasie. *Schweize Archiv für Neurologie und Psychiatrie* 15: 163–175.

Hécaen H. and Angelergues R. (1965). *Pathologie du Langage*. Paris: Larousse.

Jackson, J. H. (1878). On affections of speech from disease of the brain. *Brain* 1: 304–330.

Jones E. (1953). *The Life and Work of Sigmund Freud*. New York: Basic Books.

Lichtheim L. (1885). On aphasia. *Brain* 7: 433–485. (Originally published in *Deutsches Archiv für Klinische Medizin* 36: 204–268, 1885.)

Marie P. (1906a). Révision de la question de l'aphasie: la troisième circonvolution frontale gauche ne joue aucun rôle spécial dans la fonction du langage. *Semaine Médicale* 26: 241–247.

Marie P. (1906b). Révision de la question de l'aphasie: que faut-il penser des aphasies sous-corticales (aphasies pures)? *Semaine Médicale* 26: 493–500.

Marie P. (1906c). Révision de la question de l'aphasie: l'aphasie de 1861 à 1866: essai de critique historique sur la genèse de la doctrine de Broca. *Semaine Médicale* 26: 565–571.

Mourgue R. (1920–21). Aphasie et psychologie de la pensée. *Encéphale* 15: 649–664 (1920); 16: 26–33, 85–91 (1921).

Moxon W. (1866). On the connexion between loss of speech and paralysis of the right side. *Br. & Foreign Med. Chirurgical Rev.* 74: 481–489.

Ombredane A. (1950). *L'Aphasie et L'Élaboration de la Pensée Explicite*. Paris: Presses Universitaires de France.

Trousseau A. (1864). De l'aphasie, maladie décrite récemmment sous le nom impropre d'aphémie. *Gazettes des Hopitaux* 37: 13–14, 25–26, 37–39, 48–50.

Trousseau A. (1877). *Clinique Médicale de l'Hôtel Dieu de Paris*, ed. 5. Paris: Bailliere et fils.

Van Woerkom W. (1921). La signification de certains éléments de l'intelligence dans la genèse des troubles aphasiques. *J. Psychologie Normale Pathologique* 18: 730–751.

Van Woerkom W. (1983). Sur l'état psychique des aphasiques. *Encéphale* 18: 286–304.

Villaret A. (1888). *Handworterbuch der Gesamte Medizin*. Stuttgart: Enke.

Wernicke C. (1874). *Der Aphasische Symptomenkomplex*. Breslau, Cohn and Weigert: Breslau.

12

Pitres and Amnesic Aphasia

The concept of an amnesic (as distinct from an articulatory) type of speech disorder is a very old one. The idea can be traced back to the sixteenth century when Schenck von Grafenberg (1585) noted that "in many cases of apoplexy . . . although the tongue was not paralyzed, the patient could not speak because the faculty of memory being abolished, the words were not produced" (Benton and Joynt, 1960). Van Swieten (1742–1746) was somewhat more precise when he wrote that he had "seen many patients whose cerebral functions were quite sound after recovery from apoplexy, except for this one deficit: in designating objects, they could not find the correct names for them" (Benton and Joynt, 1960).

The system of Gall and Spurzheim (1810) included placement of an organ of the "memory of words" in the orbital area of both frontal lobes. Gall's ardent champion, J.-B. Bouillaud (1825), was the first to make a clear differentiation between amnesic and motoric forms of aphasic disorder. Emphasizing the necessity for distinguishing between the capacity to utilize words as signs of ideas and the capacity to articulate them, Bouillaud wrote that

> the nervous system which directs the formation of signs is not identical with that which produces the movements of the organs of speech, for it is not uncommon to observe suspension of speech sometimes because the tongue and its congenerous organs refuse the pronunciation of words and sometimes because the memory of these words escapeus. . . . It is important to distinguish clearly between these two causes which can lead to loss of speech, each in its own way; one by destroying the organ of memory of words, the other by an impairment in the nervous principle which directs the movement of speech [Benton 1964].

In the 1860s many clinical descriptions, e.g., by Sanders (1866), Ogle (1867), Trousseau (1868), and Broca (1869), established the validity of the distinction

Reprinted with permission from *Aphasiology*, 1988, vol. 2, no. 3/4, 209–214.

In honor of Harold Goodglass.

between amnesic and ataxic (or aphemic) forms of aphasic disorder. Such were the beginnings of the differentiation between fluent and nonfluent types of aphasia that a century later were defined in objective terms by Goodglass et al. (1965) and Benson (1967).

However, during the same period, another trend of thought that fostered a narrower definition of amnesic aphasia as a specific disorder of naming and word finding also developed. Citing descriptions dating back to the eighteenth century but mainly on the basis of their own observations, clinicians such as Bateman (1870), Kussmaul (1876) and Banti (1886) identified patients whose most prominent (and sometimes only) disability was their incapacity to produce the names of objects and persons. Applying the old term "amnesic aphasia" to this symptom-picture, they regarded it as a distinctive type of speech impairment and included it as such in their classification of the aphasic disorders. Broadbent (1878) proposed that amnesic aphasia resulted from destruction or dysfunction of a "naming centre" in the posterior region of the left hemisphere, and Mills and McConnell (1895) localized this centre in the third and second temporal gyri.

Yet it was difficult to find a place for this concept of a specific type of aphasia characterized predominantly by a failure in producing names and with an identifiable lesional localization in the prevailing classifications of aphasic disorders and the symptom-complex was generally regarded as a relatively mild form of sensory aphasia. Forgetting was a universal characteristic of the aphasic disorders and it seemed unwarranted to single out a specific clinical picture for the designation of "amnesic aphasia" (cf. Bernard, 1885).

Pitres

This was the ambiguous status of amnesic aphasia as a nosologic entity when Albert Pitres, Professor of Medicine at the University of Bordeaux, gave a course of lectures on the topic which were published serially in the *Progrès Médicale* and as a monograph (Pitres, 1898). He began by describing what he considered to be a case of pure amnesic aphasia. The patient was a 38-year-old woman who was seen three months after a stroke, at which time she presented a right hemiparesis and a discrete impairment in expressive speech. She understood everything said to her, had no difficulty in reading printed and cursive script aloud and understood what she read; writing was motorically impaired but linguistically correct; she was capable of conversational speech and her vocabulary was adequate. However, she often blocked as she searched for the appropriate word. Sometimes the search was successful; at other times she would give up or use a circumlocution. Confrontation naming was similarly impaired; while usually she was able to supply the names of presented objects, on occasion there would be inexplicable failure to name the most common objects, which she obviously recognized.

Pitres pointed out that the clinical picture fitted into none of the recognized primary categories of aphasic disorder and that it was clearly an example of "what was once called *amnesic aphasia*, that is to say, a form of aphasia in which difficulties of the language are determined by the forgetting of the words necessary for the expression of thoughts" (Pitres, 1898). Yet amnesic aphasia finds no place in most classifications and indeed is not even mentioned in many authoritative reviews. Then, after a detailed historical review and theoretical analysis, he offered his conception of amnesic aphasia and its pathological basis.

He distinguished between three forms of amnesic aphasia. The first is antonomasia (word substitution) in which the patient fails to recall and produce substantives within a setting of adequate conversational speech and understanding. The second is agrammatism, i.e., inability to formulate acceptable sentences. The third is differential loss of language in polyglots. The three forms are expressions of the same basic disability. The anomic patient is less severely impaired than the agrammatic patient who has difficulty in recalling verbs and connectives as well as substantives. The differential loss in polyglots is attributable to differences in the depth of a patient's knowledge of the languages. Thus Pitres's concept of amnesic aphasia was fairly broad, extending beyond anomia to encompass the lexical and syntactical impoverishment of agrammatism.

Turning to the question of the pathological basis of amnesic aphasia, Pitres rejected the idea that it was produced by destruction or dysfunction of a hypothetical naming centre. His review of autopsied cases of amnesic aphasia reported in the literature indicated that the causative lesion is most frequently found to be in the inferior parietal lobule, sometimes with extension into the angular gyrus. But there are exceptions and this region cannot be considered to be the only area serving word memory. Amnesic aphasia is produced by breaks in the outflow from psychosensory centres to the whole cortex and hence there cannot be an absolutely constant localization of the responsible lesion. Since it results from a break in the connections between cortical centres, it can be called a transcortical aphasia. However, this relatively simple concept does not account for all the clinical facts. On this view the patient with amnesic aphasia should not only experience difficulty in producing words corresponding to his ideas but also be unable to grasp the ideas represented by words said to him. But observation shows that spoken words always do evoke the corresponding ideas. One possible explanation is that the neural pathways from psychosensory areas to verbal areas are not the same as those from verbal areas to psychosensory areas. Finally, under the influence of fatigue, malnutrition or intoxication, patients without cerebral disease may be anomic and paraphasic.

Discussing paraphasia, Pitres pointed out that the level of patients' awareness of this disability varies considerably. Some are keenly aware of their paraphasic utterances while others are unaware that their utterances are inappropriate. However, given the correct name, they quickly appreciate their error and repeat the name in an effort to fix it in memory.

Pure amnesic aphasia is rare. The disorder in naming is usually accompanied by other disabilities. Repetition of words and phrases may be defective. Within the context of preserved capacity for silent reading for meaning, reading aloud is often impaired. Although automatic recitation is usually good, reciting poems or the words of a song from memory may produce paraphasic distortions.

In summary, "the existence of a clinical form of aphasia, uniquely determined by the loss of the evocation of words," cannot be questioned. Observation demonstrates it to be a reality. The syndrome cannot be identified with any major category in current classifications and its autonomy should be recognized. It is an associative aphasia that may be placed between the motor or emissive and the sensory or receptive aphasias.

The Fate of Amnesic Aphasia

The legacy of Pitres might be described as follows. Although he insisted that amnesic aphasia was a distinctive and autonomous form of aphasia, he acknowledged that pure cases of the disorder were rare, that it did not have a fixed lesional localization and that under some conditions even patients without brain disease might show the symptom-picture. His concept evoke varied reactions.

Wernicke (1903) discussed Pitres's amnesic aphasia at considerable length and concluded that word-finding disturbance represented "nothing other than a special form of transcortical motor aphasia." Thus, discounting the "nothing other," he agreed with Pitres that amnesic aphasia was indeed an identifiable symptom-picture and that it could be classified as a transcortical or associative type of disorder. On his part, Dejerine (1900) completely rejected the concept and insisted that the cases reported by Pitres were merely instances of mild sensory or motor aphasia. Other authorities recognized the clinical pictures as one with neurological significance. For example, Von Monakow (1905) described amnesic aphasia as an early sign of parieto-temporal disease of the dominant hemisphere.

A later generation of neurologists treated amnesic aphasia in very different ways. Head (1926) totally ignored the concept and indeed did not mention Pitres in his detailed history of thought in the field of aphasia. Nor did his category of "nominal aphasia," which is described as involving serious defects in verbal understanding, calculation and reasoning, correspond to the clinical picture of amnesic aphasia. If anything, his category of "verbal aphasia," was closer to Pitres's symptom-complex. Goldstein (1924) did recognize amnesic aphasia but interpreted it as a primary impairment in abstract thinking rather than a strictly linguistic disorder. However, his unusual conception could not survive demonstrations that patients with amnesic aphasia tended to be less impaired cognitively than were other classes of aphasics (Isserlin, 1932; Lotmar, 1933). The historical introduction of Weisenburg and McBride's (1935) *Aphasia: A Clinical and Psychological Study* does not mention the contribution of Pitres. Yet, having classified their aphasic cases into three major categories (expressive, receptive, expressive-receptive), they encountered

> a smaller number of patients whose expression was not disturbed by defects in word-formation, but by difficulties in evoking words as names of objects, conditions, or qualities. Logically patients of this type belonged to the predominantly expressive group. Psychologically, however, their disorder was so different in nature that they could not well be classified with that group. Neither did they belong to the predominantly receptive group, for their understanding remained always relatively superior. A fourth group was therefore created, and designated as the *amnesic*.

Thus, their empirical analyses, based mainly on patterns of test performance, generated a symptom-picture that was quite similar to Pitres's amnesic aphasia.

Amnesic or anomic aphasia has figured prominently in modern classifications of the aphasic disorders (cf. Albert, et al., 1981). However, reservations about its neuropathologic significance are often expressed and not uncommonly it is described as being 'merely' a symptom-complex that appears in the course of recovery from a more pervasive fluent or non-fluent aphasic disorder. Clinicopathologic correlational study has repeatedly confirmed Pitres's rather broad lesional localization (cf. Gloning et al., 1968; Newcombe et al., 1971).

The Problem

One can detect a dual character in the response to Pitres's concept of amnesic aphasia. On the one hand, clinical observation forced recognition of a symptom-complex in which disability in naming was the most prominent component. Yet there was strong resistance to the idea that it represented the autonomous disorder that Pitres claimed it was. Instead, it was conceived as being "nothing more" than a particular manifestation of sensory, motor or transcortical aphasia or a stage in the recovery from major aphasic disability.

A number of factors have contributed to this ambivalence or confusion. One is failure to discriminate between diverse types of disability in naming. Wernicke (1903), in discussing amnesic aphasia, suggested that it would be advantageous to differentiate between simple failure to produce names as contrasted to the production of paraphasic utterances. Simple failure is very common and not necessarily related to brain disease while paraphasia is of a truly aphasic nature. Later authors, such as Geschwind (1967) and Benson (1979), have distinguished between various types of misnaming and discussed their clinical significance.

A second source of confusion is the failure to recognize that, even if amnesic aphasia is only a special form of a broader diagnostic category, it may still possess a specific neuropsychological significance. Moreover, the symptom-complex has rarely been defined on an objective basis so that what is one clinician's "amnesic aphasia" is another's "mild Wernicke aphasia" or even "attenuated Broca aphasia." Finally, modern neurodiagnostic techniques have yet to be brought to bear on the question of lesional localization and underlying neurological mechanisms. Thus, whether or not Pitres's amnesic aphasia is a useful and meaningful neuropsychological concept remains to be determined.

References

Albert M. L., Goodglass H., Helm N. A., Rubens A. B., and Alexander M. B. (1981). *Clinical Aspects of Dysphasia*. New York: Springer-Verlag.

Banti G. (1886). *Afasia e sue Forme*. Firenze (Florence): Tipografia Cenniniana.

Bateman F. (1870). *On Aphasia or Loss of Speech*. London: John Churchill and Sons.

Benson D. F. (1967). Fluency in aphasia. Correlation with radioactive scan localization. *Cortex* 3: 373–394.

Benson D. F. (1979). Neurologic correlates of anomia. In H. Whitaker and H. A. Whitaker (eds.), *Studies in Neurolinguistics*, Vol. 4. New York: Academic Press.

Benton A. L. (1964). Contributions to aphasia before Broca. *Cortex* 1: 314–327.

Benton A. L. and Joynt R. J. (1960). Early descriptions of aphasia. *Arch. Neurol.* 3: 205–222.

Bernard D. (1885). *De l'Aphasie et de ses Diverses Formes*. Paris: Lecrosnier et Babé.

Bouillaud J.-B. (1825). Recherches cliniques propres à démontrer que la perte de la parole correspond à la lésion des lobules antérieurs du cerveau. *Arch. Gén. Méd.* 8: 25–45.

Broadbent W. M. (1878). A case of peculiar affection of speech. *Brain* 1: 484–503.

Broca P. (1869). Sur le siège de la faculté du langage articulé. *Tribune Médicale* 3: 254–256, 265–269.

Dejerine J. (1900). Sémiologie du système nerveux. In Bouchard, C. (ed.), *Traité de Pathologie Générale*, Vol. 5. Paris: Masson.

Gall F. J. and Spurzheim G. (1810). *Recherches sur le Système Nerveux en Général et sur Celui de Cerveau en Particulier*. Paris: Schoell.

Geschwind N. (1967). The varieties of naming errors. *Cortex* 3: 97–112.

Gloning I., Gloning K., and Hoff H. (1968). *Neuropsychological Symptoms and Syndromes in Lesions of the Occipital Lobe and the Adjacent Areas*. Paris: Gauthier-Villars.

Goldstein K. (1924). Das Wesen der amnestischen Aphasie. *Schweizer Archiv fuer Neurologie und Psychiatrie*, 15: 163–175.

Goodglass H., Quadfasel F. A., and Timberlake W. H. (1965). Phrase length and the type and severity of aphasia. *Cortex* 1: 133–153.

Head H. (1926). *Aphasia and Kindred Disorders of Speech*. London: Cambridge University Press.

Isserlin M. (1932). Ueber Sprache und Sprechen. *Nervenarzt* 5: 1–7.

Kussmaul A. (1876). *Die Stoerungen der Sprache*. Leipzig: Vogel.

Lotmar F. (1933). Zur Pathophysiologie der erschwerten Wortfindung bei Aphasischen. *Schweizer Archiv fuer Neurologie und Psychiatrie* 30: 86–158; 322–379.

Mills C. K. and McConnell J. W. (1895). The naming centre, with the report of a case indicating its location in the temporal lobe. *J. Nerv. Ment. Dis.* 22: 1–7.

Newcombe F., Oldfield R. C., Ratcliff C. G., and Wingfield A. (1971). The recognition and naming of object-drawings by men with focal brain wounds. *J. Neurol. Neurosurg. Psychiatry* 34: 329–340.

Ogle W. (1867). Aphasia and agraphia. *St George's Hospital Reports* 2: 83–122.

Pitres A. (1898). *l'Aphasie Amnésiques et ses Variétés Cliniques*. Paris: Alean.

Sanders W. R. (1866). Case illustrating the supposed connection of aphasia (loss of the cerebral faculty of speech) with right hemiplegia and lesions of the external frontal convolution of the brain. *Edinburgh Medical Journal* 11: 811–823.

Trousseau A. (1868). *Clinique Médicale de l'Hôtel-Dieu de Paris*, 3rd Ed. Paris: Baillière.

Von Monakow C. (1905). *Gehirnpathologie*, 2nd ed. Vienna: Holder.

Weisenburg T. and McBride K. E. (1935). *Aphasia*. New York: Commonwealth Fund.

Wernicke C. (1903). Der aphasische Symptomencomplex. *Deutsche Klinik* 10: 487–556.

Part III

METHODOLOGY AND ASSESSMENT

13

The Interplay of Experimental and Clinical Approaches in Brain Lesion Research

Our knowledge of the effects of brain lesions on behavior has been gained through two approaches. The first is the experimental method in which structural or functional alteration of the central nervous system is deliberately induced and its behavioral outcome noted. The second is the clinical method in which the behavioral consequences of the lesions produced by disease are observed.

If the two approaches are compared, the experimental method is seen to have significant advantages in that the investigator can exercise some control over the size and locus of the lesion he produces, the degree of control being dependent upon a number of factors such as the prevailing state of surgical technology and the depth of understanding of the structural characteristics of the brain and the anatomic relationships between its parts. Theoretically the experimental investigator has an unlimited number of animals at his disposal so that he can proceed systematically to compare the effects of lesions of different locus and size. He can also exercise a considerable degree of control over the genetic characteristics and life history of his animals as well as over other variables, such as age, that interact with experimental interventions to determine the consequences of these interventions. The clinical investigator enjoys none of these advantages. He must take the lesions as he finds them and, while some may approximate experimental lesions in discreteness, the majority are associated with one or more confounding factors that may make it difficult to draw confident conclusions about the relationship of the lesion to the behavior of the patient. Nor can the clinical investigator exercise direct control over extralesional factors such as age, health status,

Reprinted with permission from S. Finger (Ed.), *Recovery from Brain Damage*. New York: Plenum Press © 1978. Kluwer Academic/Plenum Publishers.

and the life history, although to some degree he may be able to reduce variability in these respects by an appropriate selection of cases.

But not all the advantages are on the side of the experimentalist. Detailed study of the behavioral aspects of the brain–behavior relationship is much more easily accomplished in human subjects. Animals must be trained to respond in the laboratory situation, human subjects need only to be asked to. It is a commonplace observation that animals often behave in an inexplicably stupid manner in the unnatural environment of the laboratory, quite unlike their appropriate real-life behavior. The human subject can report what he sees, the animal cannot. The cognitive capacities of the human subject are incomparably greater, offering opportunities for the analytic study of diverse aspects of mentation, which are not possible with animals.

Thus, each approach has its reciprocal strengths and weaknesses and complement each other well in the total research effort on the effects of brain lesions on behavior. Historical study shows that, in line with this complementarity, there has usually been a constant interaction between the two methods in pursuing a particular line of inquiry. In this chapter I shall illustrate the interplay of the two approaches as they were brought to bear on specific questions about brain–behavior relationships and try to show how they coalesced to provide some answers to these questions. The early history of two topics that have been investigated through both experimental and clinical brain lesion research will be sketched. The first is the evolution of our knowledge of cortical localization of visual function. The second deals with the method of double sensory stimulation, which has become a standard feature of the clinical neurological examination. As will be seen, in both instances relevant findings were first generated by experimental investigation on animals and these led to analogous and more refined study of human patients.

Cortical Localization of Visual Function

Ferrier, Munk, and the Clinicians

A detailed description of the early history of this topic may be found in the first two chapters of Polyak's (1955) monumental volume on the vertebrate visual system. As he states, "As far back in the human past as there is a record, the supreme importance of vision and of its instrument, the eye, has been recognized." Up to 1800, for practical reasons, investigation was primarily directed to the eye and its diseases. Nevertheless, the role of the brain in visual-information processing was also fully appreciated. The fact that there were structural connections between the eyes and the brain, in the form of "nerves," "ducts," or "tubes," was established very early. However, up to the middle of the nineteenth century, knowledge of details was scanty and often inaccurate. The cerebral center for vision was almost invariably placed below the cerebral hemispheres—in the lateral ventricles (Galen), the brainstem (Willis), the pineal body (Descartes), and other sites.

One reason for this was technical in nature. The limitations inherent in gross anatomical study made it very difficult indeed to trace the visual pathways beyond the optic tract. But an even more important reason was of a conceptual nature. The dominating influence of Flourens's doctrine of the equipotentiality of the cerebral hemispheres made it seem pointless to look for a focal center for vision above the level of the thalamus.

However, Flourens's dogma was challenged by two contributions in the 1850s, one of an anatomical nature and the other consisting of experimental and clinical observations, and these laid the groundwork for the subsequent identification of a cortical center for vision. By means of careful dissection of fixed specimens, Gratiolet (1854) was able to demonstrate the optic radiations arising from the lateral geniculate nuclei and fanning out to the cortex of the occipital and parietal lobes. He described the radiations as "expansions of the optic nerve terminating in a specific region of the cortex of the hemispheres." A year later, Gratiolet's anatomical discovery was complemented by the observations of Panizza (1855), who established a rough correlation between lesions in the occipitoparietal area and visual impairment, both in human case material and in dogs subjected to experimental ablations. Panizza reported that bilateral destruction of this area resulted in complete blindness while unilateral damage caused blindness in the opposite eye. A clinicopathologic study by Chaillou (1863) of a patient with extensive destruction of the "posterior" lobes and concomitant visual impairment provided an additional bit of evidence in support of Panizza's correlation. Similarly, Meynert's (1869) description of the course of the optic radiations from the thalamic level to the occipital and temporal lobes partially substantiated the observations of Gratiolet.

A more intensive search for the site of the cortical center for vision, as well as for the other senses, followed upon the discovery of the motor area of the cortex by Fritsch and Hitzig (1870). Ferrier (1876, 1878, 1890) carried out a long series of studies involving both destruction and stimulation of different cortical areas in animals, primarily the monkey, and sought confirmation of his experimental findings in relevant clinical observations. He concluded that the angular gyrus was the site of the cortical visual center since its "unilateral destruction has the effect of causing temporary blindness of the opposite eye, while bilateral destruction causes total and permanent blindness in both eyes" (Ferrier, 1878, p. 122). Confronted by a substantial amount of contradictory evidence from the studies of other investigators, he later modified his position and conceded that the visual center occupied the territory of *both* the angular gyrus and the occipital lobes. But he still insisted that "the angular gyrus is the special region of clear or central vision of the opposite eye, and perhaps to some extent also of the eye on the same side" (Ferrier, 1886, p. 288). And he maintained that the occipital lobes "can be injured, or cut off bodily, almost up to the parieto-occipital fissure, on one or both sides simultaneously, without the slightest appreciable impairment of vision" (Ferrier, 1886, p. 273).

What could have led Ferrier to these inaccurate inferences? Given his crude surgical techniques, the suggestion by Starr (1884) and Schäfer (1888) that Ferrier had destroyed fibers of the underlying optic radiations in his angular gyrus ablations is probably correct. His notion that the opposite eye was affected by unilateral destruction of the angular gyrus rested on the conception (still held at the time by some experimentalists and clinicians including Charcot) that those retinogeniculate fibers which did not decussate at the optic chiasm crossed over to the opposite hemisphere though the colliculi so that the whole retina of a single eye was represented in a single lateral cortical area.

Studies by a number of experimentalists and clinicians in the 1870s and 1880s generated unassailable evidence that the locus of the cortical center for vision was to be found in the occipital lobes. The preeminent experimentalist of the period was the Berlin physiologist Hermann Munk, a painstaking investigator, whose studies on the dog and the monkey were technically and methodologically superior to those of most of his contemporaries. He was able to keep some of his operated animals alive for years and to study them thoroughly. Thus, he had the opportunity to note restitution of function, when it occurred, as well as certain peculiarities in visual behavior that could not be observed in the acutely operated animal. In 1876 he initiated a series of studies designed to elucidate the cortical basis of sensory and motor functions, the results of which were reported in detail in 16 lengthy communications (Munk, 1890).

With respect to vision, Munk demonstrated beyond reasonable doubt that, at least in dogs and monkeys, complete destruction of both occipital lobes produced permanent loss of vision, a condition which he designated as "cortical blindness." He also showed that complete destruction of a single occipital lobe produced a contralateral hemianopia and not blindness in the opposite eye, as supposed by Ferrier and others. Thus, he established that in the animals which he had studied the cortical "center" for vision was located in the occipital lobes.

Munk's early reports encountered a skeptical reception from other animal experimentalists, particularly on the part of antilocalizationists such as Goltz and close rivals such as Ferrier. But clinicians, already prepared by case reports such as those of Levick (1866) and Pooley (1877), which had raised the possibility of an association between hemianopia and occipital lobe disease, viewed his conclusions much more favorably. Only a year after the publication of Munk's first communication, Baumgarten (1878) described a patient with persistent left homonymous hemianopia and no other signs of brain disease in whom autopsy disclosed a large cyst in the right occipital lobe. He commented that, despite the clear association between the occipital lesion and the hemianopia, he would hesitate to infer a causal connection on the basis of a single case, if it were not for the observation of Munk, who "has been able to produce a lateral hemianopia (corresponding to our case) in monkeys by unilateral extirpation of the cortex of the occipital lobe." A year later, a very similar case was reported by Curschmann (1879). His patient, with a left homonymous hemianopia persisting until death, showed no other signs of brain disease. A focus of softening in the right occipital lobe was found on autopsy, leading Curschmann to conclude that his case confirmed Munk's correlation and to remark with some pride that "in view of the absence of other focal brain symptoms, it has the status of an experiment in man."

Within a few years, Munk's occipital localization of vision was widely accepted, although some of his more specific ideas proved to be incorrect. Reviewing Munk's work through 1883, Starr (1884) concluded that "the large number of animals used, the uniform results of the experiments in all cases, the length of time during which the symptoms persisted, and the minute care displayed in the observations combine to establish the truth of the conclusions reached." Starr added that "it remains for the pathologist to determine whether these facts which are true in the case of monkeys, are true also in the case of man." He proceeded to do this by means of a review of the relevant literature.

In fact, analyses of the evidence bearing on the question had already been published. The first of these was by Exner (1881) in his monograph on cortical localization of function in man. In his review of the findings in 167 autopsied cases reported in the literature through 1879, Exner distinguished between "absolute" cortical fields, lesions of which almost always produced a particular defect, and "relative" cortical fields, lesions of which produced the defect with notable frequency but not invariably. Thus, he classified a major part of the precentral gyrus as an absolute cortical field for motor function in the contralateral limbs since lesions in that area produced impairment in close to 100% of the cases. A larger surrounding territory was designated as a relative cortical field since lesions there produced contralateral motor impairment in 40–90% of the cases.

Although Exner's series was a large one, in only six cases were visual disturbances mentioned. (In contrast, no less than 100 cases presented with motor impairment of an upper extremity.) He was not able to identify an absolute cortical field for vision in that he found no area in which lesions always produced visual disturbances. However, he did find that lesions in a number of loci on the lateral and medial surfaces of the occipital lobes did produce impairment with frequencies ranging from 33–75% and hence he classified the occipital lobes as a relative field for vision. The highest frequency (60–75%) was associated with lesions in the superior part of the first occipital gyrus, leading to his designation of this area as the most "intensive" part of the relative cortical field for vision. Conversely, he found that lesions in the territory of the angular gyrus were associated with visual defect in only about 12% of the cases.

Insofar as vision was concerned, the weakness of Exner's review lay in the fact that even the very few cases with visual disturbance in his series were poorly described and of a heterogeneous character. [Neither Baumgarten's (1878) case nor that of Curschman (1879) was included in his series, although both were published before 1880.] His sparse data could show only that the occipital lobes appeared to be more important than other regions of the cerebral hemispheres in the mediation of visual function. The subsequent analyses of Marchand and Starr of the site of lesion in patients with hemianopic defects were far more informative and convincing.

Marchand (1882) reviewed 22 cases, 11 with a right hemianopic defect and 11 with a left hemianopic defect. Within each subgroup, autopsy study showed involvement of the opposite thalamus or optic tract in five cases, the lesions being for the most part tumors. In the remaining six cases in each subgroup, lesions in the opposite occipital lobe were invariably found, the majority of these being vascular in origin. Stressing the importance of small, circumscribed vascular lesions for the study of cerebral localization, Marchand described a patient with a complete left hemianopia following a stroke whom he studied in 1876. Autopsy disclosed only an area of necrosis in the right occipital lobe. The unsuspected absence of a lesion at the level of the thalamus or the optic tract was at the time quite puzzling and "only after Munk's discoveries did this case gain clarity and interest."

Starr's (1884) case material consisted of 32 cases presenting a right (15 cases) or left (17 cases) hemianopia, either in isolation or as part of an ensemble of deficits. With one exception, all the cases had come to autopsy, the pathology in the exceptional case having been described during the course of surgical intervention. Of the 32 cases, five involved unilateral lesions at the thalamic level, two of these being neoplastic lesions also extending into the occipital lobe. Thirteen cases of right hemianopia were found to have lesions in one of another part of the left occipital lobe. In two of these cases, the field defect had been the only permanent symptom. Similarly, a lesion of the right occipital lobe was found in 14 cases with a left hemianopia, as part of an ensemble of defects in nine, as the only symptom in four, and as the only permanent symptom in one case. Starr concluded that "anatomical research, physiological experiment, and pathological observation unite in assigning to the occipital lobes of the brain the function of sight. The right occipital lobe receives impressions from the right half of both eyes, and the left occipital lobe receives impressions from the left half of both eyes. The visual area of the brain lies in the occipital lobes."

Precise Localization of the Visual Center

From his ablation studies, Munk reached the conclusion that, although complete removal of the occipital lobes was required to produce cortical blindness (and complete removal of one lobe to produce a contralateral hemianopia), their upper convex surface represented the center of clearest vision. He proposed the idea that this area was the site of termination of the pathways from the foveal region of the retina but did not undertake any anatomical studies to demonstrate the point. This was as far as Munk was able to go and, as will be seen, a certain amount of confusion was engendered by his contention that lesions of the same area were also responsible for the production of another type of visual defect which he called "mindblindness." Munk, in 1879, was also the first investigator to propose that there was a fixed relationship between elements of the retina and corresponding loci in the occipital lobe.

The evidence that the primary cortical center for vision was to be found in the calcarine region of the mesial surface of the occipital lobes came from clinicopathologic correlations in patients with discrete lesions in that area. The first case of this type, reported by Huguenin (1881; Haab, 1882), concerned an 8-year-old tubercular girl who developed a left homonymous hemianopia during the course of an illness of 5 months duration. She suffered from headache, convulsions, and general mental impairment, but showed no motor, auditory, somatosensory, or speech defects. Autopsy disclosed two discrete neoplastic lesions, a small one in the left prefrontal area and a slightly larger one on the mesial surface of the right occipital lobe. Since the small left prefrontal lesion could be safely dismissed as the cause of the hemianopia, it was evident that the mesial occipital tumor (Fig. 13–1A) was the crucial lesion.

It was Haab (1882) who first raised the question of whether the mesial, rather than the convex, region of the occipital lobes might be the site of the cortical visual center. Commenting on the findings in Huguenin's case, he remarked: "It is of interest to see that in this case the tumor destroyed precisely the center of the cortical area in which the stripe of Vicq d'Azyr is found. Has this peculiarly structured cortex perhaps specific connections with the visual sense?" (Haab. 1882, p. 149). He went on to describe the findings in a second case which reinforced this possibility. It was that of a 61-year-old man with a left homonymous hemianopia in whom autopsy study again disclosed a lesion in the mesial area of the right occipital lobe. The visual field defect and a slight awkwardness in moving the right arm and leg were the only symptoms shown by this intelligent patient 5 months after a stroke. The hemianopia persisted until the patient's death 3 years later. The only lesion found on autopsy was an area of necrosis surrounding the calcarine fissure in the right occipital lobe (Fig. 13–1B).

An even more precise localization of the cortical visual center in a specific area of the occipital lobe was indicated by the subsequent case report of Hun

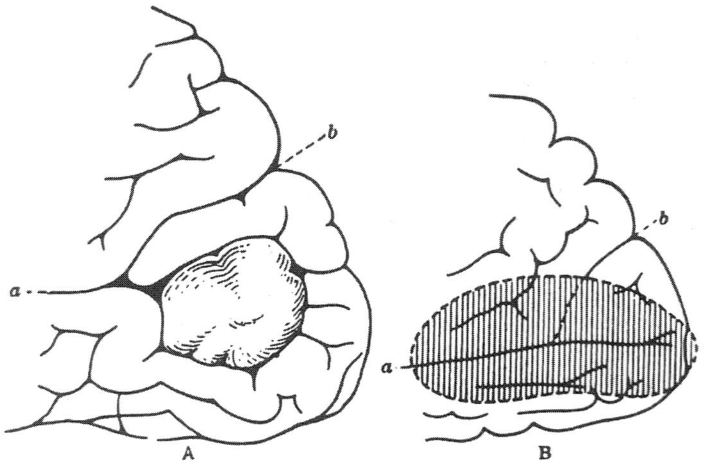

FIGURE **13.1.** **A** Site of lesion on the mesial surface of the right occipital lobe in the case of Huguenin (1881); **B** in the case of Haab (1882). Both patients showed a left homonymous hemianopia during life.

(1887), describing a 57-year-old patient with a left homonymous inferior quadrantanopia of about 2 years duration. The only finding on autopsy, apart from slight dilatation of the lateral ventricles, was a circumscribed atrophic area of cortex just above the calcarine fissure in the right occipital lobe, i.e., in the lower part of the cuneus.

> In this case there is a lesion which destroys the lower half of the right cuneus, and there is one constant symptom which is present during the whole course of the disease: a blindness limited to the lower left quadrant of the field of vision of each eye. In the absence of any other cerebral lesion the destruction of the lower half of the right cuneus must be regarded as the cause of the blindness in the lower left quadrant of each field of vision. . . . This case makes it probable that the fibres from the right upper quadrants of each retina terminate in the lower half of the right cuneus [Hun, 1887. pp. 144–145].

Hun's anatomic inference (or guess) that there was a topographic representation of the retinae onto the mesial surface of the occipital lobes was fully supported by subsequent investigators. Their work has been so well described by Brouwer (1936, pp. 459–482) and Polyak (1955, 179–203) that there is no point in reviewing it once again. It need only be pointed out that the leading investigators of the period, Wilbrand (1887, 1890; Wilbrand and Saenger, 1904, 1917) and Henschen (1890–1896), were primarily clinical researchers who correlated the perimetrically defined visual field defects shown by patients during life with autopsy findings. On the basis of an enormous case material, they were able to demonstrate that there was indeed a "cortical retina," as Henschen called it, on the mesial aspect of the occipital lobes, reflecting a point-to-point correspondence between the receptor surface and the cortical area.

Thus, clinicopathologic study of patients, rather than animal experimentation, provided the first indications of the locus and organization of the cortical visual center. The experimental demonstration that the calcarine region was the primary cortical end-station for vision was made by Minkowski (1911). He first showed that ablation of the cortical area on the convex surface that Munk had designated as the center for foveal vision produced no visual disturbances at all in the dog. He surmised that Munk's results were obtained because of inadvertent injury to the visual radiations which course directly under the cortex of the second and third occipital gyri, and in fact he showed by study of serial sections that, when an ablation presumably limited to the cortex did led to visual defects, the radiations had been invariably injured. Minkowski went on to make complete and partial ablations of the striate area and found, in line with expectations, that complete bilateral destruction caused by permanent blindness, complete unilateral ablation produced a contralateral hemianopia, and partial ablations of the superior and the inferior surface of the striate area produced an inferior and a superior surface of the striate area produced an inferior and superior hemianopia, respectively. Hence, he felt confident in concluding that the striate area constituted the cortical center for vision in the dog and that within this area there was a fixed correspondence between retinal loci and cortical loci.

Visual Agnosia

If locus A, of the cerebral cortex of a dog is extirpated on both sides a peculiar disturbance in vision is noticeable 3–5 days after the injury, at a time when the inflammatory reaction has passed and no abnormality of hearing, smell, taste, movement, and sensation in the animal is present. The dog moves quite freely and easily indoors as well as in the garden without bumping against a single object. If obstacles are placed in his path, he regularly goes around them or, if a detour is not possible, he overcomes them adroitly, e.g., by crawling under a stool or carefully climbing over the man's foot or the animal's body which obstructs his path. But now the sight of people whom he had always greeted joyfully leaves him cold, as does the company of other dogs with whom he used to play. He may be so hungry and thirsty that he is overactive: yet he no longer looks for food in the part of the room where he used to find it. And if the bowl of food and bucket of water are placed directly in his path, he repeatedly goes around them without paying attention to them. Food presented to him visually evokes no response as long as he does not smell it. A finger or fire brought close to the eye no longer makes him blink. The sight of a whip, which invariably used to drive him into a corner, no longer frightens him at all. He had been trained to present the ipsilateral paw when one waved a hand in front of an eye. Now one can wave one's hand indefinitely, the paw remains at rest until one says, "paw." And there are other observations of this nature. There can be no doubt about their interpretation. As a

> result of the extirpation, the dog has become mindblind, i.e., he has lost the visual ideas which he possessed, his memory images of previous visual perceptions, so that he does not know or recognize what he sees. However, the dog sees. Visual sensations reach consciousness and the stage of perception. They make it possible for ideas about the presence, form, and location of external objects to arise so that new visual ideas based on new memory images of the visual perceptions can be acquired.

Thus Munk (1878, pp. 162–163; 1890, pp. 21–22) described for the first time the condition to which he gave the name "mindblindness," and which later came to be designated as "visual agnosia" or "optic agnosia." Concomitantly, he offered an explanation for the condition. The animal had lost his "memory images" of previously perceived stimuli. Consequently, he could not relate current experience to past experience and hence failed to grasp the "meaning" of a perceived stimulus.

But Munk found that mindblindness was only a temporary condition. Within a few weeks, the dog once again could recognize his master and other dogs and once again responded in a normal fashion to them. His explanation was that during the course of postoperative experience, new memory images were laid down in parts of the occipical cortex other than locus A_1. It will be recalled that Munk had specified that locus A_1 was the cortical center for foveal vision as well as the depository of memory images:

Munk's concept received a mixed reception. The fact that mindblindness appeared after a relatively superficial lesion in the very same area that subserved foveal vision and that it was a temporary condition made it seem probable that the animal's impaired behavior was due simply to loss of central vision. His notion that the mindblind dog was reduced to the status of a puppy without a store of visual memory images who could now deposit new images in another part of the occipital cortex seemed quite farfetched. Even his assumption that the mindblind dog's behavior was clearly deviant was questioned. Minkowski (1911), having removed Locus A_1 from dogs without finding either a loss of central vision or signs of "mindblindness," remarked that he had often observed normal dogs to behave "unintelligently" in the face of visual stimuli, showing no response to the brandishing of a whip or sticking their paw in a piece of burning wood.

Consequently a substantial number of investigators, the earliest of whom was Mauthner (1881), interpreted mindblindness as the product of defective central vision perhaps coupled with postoperative mental blunting. For example, Siemerling (1980) studied a patient with mindblindness and was able to demonstrate a reduction in both visual acuity and color sensitivity which he concluded was responsible for the impairment in visual recognition.

But Munk's concept of mindblindness was accepted by other clinicians who observed a similar condition in some of their patients. Wilbrand (1887) and

Lissauer (1890) described such patients who did not recognize objects or persons despite seemingly adequate visual acuity, and they related the condition to focal disease of the occipital lobes. Wilbrand agreed with Munk in attributing the defect to a loss of visual memory images but deviated from his thinking by postulating the existence of a discrete occipital cortical area, separate from the center for visual perception, which he designated the "visual memory field."

For his part, Lissauer (1890) not only presented a detailed description of the behavior of a patient with mindblindness but also offered a thoughtful discussion of the mechanisms that might be operating to produce the defect. The complete act of recognition involves two processes. The first is apperception, i.e., the conscious perception of an object, person, or event, implying the integration of the received sensory data into a unity or entity. The second process is the linking of the content of the perception with past experiences, implying associative activity and conferring meaning on the perception. Theoretically a patient might be rendered mindblind by a defect in one or the other mechanism. In practice, every patient suffering from mindblindness probably suffers from defects in both mechanisms because of the intimate interactive relationship between them. However, the severity of impairment in each might differ significantly. Thus, Lissauer felt that his patient exhibited a primarily associative type of mindblindness since a number of test performances indicated that he had excellent visual discriminative capacity.

One of the points made by Freud (1891) in his monograph on aphasia was the necessity for distinguishing between defects in naming objects and defects in recognizing them if clarity of thinking about the aphasic disorders was to be achieved. He therefore proposed that the term "agnosia" be employed to denote impairment in recognition within the context of adequate basic sensory capacity. His suggestion was generally adopted and "mindblindness" was discarded in favor of "visual agnosia" or "optic agnosia."

Up to this time, the structural characteristics of the occipital lobes and their connections with other hemispheric regions had received little attention. This gap was now filled by detailed anatomic study. Smith (1907) distinguished between morphologically differentiated striate and extrastriate occipital cortex, subdividing the latter into parastriate and peristriate areas. Brodmann (1909) similarly divided extrastriate cortex into an area 18 immediately surrounding striate cortex (area 17) and an outlying preoccipital area 19, a parcellation roughly corresponding to Smith's classification. At the same time, beginning with the work of Flechsig (1901), the connections of the occipital lobes with other cortical areas were investigated. Short association fibers connect area 17 with areas 18 and 19, from which arise longer association tracts leading to other parts of the cerebral hemispheres. These findings provided an anatomical framework for inferences about the lesional basis for disturbances in visual performance. Area 17 was the center for elementary visual experience. Elaboration of that experience into meaningful percepts required the functional integrity of areas 18 and 19, for these regions were the essential link between the primary visual center and the rest of the cortex. Thus, visual agnosia could be conceived as the outcome of lesions in area 18 and 19 which prevented the transmission and eventual integration of information arriving in area 17.

The concept of visual agnosia had had a checkered career since its introduction by Munk and the early studies of human subjects. On the one hand, the "reductionist" interpretation of Mauthner and Siemerling that the disorder is not a higher-level impairment in perceptual integration, association, or memory but only the expression of basic sensory deficit has been supported by some outstanding experimentalists and clinical investigators. The issue is, of course, whether or not the agnosic animal or patient does in fact have at his disposal the sensory information necessary for an accurate cognitive response. For example, Pavlov (1927, 1928) interpreted the mindblindness of Munk not as a higher-level psychological impairment but simply as loss of the capacity to make fine visual discriminations, and he suggested that the classical formula, "the dog sees but does not understand," should be reversed to read "the dog understands but does not see sufficiently well" (Pavlov, 1927, p. 343). Similarly, Bay (1950, 1953, 1954) contended that visual agnosia in patients is explainable in terms of certain defects in visuosensory capacity, these defects typically occurring within the context of general mental impairment which itself hampers the process of drawing conclusions on the basis of inadequate visual information. He placed particular stress on alterations in rate of sensory adaptation as the defect which may underlie the type of behavior called "visual agnosia." Critchley (1964) and Bender and Feldman (1965) also have advanced the view that visual agnosia is essentially the outcome of defective sensory capacity coupled with an overall decline in intellectual level. The "reductionists" have supported their position by citing the fact that practically every patient with visual agnosia is found to have *some* type of visual impairment, such as a field defect, inadequate visual scanning, or a disturbance in ocular fixation.

But the concept of visual agnosia as a "higher-level" disorder was fully accepted by other clinical investigators who described different subtypes of visual agnosia. The rather gross disability shown by Munk's dogs and Lissauer's patient was designated as "visual object-agnosia" while less pervasive disabilities involving one or another aspect of visual perception such as "visual form agnosia," "facial agnosia," and "visuospatial agnosia" were singled out for special study. Countering the argument that these disorders merely represent a partial impairment in basic sensory capacity, the "antireductionists" have pointed to the innumerable cases of severe visual defect that do not show the perceptual–integrative or associative disturbances characteristic of the agnosic patient.

The Method of Double Sensory Stimulation

Jacques Loeb

In 1884, the physiologist Jacques Loeb, who had worked with Goltz in Strasbourg, published a paper on the visual disturbances that follow experimental ablations of the brain in dogs. In it and two subsequent papers (Loeb, 1885, 1886), he described for the first time the responses of operated animals to double bilateral visual stimulation. Having noted that the most frequent immediate effect of unilateral destruction of one cerebral hemisphere is to produce a contralateral hemiamblyopia in which the animal is completely nonresponsive to visual stimulation on that side, he then described the course of recovery from the defect. In the first stage, the dog still does not perceive objects brought slowly into the affected field of vision but may respond to oscillating objects or to those that are rapidly introduced into the field. Further recovery of function then occurs.

> The intensity of stimulus in the crossed visual half-field, which is necessary to elicit a reaction on the part of the dog, decreases steadily. After a time, if a single piece of meat is presented to the dog, he will react to it, even if it is not moved. In addition, when the meat is moved or thrown to the right, the dog follows it just as he would if it were moved or thrown to the left. It would appear from these from these tests that a visual disturbance is no longer present. However, if two pieces of meat are suddenly presented simultaneously to the dog, one in the right and the other in the left visual field, the animal who has been operated in the left hemisphere will without exception take the piece of meat to the left (Loeb. 1886, p. 294).

He then pointed out that such an impairment in response to double visual stimulation may be the only functional outcome of a less destructive cerebral lesion.

> These findings record the course of a rather severe hemiamblyopia from the time of operation to the restitution of visual capacity; however, after superficial lesions and favorable conditions of operation and recovery, the initial disturbance is not as severe as here described. In the majority of cases, only the last described stage is present from the very beginning: the dog takes single pieces of meat under all conditions and favors that situated on the side of the lesion only upon simultaneous presentation of two pieces of meat (Loeb. 1886. pp. 275–276).

Seeking a physiological explanation of this pattern of responsiveness in which stimulation in the affected field is perceived when it is presented in isolation but not reacted to when presented in combination with concurrent stimulation in the healthy field, Loeb postulated that a unilateral hemisphere lesion produced impaired conduction in the involved neural pathways. As a consequence, the reactions mediated by these pathways are slower and weaker than those mediated by the neural connections of the intact hemisphere. In support of this interpretation, he cited the observation that if, under a condition of double stimulation, the intensity of the stimulus in the affected field is augmented to a sufficient degree, it would be perceived along with the stimulus to the healthy field.

Clinical Application

Loeb demonstrated the behavior of his dogs to the clinical neurologist Hermann Oppenheim, who immediately applied the method of double sensory stimulation to patients with brain disease and found some who showed the predicted pattern of responsiveness (Oppenheim, 1885). Thus, two patients who perceived tactile stimulation on their affected side when it was presented in isolation failed to perceive it in combination with stimulation on the healthy side. Another patient showed failure to respond to tactile or visual stimuli when each was paired with corresponding stimulation on the healthy side. Still another patient showed failure to respond adequately to double simultaneous tactile or auditory stimulation. Confirming Loeb's observations on dogs, Oppenheim also reported that augmentation of the intensity of the stimulus on the affected side could lead to the normal perception of both stimuli on the part of a patient.

Finding that the procedure was of clinical value in an occasional case, Oppenheim adopted it as a diagnostic maneuver and described it in his famous textbook of neurology.

> In certain cerebral diseases, which lead to unilateral sensory disturbances, I have often employed the following method of examination: two symmetrical locations on both sides of the body are simultaneously stimulated with touching by a brush or by pinpricks: under these conditions it happens that the patient invariably perceives only the stimulus which has been applied to the healthy side, while with single stimulation he feels every stimulus on the affected side. We shall designate this mode of examination as the method of double stimulation (Oppenheim, 1898, p. 51).

Subsequently the method of double sensory stimulation was utilized for investigative purposes in patients with suspected unilateral lesions by a few neurologists. Poppelreuter (1917) designated defective responsiveness to double visual stimulation as a "hemianopic weakness of attention." Thiébaut and Guillaumat (1945) called the deficit a "relative hemianopsia." The phenomenon was studied in detail by Bender and his co-workers (Bender and Teuber, 1946; Bender et al., 1950; Bender, 1952; Bender and Feldman, 1952), who showed that it occurred in the different sensory modalities, gave it the name of "extinction," and described the diverse forms it may take. It was possible to show with human patients, who could give a verbal report of their experience, that partial extinction of response in the double stimulation paradigm may occur, i.e., the patient perceives the stimulus on the affected side or field but experiences it as weaker than when the stimulus is presented in isolation. Bender called this phenomenon "obscuration."

Utilizing a method of subjective magnitude estimation. Benton and Levin (1972) were able to produce the "obscuration" response in normal subjects by appropriate manipulation of the relative strength of competing tactile stimuli. Another type of deviant response, originally described by Jones (1907), was a tendency on the part of patients with unilateral lesions to report that both limbs had been touched when in fact stimulation had been applied only to the ipsilateral limb.

Eighty years after Loeb's pioneer studies, extinction to bilateral sensory stimulation was once again investigated experimentally in animals by Schwartz and Eidelberg (1968). Having been trained to respond differentially to electrical stimulation of the right, left, and both hands, monkeys were subjected to unilateral parietal and frontal ablations. Postoperatively a tendency to respond to double tactile stimulation as if single stimulation had been delivered to the hand ipsilateral to the side of lesion was observed. Daily fluctuations in the relative frequency of extinction responses, noted by Bender in patients, were also noted. Moreover, some animals showed the phenomenon of "synchiria" reported by Jones in patients, i.e., they responded to single stimulation of the limb ipsilateral to the side of the lesion as if double stimulation had been applied.

Concluding Comments

This sketch of the successive stages in the development of investigative work on two topics in the area of brain lesion research indicates how the experimental and clinical approaches interacted to advance understanding of the specific problem. As was mentioned earlier in the chapter, the initial observations were made on animals and these provided the impetus for analogous and more refined study of human subjects. In turn, the results of clinical study led to more detailed experimental investigation in animals. Thus, Munk's conclusion that the cortical mechanisms mediating visual function were located in the occipital lobes received a much more favorable reception from clinicians than from his fellow experimentalists, whose own preconceptions hindered acceptance. In contrast, as Marchand and others pointed out, clinicians found Munk's results helpful in explaining previous observations, the significance of which had not been at all clear. Once Munk's experiments showed clinicians where to look for the cortical lesions producing visual impairment, they took full advantage of the experiments of nature that came their way and they were able to go far beyond the experimentalists of the period in establishing precise anatomical–behavioral correlations. Given this background of knowledge, Minkowski could once again investigate the problem in greater depth and provide experimental confirmation of the clinical correlations.

Is it the rule that the interplay of experimental and clinical research on a brain–behavior problem is likely to be initiated by observations in animals? There is probably no such rule. The choice of a starting point in recounting the history of investigative work on a particular topic is largely determined by one's perception of whose work was particularly influential in determining the direction of subsequent research. With respect to vision, the experiments of Ferrier and Munk certainly meet this criterion and, hence, one regards them as pioneers. But their efforts were surely inspired by the discovery of the excitable motor cortex by Fritsch and Hitzig, who, on their part, cited earlier clinical observations relating discrete paralyses to focal brain lesions in support of the principle of cortical localization of motor function.

As early as 1874, Jackson advanced the concept that the posterior area of the right hemisphere subserved visual recognition and visual memory in human subjects. Subsequently, he published a case report in support of it (Jackson, 1876). Ferrier was quite familiar with Jackson's ideas along these lines and indeed referred to them as "hypotheses deserving consideration and further investigation" (Ferrier, 1878, p. 119). Thus, one could consider that Jackson was the "real" pioneer in pointing to a posterior representation of visual function or even Panizza (1855), whose early contribution seems to have been completely ignored at the time of its publication. Attention was called to it only after the publication of Munk's research (cf. Tamburini, 1880). And Panizza reported both experimental findings and clinical observations to make his point.

Thus, it seems rather fruitless to attempt to determine a starting point in an absolute sense and to ask whether this was represented by animal experimentation or clinical observation. The important fact is that, generally speaking, both the experimentalists and the clinicians kept themselves informed about developments in the others' field and took full advantage of these developments.

References

Baumgarten P. (1878). Hemiopie nach Erkrankung der occipitalen Hirnrinde. *Centralblatt für die Medicinischen Wissenschaften* 16: 369–371.

Bay F., (1950). *Agnosie und Funktionswandel.* Berlin: Springer-Verlag.

Bay F., (1953). Disturbances of visual perception and their examination. *Brain.* 76: 515–550.

Bay F., (1954). Optische Faktoren bei den räumlichen Orientierungsstörungen. *Deutsche Zeitschrift für Nervenheilkunde* 171: 454–459.

Bender M. B. (1952). *Disorders in perception.* Springfield. Ill.: Charles C. Thomas.

Bender M. B. and Feldman D. S. (1952). Extinction of taste sensation on double simultaneous stimulation. *Neurology* 2: 195–202.

Bender M. B. and Feldman M. (1965). The so-called "visual agnosias." *Proceedings, VIII International Congress of Neurology* pp. 153–156.

Bender M. B. and Teuber H. I., (1946). Phenomena of fluctuation, extinction and completion in visual perception *Arch.* Neurol. Psychiatry 55: 627–658.

Bender M. B., Teuber H.-I., and Battersby W. S. (1950). Discrimination of weights by men with penetrating lesions of parietal lobes. *Trans. Am. Neurolog. Assoc.* 75: 252–255.

Benton A. I., and Levin H. S. (1972). An experimental study of "obscuration." Neurology 22: 1176–1181.

Brodmann K. (1909). *Vertgleichende Lokalisationslehre der Grosshirnrinde.* Leipzig: J. A. Barth.

Brouwer B. (1936). Chiasma. Tractus opticus. Sehstrahlung and Sehrinde. In Bumke O. and Foerster. (eds.), *Handbuch der Neurologie*, Vol. 6. Berlin: Springer-Verlag.

Chaillou F. H. (1863). Ramollissement multiple du cerveau. *Bulletin de la Société Anatomique de Paris* 8 (2nd Ser.): 70–73.

Critchley M. (1864). The problem of visual agnosia. *J. Neuro. Sci.* 1: 274–290.

Curschmann H. (1879). Die lehre von der Hemianopsie und von den cerebralen Centren des Gesichtssinnes. *Centralblatt für Praktische Augenheilkunde* 3: 181–182.

Exner S. (1881). *Untersuchungen uber die Localization-der Functionen in der Grosshirnrinde des Menschen.* Wien: Wilhelm Braunmüller.

Ferrier D. (1878). *The Localisation of Cerebral Disease.* London: Smith, Elder and Co.

Ferrier D. (1876)The Functions of the Brain. London: Smith. Elder and Co.(2nd ed., 1886).

Ferrier D. (1890). *The Croonian Lectures on Cerebral Localisation.* London: Smith. Elder and Co.

Flechsig P. (1901). Developmental (myelogenetic) localisation of the cerebral cortex in the human subject. *Lancet* 2: 1027–1029.

Freud S. (1891). *Zur Auffassung der Aphasien.* Leipzig und Wien: Deuticke.

Fritsch G. and Hitzig E. (1870). Ueber die elektrische Erregbarkeit des Grosshirns. *Archiv fur Anatomie. Physiologie und Wissenschaftliche Medizin* (Leipzig) pp. 300–332.

Gratiolet P. (1854). Note sur les expansions des racines cérébrales du nerf optique et sur leur terminaison dans une région determinée de l'écorce des hémisphères. *Comptes Rendus de l'Académie des Sciences* (Paris) 29: 274–278.

Haab O. (1882). Ueber Cortex-Hemianopie. *Klinische Monatsblätter für Augenheilkunde* 20: 141–153.

Henschen S. E. (1890–96). *Klinische und anatomische Beiträge zur Pathologie des Gehirns*, Parts 1–3. Upsala: Almquist and Wiksell.

Huguenin G. (1881). Ueber Hemiopie. *Korresponden-Blatt für Schweizer Aerzte* 11: 43–44.

Hun H. (1887). A clinical study of cerebral localization, illustrated by seven cases. *Am. J. Med. Sci.* 93: 140–168.

Jackson J. H. (1874). On the nature of the duality of the brain. *Medical Press and Circular* 1874 (reprinted in *Brain* 38: (1915), 80–103).

Jackson J. H. (1876). Case of large cerebral tumour without optic neuritis and with left hemiplegia and imperception. *Royal Ophthalmic Hospital Reports* 8: 434–444.

Jones F. (1907). The precise diagnostic value of allochiria. *Brain* 30: 490–532.

Levick. (1866). Abscess of brain. *Am. J. Med. Sci.* 52: 413–414.

Lissauer H. (1890). Ein Fall von Seelenblindheit nebst einem Beitrag zúr Theorie derselben. *Archiv für Psychiatrie und Nervenkrankheiten* 21: 222–270.

Loeb J. (1884). Die Sehstörungen nach Verletzung der Grosshirnrinde. *Pfluger's Archiv für die Gesamte Physiologie* 34: 67–172.

Loeb J. (1885). Die elementaren Störungen einfacher Functionen nach oberflächlicher, umschriebener Verletzung des Grosshirns. *Pfluger's Archiv für die Gesamte Physiologie* 37: 51–56.

Loeb J. (1886). Beiträge zur Physiologie des Grosshirns. *Pflüger's Archiv für die Gesamte Physiologie* 39: 265–346.

Marchand F. (1882). Beitrag zur Kenntnis der homonymen bilateralen Hemianopsie und der Faserkreuzung im Chiasma opticum. *Graefe's Archiv für Ophthalmologie* 28: 63–96.

Mauthner L. (1881). *Gehirn und Auge*. Wiesbaden: Bergmann.

Meynert T. (1869). Beiträge zur Kenntnis der centralen Projection der Sinnesoberflächen. *Sitzungsberichte der Kaiserlichen Akademie der Wissenschaften, Mathematisch-Naturwissenschaftliche Classe* (Wien) 60: 547–566.

Minkowski M. (1911) Zur Physiologie der corticalen Sehsphäre. *Deutsche Zeitschrift für Nervenheilkunde* 1: 109–118.

Munk H. (1878). Weitere Mittheilungen zur Physiologie der Grosshirnrinde. *Archiv für Anatomie und Physiologie* 2: 162–178.

Munk H. (1879). Weiteres zur Physiologie der Sehsphäre der Grosshirnrinde. *Archiv für Anatomie und Physiologie* 3: 581–592.

Munk H. (1890). *Ueber die Functionen der Grosshirnrinde*. Berlin: August Hirschwald.

Oppenheim H. (1885). Ueber eine durch eine klinisch bisher nicht verwerthete Untersuchungs-methode ermittlete Form der Sensibilitätsstörung bei einseitigen Erkrankungen des Grosshirns. *Neurologisches Zentralblatt* 4: 529–533.

Oppenheim H. (1898). *Lehrbuch der Nervenkrankheiteu fur Aerzte und Studirende*, II Aufl. Berlin: Karger.

Panizza B. (1855). Osservazioni sul nervo ottico. *Giornale, Istituto Lombardo di Scienze e Lettere*, 7: 237–252.

Pavlov I. P. (1927). *Conditioned Reflexes*. London: Oxford University Press.

Pavlov I. P. (1928). *Lectures on Conditioned Reflexes*. New York: International Publishers.

Polyak S. (1955). *The Vertebrate Visual System*. Chicago: University of Chicago Press.

Pooley T. R. (1877). Rechtseitige binoculare Hemiopie bedingt durch eine Gummigeschwulst im linkeren hinteren Gehirnlappen. *Archiv für Augen und Ohrenheilkunde* 6: 27–29.

Poppelreuter W. (1917) *Die psychischen Schädigungen durch Kopfschuss im Kriege 1914–1916: die Störungen der niederen und höheren Sehleistungen durch Verletzungen des Okzipitalhirns* Leipzig: Voss.

Schäfer E. A. (1888). Experiments on special sense localisation in the cortex cerebri of the monkey. *Brain* 10: 362–380.

Schwartz A. S. and Eidelberg, E. (1968). "Extinction" to bilateral simultaneous stimulation in the monkey. *Neurology* 18: 61–68.

Siemerling E. (1890). Ein Fall von sogenannter Seelenblindheit nebst anderweitigen cerebralen symptomen. *Archiv für Psychiatrie und Nervenkrankheiten* 21: 28–299.

Smith G. E. (1907). New studies on the folding of the visual cortex and the significance of the occipital sulci in the human brain. *J. Anat.* 41: 189–207.

Starr M. A. (1884). The visual area in the brain determined by a study of hemianopsia. *Am. J. Med. Sci.* 87: 65–83.

Tamburini A. (1880). Rivendicazione al Panizza della scoperta del centro visivo corticale. *Revista Sperimentale di Freniatria e Medicina Legale* 6: 153–154.

Thiébaut F. and Guillaumat L. (1945). Hémianopsie relative. *Rev. Neurol.* (Pavis) 77: 129–130.

Wilbrand H. (1887). *Die Seelenblindheit als Herderscheinung und ihre Beziehungen zur homonymen Hemianopsie*. Wiesbaden: J. F. Bergmann.

Wilbrand H. (1890). *Die hemianopischen Gesichtsfeld-Formen und das optische Wahrnehmungszentrum*. Weisbaden: J. F. Bergmann.

Wilbrand H. and Saenger A. (1904, 1917) *Die Neurologie des Auges*. Vol. 3 (1904), Vol. 7 (1917). Wiesbaden: J. F. Bergmann.

14

Basic Approaches to Neuropsychological Assessment

The term "neuropsychological assessment" refers to the objective evaluation of the cognitive, linguistic, perceptual, and psychomotor performances of a person with the aim of relating the status of his performances to the structural and functional condition of his brain. Within this broad aim, two specific purposes can be discerned. On the one hand, given a patient with an identified brain lesion, neuropsychological assessment is utilized to define the behavioral consequences of the lesion. On the other hand, given a patient in whom there is a question about the presence or extent of brain disease, neuropsychological assessment is utilized for the purpose of inferring brain status and hence as an aid in resolving the question.

Neuropsychological assessment originated in the attempts by physicians in the late nineteenth century to evaluate the behavioral capacities of patients with brain disease more reliably and more comprehensively than was possible from the superficial observations in the conventional clinical examination of that period. Called upon to answer important practical questions such as the legal competence of an aphasic patient or the vocational capabilities and eligibility for a pension of a patient with a head injury, they found themselves poorly equipped to meet this responsibility. It was within the context of a search for more adequate answers to these questions that tests for assessing diverse cognitive functions were first developed. At the same time, scientific developments during the 1870s and 1880s (the "golden age of cerebral localization") provided an impetus for the application of experimental findings to clinical practice. For example, the 'mindblindness' resulting from partial occipital lobe ablations in dogs de-

Reprinted with permission from S. R. Steinhauer, J. H. Gruzelier, and J. Zubin (eds.), *Handbook of Schizophrenia, Vol. 5: Neuropsychology, Psychophysiology and Information Processing*. © Elsevier Science Publishers B.V., 1991.

scribed by the physiologist Hermann Munk (1878) impelled clinicians to look for the same type of "higher-level" visuoperceptive deficit in patients and to relate its presence to occipital lobe disease (Wilbrand, 1887; Lissauer, 1890). Similarly, the method of double simultaneous sensory stimulation devised by Jacques Loeb (1884, 1885) to elicit evidence of lateralized inattention or "neglect" in dogs with focal cerebral ablations was quickly adopted and expanded by the clinical neurologist Hermann Oppenheim (1885) as a test for the presence of a unilateral lesion in patients.

The first systematic neuropsychological test battery was published in 1888 by the Würzburg neuropsychiatrist Conrad Rieger (1888). His comprehensive battery, which took several hours to give, consisted of about 40 tests assessing diverse cognitive and perceptual capacities, as well as language functions and motor skills. It is doubtful that this lengthy examination was used very much outside the Würzburg University Psychiatric Clinic but it did serve as a model for the later more widely employed test batteries and mental status outlines assembled by Heilbronner (1905), Rossalimo (1911), Poppelreuter (1917), Franz (1919), Gelb and Goldstein (1920), and Lipmann (1922). During the same period, single-purpose tests for assessing one or another cognitive function, e.g., the "absurdities" test of Liepmann (1905) and the visual memory test of Sapas (1918), were also developed in a number of clinics. In addition, intelligence test scales (most notably the Binet and the Wechsler tests) were widely used for purposes of neuropsychological assessment.

By 1943 a large variety of single tests and a number of test batteries (Conkey, 1938; Shipley, 1940; Benton and Howell, 1941; Goldstein and Scheerer, 1941; Wells and Reusch, 1948; Hunt, 1943) were available to the clinical examiner and researcher for assessing the cognitive capacities (in the broadest sense) of neurological and psychiatric patients. These resources provided the background for the neuropsychological assessment procedures that were developed after World War II and are in current use.

The Nature of Neuropsychological Assessment

Neuropsychological assessment is distinguished from more global and impressionistic approaches to behavioral evaluation by its more objective character, i.e., by its employment of the "method of tests" to generate information that can serve as a basis for clinical judgment. The method of tests differs from the other approaches in a number of respects. A test is a restricted form of behavioral observation in which a specific type of behavior (e.g., verbal repetition, execution of a motor act on verbal command, copying a specific design, naming a visually presented object) is elicited under controlled stimulus conditions and described in objective and quantitative language. Control of stimulus conditions is achieved by presenting a defined task or stimulus-complex in a standard manner to every patient. The task or stimulus-complex is designed in such a way that the examiner is able to record the patient's responses in more or less precise quantitative terms. Additionally, by the use of instrumentation, the method of tests permits the study of behavioral phenomena that are difficult (and sometimes impossible) to observe clinically, e.g., speed of perception through tachistoscopic study, visuoconstructional performance through special tasks, capacity for abstract thinking through sorting tests. Finally, by appropriate manipulation of stimulus conditions and response requirements, the method of tests provides the opportunity to analyze the components of a performance and thus to identify the basic disability underlying a detective performance. For example, given a patient who exhibits slowed behavior and about whom the question of whether his slowness reflects motor retardation (bradykinesia) or slowness in thinking (bradyphrenia) has been raised, the combined administration of simple and complex reaction time tasks may serve to identify his basic disability as being primarily motoric in nature or, in contrast, primarily on the level of decision-making.

It is evident that neuropsychological assessment differs from conventional clinical observation in a number of respects. It is certainly more objective and more quantitative and these characteristics sometimes have led to its categorization as a "laboratory procedure" in the same class as serology, clinical chemistry, neuroradiology and electroencephalography. This is a misconception of its nature. Neuropsychological assessment consists essentially of a set of clinical examination procedures and hence does not differ in kind from conventional clinical observation. Both neuropsychological assessment and clinical observation deal with the same basic data, namely, the behavior of the patient. Neuropsychological assessment may be viewed as a refinement and extension of clinical observation—a refinement in that it describes a patient's performances more precisely and reliably and an extension in that, through instrumentation and special test procedures, it elicits types of performance that are not accessible to the clinical observer.

Nor do neuropsychological tests differ in kind from other behavioral tests. A neuropsychological test is defined by the use to which it is put, namely, to relate behavior to brain status, not by its intrinsic nature. Indeed, by focusing on different aspects of a subject's performance, the same test may be used as a neuropsychological measure to probe for the presence of cerebral dysfunction, as a personality test to bring to light emotional dispositions and conflicts, as a measure of "general intelligence," or even as a test of vocational aptitude. The Rorschach test (Goldfried et al., 1971) and the Wechsler scales (Matarazzo, 1972) have been used for all these purposes.

A related consideration is that all specific behaviors (including task performances) have multiple determinants and hence that failure on a neuropsychological test may be produced by factors of a diverse nature. Thus, when performance deficits are elicited in a neuropsychological examination, other possible determinants of the failure must be considered before the inference of cerebral abnormality is made. Among these determinants are poor cooperation and effort on the part of apathetic, preoccupied, hostile, asocial or paranoid patients, lack of energy in patients who are depressed or who are depleted by systemic extracerebral disease, inattention associated with preoccupation or anxiety, simulation or exaggeration of mental incompetence, and poor understanding and task adjustment on the part of culturally handicapped patients. These considerations apply with considerable force to the neuropsychological assessment of psychiatric patients, who by definition exhibit one or another form of behavioral deficit.

The Validation of Neuropsychological Tests

The question of how accurately neuropsychological assessment procedures reflect the status of underlying cerebral mechanisms is not an altogether simple one. The administration of neuropsychological tests to patients with the aim of inferring the presence or absence of brain pathology represents the clinical application of the knowledge and assumptions about human brain–behavior relationships at a given point in time. As advances in knowledge are achieved (and old assumptions discarded) as a result of systematic clinicopathologic correlations, basic concepts change and with them the interpretation of neuropsychological test performances. For example, block design and stick-construction test performances were once regarded as measures of the "abstract attitude," with failure on these tasks being particularly related to frontal lobe dysfunction (Goldstein and Scheerer, 1941). But subsequent clinicopathologic study established that defective performance reflected visuoperceptive disability and was more closely related to posterior right hemisphere disease. The interpretation of patients' behavior on these tests changed accordingly (Benton et al., 1983; Lezak, 1983; Benton, 1984; Benton, 1985). Thus the validity of neuropsychological test procedures rests ultimately on the validity of the conceptions and corpus of knowledge on which they are based.

The study of brain–behavior relationships in dementia illustrates the problems in interpretation that may arise when measures of behavioral competence are correlated with measures of cerebral status derived from procedures such as autopsy, CT scan and PET scan. Autopsy findings are often regarded as the "gold standard" against which other measures, behavioral or infrabehavioral, are validated. There is some question whether the necropsy always deserves this exalted status. Examination of a dead brain months or years after the behavioral assessment, which will be correlated with it, reflects the changes produced by intervening disease and by death itself as well as the progressive behavioral and cerebral changes occurring after the time of assessment of the living patient. These extraneous factors must surely attenuate the size of observed correlations.

In any case, autopsy (and also biopsy) studies have disclosed significant correlations of moderate size between diverse measures of behavioral competence and measurements of the severity of structural brain abnormality as indexed by counts of senile plaques and neurofibrillary tangles in the cortex of patients with the diagnosis of dementia of the Alzheimer type (Blessed et al., 1968; Farmer et al., 1976; Perry et al., 1978; Wilcock and Esiri, 1982; Wilcock et al., 1982; Neary and Snowden, 1985). The reported correlation coefficients have ranged from approximately 0.25 to 0.75 in different studies utilizing a variety of measures of cognitive functions.

The widely cited studies of the Newcastle team of investigators (Blessed et al., 1968; Roth et al., 1966; Tomlinson et al., 1968; Tomlinson et al., 1970) reported relatively high correlation coefficients between mean plaque counts from sections taken from eight cortical areas and estimated severity of dementia as measured by test performances and ratings of "real-life" behavioral competence by nurses and relatives. Specifically, a correlation coefficient of 0.59 (ca. 35% common variance) was obtained for the plaque vs. test score association and 0.77 (ca. 59% common variance) for the plaque vs. "real-life" competence association. However, the subsequent study of Wilcock and Esiri (1982) found a smaller correlation coefficient between plaque count and estimated severity of dementia (ca. 0.40) but, in contrast, a somewhat higher coefficient (ca. 0.55) between count of neurofibrillary tangles and estimated severity of dementia. The biopsy study of Neary and Snowden (1985) showed the same trend with correlation coefficients of about 0.30 between plaque counts and degree of dementia and about 0.55 between tangle counts and degree of dementia. Wilcock et al. (1982) measured choline acetyltransferase activity in autopsy samples of the brains of demented patients and found correlation coefficients ranging from −0.38 to −0.67 between activity level and estimated severity of dementia. The biopsy study of Neary and Snowden (1985) generated similar findings of correlations of modest size between degree of dementia and both choline acetyltransferase activity and acetylcholine synthesis. Finally, all studies investigating the question have found that the structural and biochemical measures are intercorrelated to a modest degree, e.g., about 0.30 between plaques and tangles (Wilcock and Esiri, 1982); about −0.22 between plaques and choline acetyltransferase activity (Wilcock et al., 1982); about −0.26 between plaques and acetylcholine synthesis (Neary and Snowden, 1985); and about −0.44 between tangles and choline acetyltransferase activity (Wilcock and Esiri, 1982).

The substantial number of studies investigating the association of computed axial tomography (CT) and magnetic resonance imaging (MRI) measures with cognitive functions in elderly and demented patients have yielded correlations of the same size and in the same range as are found in autopsy studies (Earnest et al., 1979; Kaszniak et al., 1979; Wu et al., 1981; Delcon et al., 1980; Bird et al., 1986). The report of Wu et al. (1981) may serve as a representative example. Fifty-five male patients in the age range of 50–77 years who had been referred for CT scan because of mental impairment, headache, seizures and a number of other complaints were given a battery of tests assessing orientation and memory and the Wechsler Adult Intelligence Scale (WAIS). Computed tomography scans showing focal disease had been excluded from consideration. Two indexes, a composite measure of frontal, caudate and sulcal measurements and a "subjective" six-point rating of the scans ranging from "normal" through "moderate atrophy" to "severe atrophy," were used in the main correlational analyses. The obtained correlation coefficients (corrected for age and educational level of the patients) with the cognitive measures ranged from −0.09 to −0.45 for the composite index and from −0.24 to −0.46 for the "subjective" rating. The correlation coefficients between both measurements and WAIS score were practically equal (−0.36 and −0.37). Not surprisingly, the two CT measures were substantially intercorrelated ($r = 0.77$).

The overall results of these correlational studies are clear enough. Relationships between the severity of behavioral impairment and the severity of structural or functional cerebral abnormality have been firmly established. But, from a quantitative standpoint, the observed correlations are at best moderate in size and they account for only a small part of the common variance of the behavioral and cerebral measures. There are, of course, many possible reasons for these rather unimpressive findings. The newer neurodiagnostic techniques are still in a rapid stage of development and it is evident that in their present state their capacity to disclose cerebral abnormality is limited with specific limitations associated with specific procedures. For example, MRI is capable of disclosing multifocal and white matter lesions in cases of "diffuse" closed head injury that are not detected by CT scan (Gandy et al., 1984; Han et al., 1984; Levin et al., 1985a, b). On the other hand, some types of lesion (e.g., punctate foci of calcification) are better visualized in CT scans (Brant-Zawadzki et al., 1983). Needless to say, these comparative observations hold only for the particular stage of technical development and clinical sophistication at which they were made.

There is also the factor of the still relatively limited experience with these procedures on the part of radiologists, neurologists, and other experts who are still learning to discriminate true abnormality from artifact and to identify the changes of major clinical significance. Finally, there is a question of whether the most commonly employed psychological test procedures provide optimal behavioral measures of the behavioral functions mediated by cerebral neural networks. On the one hand, there is the finding of the Newcastle team (Blessed et al., 1968) that ratings of "real-life" behavioral competence correlated more closely ($r = -0.77$) with plaque counts than did scores on their test battery ($r = -0.59$). On the other hand, in the study of Neary and Snowden (1985), performance on a continuous visual reaction time task correlated as closely with neurofibrillary tangle counts as did scores on the more complex WAIS and Token tests. The early literature includes many studies that evaluated the ability of various tests to discriminate between brain-diseased and control patients (Spreen and Benton, 1965). But there is a death of comparable "second generation" studies of this type assessing the sensitivity of diverse behavioral measures to the extent and type of brain change as disclosed by the newer neurodiagnostic techniques.

The rapidly changing status of both neuropsychological and neuropathological–biochemical diagnostic procedures indicates that at the present time it is not possible to draw any firm conclusions about the validity of neuropsychological assessment, as defined by its agreement with criterion measures, since the criterion measures themselves have still to be defined. Indeed, in the pathological–biochemical studies of dementia which have been cited, the criterion measure against which the neurodiagnostic techniques are evaluated is the behavioral status of the patient as defined by neuropsychological test performances or ratings of behavioral competence.

Neuropsychological Assessment in Clinical Diagnosis

As has been noted, neuropsychological test procedures represent a refinement and extension of clinical observation. Possibly it is best conceived as a special form of clinical observation that provides a distinctive set of data to be considered separately from the information emerging from the conventional clinical examination and to be integrated with it in reaching a diagnostic judgment.

The usefulness of the distinctive set of data generated by neuropsychological assessments can scarcely be questioned. It can confirm or negate clinical impressions, bring to light new facts and suggest relationships that were not suspected. The scope of application of neuropsychological test procedures has extended far beyond the fields of neurology, neurosurgery, and psychiatry. Their employment in clinical pharmacology is, of course, well known. In addition, they have been utilized to advantage in anesthesiology, toxicology, cardiac surgery, and internal medicine where neuropsychological test findings have proved to be indispensable in addressing unresolved questions such as, for example, the effects of environmental toxins, the neuropsychiatric sequelae of open heart surgery, the effects of hemodialysis on cognitive functions and the intellectual changes associated with metabolic diseases. In these instances, the objective quantitative information from the tests has provided the core data required to clarify controversial issues.

One of the strengths of neuropsychological assessment is that for the most part their development and application are based on empirically derived normative determinations rather than on subjective impressions of what constitutes a normal performance. Adequate standardization of a test requires not only that a sufficient number of subjects be assessed in order to establish the range of normal variation but also that the influence of age, educational level, and sex on performance be ascertained so that the score of an individual patient can be correctly interpreted. Subjective impression of what constitutes a normal performance carries with it the risk either of ignoring the significance of factors such as age and educational background or, conversely, of overestimating their influence. There is also the uncontrolled factor of interindividual variation in judgment among clinical examiners.

The assessment of temporal orientation in patients provides an illustration of how empirically based normative information may differ from clinical impressions of "normality." The evaluation of accuracy of temporal orientation is, of course, a stable feature of the mental status examination. Yet most textbooks of neurology and psychiatry and manuals for the mental status examination, which direct the reader to ask the patient to state the year, month, day of month, day of week and time of day, do not give any indication of the range of normal performance. Thus it is left to the examiner to decide how great a deviation (if any) from a perfect performance should be interpreted as indicative of impaired temporal orientation.

Empirical studies of temporal orientation in normal subjects, patients with brain disease and psychiatric patients have established the range of normal performance as well as the frequency of defective performance in different diagnostic groups (Benton et al., 1964; Levin and Benton, 1975; Joslyn and Hutzell, 1979; Natelson et al., 1979). Briefly stated, the findings from a structured interview indicated that 95% of normal subjects made either perfect or near-perfect performances, e.g., misstating the day of the month by 1 or 2 days or misstating the day of week by 1 day. None misstated the year or the month. With these normative data as a basis for comparison, it was found that 24% of a sample of non-aphasic patients with brain disease performed defectively, 9% on a moderately defective level (poorer than 95%–99% of controls) and 15% at a severely defective level (poorer than 99.5% of controls). Comparison of these findings with notations in the patients' charts disclosed that, while almost all of the severely disoriented patients had been identified on clinical examination, none of the patients with moderately defective orientation had been detected. Further investigation indicated that the probable reason why the moderately disoriented patients had been described as "oriented for time, place, and person" was that clinical neurologists' estimates of the range of normal variation tend to be too broad. Thus, in response to a questionnaire, their median estimates were that 2 in 100 normal subjects would misstate the year and that 5 in 100 would misstate the month, whereas the normative data showed that these errors are not found in normal subjects. The clinical significance of this discrepancy between objective determinations and clinical judgments of "normality" is reflected in the finding that moderate impairment in temporal orientation is a useful sign of early dementia (Eslinger et al., 1985).

Another characteristic of neuropsychological assessment is that a well-constructed test is so designed that it can define the boundaries of a specific cognitive ability, i.e., the level at which a patient performs fully adequately and the level at which he fails. To achieve this aim it may be necessary to standardize a test (or different versions of it) on different diagnostic groups, e.g., normal subjects, non-aphasic brain-diseased patients, aphasic patients, so that not only will the limits of a patient's capacity be defined but also his placement within his own diagnostic group.

A study of visual confrontation naming, a capacity that is assessed in every examination of a patient with suspected aphasia or dementia, will be cited to illustrate the first point that a test of appropriate difficulty level is required to arrive at a correct evaluation. In this study (Benton, 1973), the naming performances of a group of clinically aphasic patients were assessed by both the conventional procedure of the clinical examination of having him name a few common objects (or pictures of them) and by a standardized and more demanding test of the capacity. As shown in Table 14–1, the clinical test consisted in the presentation of six objects to be named while the standardized test consisted in the presentation of 30 pictures. It will be noted that all control patients performed perfectly on the object naming test while the more demanding picture naming test produced a range of scores. When defective performance was defined as a score below that of the poorest control patient, the object naming test identified only 29% of the aphasics as impaired, presumably leading to the conclusion that the "naming function" was essentially intact in 71%. But the picture naming test, which was more effective in defining the limits of naming capacity, identified 83% of the aphasics in this sample as defective, a result which is more in accord with clinical experience. Thus the findings of the study demonstrated

TABLE 14–1. Visual Confrontation Naming: Performances of Control and Aphasic Patients*

TEST	CONTROLS RANGE OF SCORES	APHASICS DEFECTIVE PERFORMANCES
Six objects†	(All perfect performance)	29% (scores below 6)
Multilingual aphasia examination: visual naming	40–60	83% (scores below 40)

*Benton (1973).

†Key, pencil, comb, knife, ring, plate.

fairly conclusively that a test of appropriate difficulty level is necessary to elicit evidence of defective naming in all but the most severely disabled patients. Since it is the patient with only a mild or moderate degree of disability who is likely to present a diagnostic problem, the clinical importance of utilizing an adequate test for the assessment of naming ability is obvious.

Visual confrontation naming may also serve as an example of the clinical utility of multiple standardizations of a neuropsychological test. In addition to its standardization on a normative sample of control patients (i.e., without history or evidence of brain disease), the visual naming test mentioned above was also standardized on a "reference" group of aphasic patients formed on the basis of certain restrictive criteria (Benton and Hamsher, 1983). The percentile ranks of the scores of these patients as defined by the score distributions of both the control patients and the aphasic patients are shown in Table 14–2. Inspection of the table shows that 60% of the aphasics scored below the entire distribution of the control patients. Thus utilization of normative standards based on the performances of control patients would be of no value for monitoring the course of the disorder or evaluating the effects of therapy in many of these patients in whom significant changes in performance level would not be reflected in changes in percentile ranks. On the other hand, utilization of the standards for the aphasic reference group would reflect even modest changes in performance level. Conversely, norms for the aphasic reference group would scarcely be appropriate for detecting a modest decline in naming ability in a suspected beginning aphasia or dementia.

The distinctive clinical utility of neuropsychological assessment, i.e., the de-

TABLE 14–2. Visual Naming: Distribution of Scores of Aphasic Patients*

SCORE	N	PERCENTILE	CORRESPONDING PERCENTILE OF CONTROL SUBJECTS
60	—		
58	—		
50–56	5	92–100	27–64
48	2	88–90	18
44–46	7	74–86	7–12
40–42	6	62–72	2–5
32–38	5	52–60	0
24–30	7	38–50	0
16–22	7	24–36	0
8–14	4	15–22	0
0–6	7	0–14	0

*Benton and Hamsher (1983).

gree to which it can contribute *new* information to the diagnostic workup, can be evaluated most directly in situations where the findings of the clinical examination and the neuropsychological assessment are not congruent, e.g., where one approach has yielded positive findings and the other negative or questionable findings. An example of this type of situation was described by Poitrenaud and Barrere (1973) of the Centre de Gérontologie Claude Bernard in Paris. Their study evaluated the predictive significance of a battery of tests given to 46 ambulatory patients who were judged not to be demented but who nevertheless were referred for neuropsychological assessment because of equivocal findings on clinical examination or their own complaints of mental difficulties. Five years later their status was again evaluated to determine whether or not the initial neuropsychological assessment had any prognostic significance. The essential findings of the study are shown, in Table 14–3. As will be seen, of the 46 patients, 31 performed normally on the test battery while 15 performed defectively. At the 5-year follow-up, 30 were judged to be mentally intact and 16 to be demented. Of the 31 patients who had performed normally on the initial neuropsychological assessment, only two were judged to be demented 5 years later. In contrast, of the 15 patients who had performed defectively, 14 proved to be demented at follow-up examination. It is clear that there was a close relationship between the initial test findings and subsequent mental status as judged clinically, the proportion of correct predictions being 93%.

The superiority of standardized neuropsychological assessment to impressionistic clinical evaluation can be demonstrated in many situations. Yet perhaps the advantage is not always on the side of formal assessment. During the course of his examination, the experienced and perceptive clinician may elicit evidence of failing memory, poor practical judgment, or thought disorder that is not brought out in the more structured and impersonal context of neuropsychological testing. For example, a seemingly competent patient may repeat an observation or opinion that he expressed only 3 minutes previously. And if the clinician returns to the same topic, the patient may once again repeat the observation or opinion, thus disclosing his inability to keep track of ongoing events. Or, on

TABLE 14–3. Prediction of Mental Decline in Older Subjects*

	CLINICAL STATUS (1972)	
TEST SCORE (1967)	NORMAL	DEMENTED
Normal	29	2
Impaired	1	14
Proportion of correct prediction = 93%		

*Poitrenaud and Barrere (1973).

subtle questioning, a patient may make outlandish comments about his wife or children, thus betraying poor social judgment, blunted affect, or thought disorder. Behaviors such as these are more likely to be manifested in the conversational setting of a clinical examination than in the more impersonal context of standardized neuropsychological assessment, particularly if the tests are given by a technician. The astute clinician, of course, will take account of these behaviors in reaching a diagnostic judgment.

It must also be kept in mind that test standardization is not always a reliable guide for judging the expected performance of a patient. The normative values of a test (particularly one of a verbal nature) standardized in the urban Northeastern United States may not be valid for the agricultural Southwest, let alone for the neighboring countries of Canada and Mexico. Nor can it be assumed that test norms are stable over time. Changing educational practices and cultural factors (e.g., the advent of television) may render them obsolete, sometimes within a relatively short time period. For example, a comparison of the performances of the same subjects on the Revised Wechsler Adult Intelligence Scale (published in 1981) with the first edition of the Scale (published in 1955) showed that an IQ score of 100 on the revised version corresponded to an IQ score of 108 on the older version, a difference of approximately 0.5 standard deviation (Wechsler, 1981). Similarly, follow-up studies of World War II veterans who were given intelligence tests on entry into military service and subsequently reassessed with the same tests some years after discharge have found that the men generally made higher scores on retest (Weinstein and Teuber, 1957; Schwatzman and Douglas, 1962).

Even when a test is carefully standardized, with due regard to the influence of age, educational level and sex on performance level, one sometimes finds an extremely wide range of scores within each age-educational-sex cell (e.g., 22–49-year-old male university graduates) so that two subjects scoring well within the normal range may differ quite significantly in performance level. Obviously there are other factors (e.g., family background, occupational achievement) which are correlated with performance level and which, if known, can be utilized to define the expected performance level of an individual patient. Thus a clinical examiner, who comes to know the background and achievements of a patient in some detail, may be able to make a more precise estimate of what his expected performance should be than is possible from recourse to statistical norms.

Neuropsychological Assessment and Psychopathology

The neurological approach to psychopathology is as old as scientific psychiatry itself. One needs only to recall Griesinger's dictum that all mental disease is brain disease, Meynert's definition of psychiatry as the medical specialty that deals with "diseases of the forebrain," and Kraepelin's early conviction that dementia praecox is the behavioral expression of a basic abnormality of the brain. Each succeeding decade has witnessed renewed attempts to relate cerebral abnormality, both structural and functional, to the behavioral manifestations of the major psychiatric disorders. Today this effort appears to be more promising than ever, thanks to the utilization of the newer neurodiagnostic techniques coupled with more adequate experimental designs. Neuropsychological assessment has figured prominently in recent research in this area, where the findings generated by its employment are often considered to be "behavioral markers" of an underlying cerebral status. Some conceptual and methodological issues associated with the application of neuropsychological assessment procedures to problems of psychopathology are briefly discussed in this section.

The interpretation of the neuropsychological test performances of psychiatric patients often proceeds by analogy. If a patient shows a performance deficit which has been identified in the literature of clinical neurology as the behavioral consequence of a focal brain lesion, the inference may be drawn that the patient also has the focal lesion. Of course, this approach to psychiatric symptomatology long antedates the employment of neuropsychological tests in this context. To cite only one early example, Gurewitsch (1932) noted that some of his patients (including schizophrenics) showed behavioral deficits that neurological observation had associated with posterior parietal lobe lesions (e.g., right–left disorientation, lateral neglect, distortions of the body image). He therefore concluded that it was justifiable to speak of a true parietal syndrome and to postulate a corresponding lesional localization in these patients.

A current example of the use of neuropsychological test findings to support the inference of a neurological basis for a psychopathological symptom is provided by recent studies of the Capgras syndrome ("illusion of doubles"). The nature of this bizarre, intensely affect-laden delusion, which is very often associated with a schizophrenic illness and/or paranoid ideation, was typically interpreted in terms of psychodynamic concepts (Todd, 1954; Enoch et al., 1967). It was only in the 1970s that evidence in favor of an organic etiology was adduced (MacCallum, 1973). It was then that neuropsychological tests were employed to provide objective evidence in support of both the general concept of an organic basis and a specific hypothesis of right hemisphere dysfunction. Christodoulou (1977) and Kokkema and Christodoulou (1985) reported that Capgras patients generally showed a lower WAIS Performance Scale than Verbal Scale IQ (the difference sometimes being as large as 25–29 points), Benton Visual Retention Test scores that were consistently lower than Full Scale IQ scores and generally poor performance on Rey's Figure Drawing Test. Similarly, Wilcox and Waziri (1983) described a patient whose performance on the verbal Logical Memory and Paired Associate subtests of the Wechsler Memory Scale were normal while her performance on the Visual Reproduction subtest of the scale as well as on tests of facial recognition and judgment of line orientation were defective, the profile of performance suggesting a "major disturbance in the function of the right hemisphere." Thus neuropsychological test results have implicated specific cerebral dysfunction in Capgras patients (a finding which is not necessarily incompatible with psychodynamic formulations of the genesis of the symptom).

This neurological type of interpretation of the test performances of psychiatric patients is not only quite legitimate but also advantageous in that it tends to eliminate observational bias in dealing with an unresolved question. However, it is not without its pitfalls. First there is the consideration that a failing test performance may be determined by factors other than the presence of brain damage. Thus the finding of "right-left disorientation" or "constructional apraxia" in a psychiatric patient may result from apathy, preoccupation or even negativism on his part rather than from a focal brain lesion. Secondly, the relationship of specific perceptual and cognitive defects to focal lesions is in fact not nearly as close as most summaries of the neurological literature would imply. On the one hand, cases that do not conform to an accepted lesional localization are not particularly rare. For example, visuospatial disability may be encountered in patients with anterior lesions in either hemisphere as well as in those with right posterior parietal disease and "finger agnosia" in patients with right, as well as left, hemisphere disease (Benton, 1985; Gainotti et al., 1972). On the other hand, negative cases in which an identified lesion has not produced the behavioral defect supposedly characteristic of it (e.g., a patient with a right occipitoparietal infarct who does *not* show visuospatial or visuoconstruction difficulties) are also not uncommon. But, except in the field of aphasia, these cases are seldom the subject of study.

Finally, some neuropsychological test performances are informative only if extreme values are observed. Dichotic listening, a noninvasive technique which is utilized for determining the language-dominant hemisphere, is a case in point (Springer, 1986). When applied to normal righthanded subjects, dichotic listening tests identify 70–80% as having a "right ear advantage" indicative of left hemisphere dominance for speech. There is an obvious discrepancy between this determination and the accepted value of 95–98% derived from clinical study of righthanded patients with unilateral cerebral lesions and from the results of the Wada sodium amytal test. One must conclude that performance pattern in dichotic listening is not a valid index of hemispheric dominance for speech. One reason for this lack of validity is that the technique does not generate a very reliable measure, at least not in normal young adults. Studies of the question have found test–retest reliabilities of only 0.50–0.70 (i.e., accounting for no more than 50% of the common variance) and shift of ear advantage from one ear to the other is not uncommon with about 30% of subjects showing such a shift from test to retest (Pizzamiglio et al., 1974; Blumstein et al., 1975).

Thus the dichotic listening technique, at least as it is generally employed and interpreted, does not provide a firm basis for evaluating differential hemispheric functioning in psychiatric patients. As a consequence, one finds that dichotic listening studies of schizophrenic and depressed patients have produced a disappointing set of inconsistent results (Springer, 1986).

In contrast, application of dichotic listening to patients with brain disease has been far more informative, primarily because patients with focal lesions may show extreme "between-ears" differences that can be satisfactorily explained in terms of underlying anatomical mechanisms. Right-handed "split-brain" (callosectomized) patients show an overwhelming right ear superiority with almost no reporting of stimuli presented to the left ear (Sparks and Geschwind, 1968; Milner et al., 1968; Springer and Gazzaniga, 1975; Springer et al., 1978). Patients with right temporal lobe lesions show a pronounced right ear advantage which is not quite as extreme as that seen in callosectomized patients (Sparks et al., 1970). Patients with left temporal lobe lesions may show *either* a pronounced left ear advantage *or* a pronounced right ear advantage depending upon the exact site of the lesion and the specific neural pathways interrupted by it (Sparks et al., 1970; Damasio and Damasio, 1979).

It is clear that the dichotic listening scores of moderate size that are so often encountered in samples of psychiatric patients do not have the specific neurological significance carried by extreme scores. This does not mean that moderate scores are necessarily devoid of significance. But it does suggest that their interpretation should be extremely tentative and that findings in one or another direction should be regarded as raising questions rather than as reliable indications about interhemispheric relations.

Directions of Future Development

There can be little doubt that neuropsychological assessment procedures will play an increasingly important role in the study of brain–behavior relationships in psychiatric patients. As hypotheses about the nature of these relationships become more specific, the precision and analytic power of objective assessment methods will be needed to provide crucial tests of them. Contemporary research has already established that structural abnormalities of the brain in schizophrenic patients, as indexed by CT scan, are correlated to varying degrees with diverse measures of cognitive function in these patients (Weinberger and Wyatt, 1982). A host of other findings in schizophrenics, e.g., abnormal profiles of regional cerebral blood flow and deviant EEG patterns, call for detailed neuropsychological analysis in order to elucidate their functional and clinical significance (Nasrallah, 1982).

Fixed test batteries, the most prominent of which are the Wechsler Adult

Intelligence Scale (Lezak, 1983; Wechsler, 1981), the Halstead-Reitan battery (Lezak, 1983; Ball, 1981) and the Wechsler Memory Scale (Lezak, 1983), are the most widely used instruments in both clinical practice and clinical research. Although they have proved to be useful in both settings, these batteries also have serious limitations (Lezak, 1983; Benton, 1985). First, their fixed character permits no flexibility in responding to different clinical referral or research questions; the same set of tests is given regardless of whether the question is one of dementia, specific memory impairment, visuoperceptual disability, frontal lobe dysfunction or defective interhemispheric integration. It would seem obvious that the same set of eight to ten tests cannot be expected to provide an adequate evaluation of all the specific questions that may be raised in practice or research.

Secondly, these widely used batteries can scarcely be considered to be optimal sets of tests for diagnostic purposes. As is well known, the Wechsler battery was constructed as a measure of "general intelligence." It has proved to be valuable for a variety of practical purposes such as vocational counseling, school assignment and job placement. Although it was not designed for the purpose, it has also been used advantageously in assessing patients with brain disease. But it is far from being an ideal instrument for analyzing the cognitive functioning of brain-diseased patients and relating these functions to neurological variables. For example, it does not assess short-term memory or recent memory nor does it permit making a clear distinction between linguistic and nonlinguistic capacities.

The Halstead-Reitan battery, which was explicitly designed for the assessment of patients with brain disease, is a rather unusual set of tests. Apart from the Category Test (a measure of concept formation), the reasons for the inclusion of some tests, e.g., rhythm discrimination, speech sounds perception, in preference to other more obvious possibilities are not clear. In any case, important areas of function such as memory and language capacities are not assessed. The Wechsler Memory Scale is a mélange of seven brief tests of orientation, "immediate memory," serial speech, recent memory, verbal learning, memory for paragraphs and figural memory from which a single "memory quotient" is derived. Other than as a measure of general mental competence, this "memory quotient" representing an amalgamation of scores on tests of memory and nonmemory functions has little meaning and is of no value in analytic neuropsychological assessment.

The limitations of these fixed batteries are widely recognized and in practice they are often supplemented by additional tests. Thus, the Wechsler Adult Intelligence Scale *and* the Halstead-Reitan battery, *and* the Trail Making Test (Lezak, 1983; Spreen and Benton, 1965; Reitan, 1958), or either of these batteries *and* specific tests of memory, visuoconstructional capacity and language functions (Benton et al., 1983; Buschke and Fuld, 1974; Benton, 1974; Graham and Kendall, 1960) may form part of an expanded battery which is routinely given.

Nevertheless, it is doubtful that any fixed neuropsychological test battery, however comprehensive and time-consuming it may be, can be regarded as fully adequate since it cannot possibly answer all the questions that arise in either practice or research. For example, the concept of interhemispheric dysfunction in schizophrenic patients that has come out of anatomic, physiologic, and behavioral studies (Nasrallah, 1982) requires the application of carefully constructed and standardized tests that make specific demands on the transfer of information across the hemispheres to elucidate the concept and evaluate its cogency. Thus the development of a number of such tests—visual, tactile, motor and verbal—is called for. Yet, assuming the availability of standardized tests of interhemispheric information processing, it would not be appropriate to include them in a battery that is routinely given since the "cost-benefit" ratio associated with their administration would be astronomically high.

But these tests, as well as special-purpose tests of other types, are needed if neuropsychological assessment is to fulfill its role in clinical practice and research. It is likely that, as the need for them is recognized, a number of special-purpose tests will be developed and standardized for wider use. These assessment instruments should reflect the newer concepts and advances in understanding of brain-behavior relationships in a variety of fields, e.g., memory (Squire and Butters, 1984), language functions (Marshall, 1986), and perceptual processes (DeRenzi, 1982), as they pertain to psychiatric and neurologic disorders.

Taken in their totality, these tests will form an inventory from which a selection could be made to answer research or clinical diagnostic questions. The role of specific tests in answering specific research questions is obvious. In clinical evaluation they can be utilized in response both to the referral question and to the diagnostic possibilities suggested by the patient's test performances as the neuropsychological examination proceeds. Thus their utilization will serve to define the character of clinical neuropsychological assessment as a logical, sequential decision-making process rather than as the administration of a fixed battery of tests.

It is possible that some neuropsychological test performances (more probably, patterns of test performance) will prove to be sufficiently valid that they can serve as reliable indicators of specific cerebral dysfunction, independently of any anatomic or physiologic findings. Such an achievement would mean that the clinician and researcher would have available a number of true behavioral markers of cerebral abnormality.

References

Benton A. L. (1973). The measurement of aphasic disorder. In Caceres Velasquez A. (ed.), *Aspectos Patólogicos del Lenguaje*. Lima: Centro Neuropsicologico-Patología de Lenguaje, pp. 61–78.

Benton A. L. (1974). *The Revised Visual Retention Test*, 4th ed. New York: Psychological Corporation.

Benton A. L. (1984). Constructional apraxia. *Semin. Neurol.* 4: 220.

Benton A. L. (1985a). Visuoperceptual, visuospatial, and visuoconstructive disorders. In Heilman K. M., and Valenstein, E (eds.), *Clinical Neuropsychology*, 2nd ed., *Ch. 8*, pp. 151–186. New York: Oxford University Press.

Benton A. L. (1985b). Body schema disturbances. In Heilman K. M., Valenstein E. (eds.) *Clinical Neuropsychology,* 2nd ed., Chap. 6. New York: Oxford University Press, pp. 115–129.

Benton A. L. (1985c). Some problems associated with neuropsychological assessment. *Bull. Clin. Neurosci.* 50: 11.

Benton A. L. and Hamsher K. (1983). *Multilingual Aphasia Examination*. Iowa City, IA: AJA Associates.

Benton A. L., Hamsher K., Varney N. R., and Spreen O. (1983). *Contributions to Neuropsychological Assessment*. New York: Oxford University Press.

Benton A. L. and Howell I. L. (1941). The use of psychological tests in the evaluation of intellectual function following head injury. *Psychosom. Med.* 3: 138.

Benton A. L., Van Allen M. W, and Fogel M. L. (1964). Temporal orientation in cerebral disease. *J. Nerv. Ment Dis.* 139: 110.

Bird J. M., Levy R., and Jacoby R. J. (1986). Computed tomography in the elderly. *Br. J. Psychiatry* 148: 80.

Blessed G., Tomlinson B. E., and Roth M. (1968). The association between quantitative measurements of dementia and of senile changes in the grey matter of elderly subjects. *Br. J. Psychiatry* 114: 797.

Blumstein S., Goodglass H., and Tartter V. (1975). The reliability of ear advantage in dichotic listening. *Brain Language* 2: 226.

Boll T. J. (1981). The Halstead-Reitan Neuropsychology Battery. In Filskov S. B., Boll T. J. (eds.), *Handbook of Clinical Neuropsychology,* Ch. 18. New York: Wiley-Interscience, pp. 577–607.

Brant-Zawadzki M., Davis P. L., Crooks L. E., Mills C. M., Norman D., Newton T. H., Sheldon P., and Kaufman L. (1983). NMR demonstration of cerebral abnormalities. *Am. J. Radiol.* 140: 847.

Buschke H. and Fuld P. A. (1974). Evaluating storage, retention, and retrieval in disordered memory and learning. *Neurology, 24*, 1019.

Christodoulou G. N. (1977). The syndrome of Capgras. *Br. J. Psychiatry* 130: 556.

Conkey R. (1938). Psychological changes associated with head injuries. *Arch. Psychol.* 33: 62.

Damasio H. and Damasio A. R. (1979). "Paradoxic" ear extinction in dichotic listening. *Neurology* 29: 644.

DeLeon M. J., Ferris S. H., and George A. E. (1980). Computed tomography evaluations of brain-behavior relationships in senile dementia of the Alzheimer's type. *Neurobiol. Aging* 14: 69.

DeRenzi E. (1982). *Disorders of Space Exploration and Cognition*. New York: Wiley.

Earnest M. P., Heaton R. K., Wilkinson W. E., and Manke W. F. (1979). Cortical atrophy, ventricular enlargement and intellectual impairment in the aged. *Neurology* 29: 1138.

Enoch M. D., Trethowan W., and Barker J. (1967). *Some Uncommon Psychiatric Syndromes*. Bristol: Wright.

Eslinger P. J., Damasio A. R., Benton A. L., and Van Allen M. W. (1985). Neuropsychologic detection of abnormal mental decline in older persons. *JAMA* 253: 670.

Farmer P. M., Peck A., and Terry R. D. (1976). Correlations among numbers of neuritic plaques, neurofibrillary tangles, and the severity of senile dementia. *J. Neuropathol. Exp. Neurol.* 35: 367.

Franz S. F. (1919). *Handbook of Mental Examination Methods*. Macmillan, New York.

Gainotti G., Cianchetti C., and Tiacci C. (1972). The influence of hemispheric side of lesion on nonverbal tests of finger localization. *Cortex* 8: 364.

Gandy S. E., Snow R. B., Zimmerman R. D., and Deck M. D. F. (1984). Cranial nuclear magnetic resonance imaging in head trauma. *Ann. Neurol.* 16: 254.

Gelb A. and Goldstein K. (1920). *Psychologische Analyse hirnpathologischen Fälle*. Leipzig: Barth.

Goldfried M. R., Stricker G., and Weiner I. B. (1971). *Rorschach Handbook of Clinical and Research Application*. Englewood Cliffs, NJ: Prentice-Hall.

Goldstein K. and Scheerer M. (1941). Abstract and concrete behavior. *Psychol. Monogr.* 53.

Graham F. K. and Kendall B. S. (1960). Memory-for-Designs Test. Perceptual Motor Skills, *Monogr. Suppl. No. 2*.

Gurewitsch M. (1932). Über das interparietale Syndrom bei Geisteskrankheiten. *Zeitschr. Ges. Neurol. Psychiatrie* 140: 593.

Han J. S., Kaufman B., and Alfidi R. J. (1984). Head trauma evaluated by magnetic resonance and computed tomography. *Radiology* 150: 71.

Heilbronner K. (1905). Zur klinisch-psychologischen Untersuchungstechnik. *Monatsschr. Psychiatrie Neurol.* 17: 15.

Hunt H. F. (1943). A practical clinical test for organic brain damage. *J. Appl. Psychol.* 27: 375.

Joslyn D. and Hutzell R. R. (1979). Temporal disorientation in schizophrenia and brain-damaged patients. *Am. J. Psychiatry* 136: 1220.

Kaszniak A. W., Garron D. C., Fox J. H., Bergen D., and Huckman M. (1979). Cerebral atrophy, EEG slowing, age, education, and cognitive functioning in suspected dementia. *Neurology* 29: 1273.

Kokkema A. and Christodoulou G. N. (1985). Psychometric investigation of patients with delusional misidentification syndromes. In Pichot P., Berner P., Wolf R., and Thau K (eds.), *Psychiatry: The State of the Art, Vol. 1*, pp. 841–849. New York: Plenum.

Levin H. S. and Benton A. L. (1975). Temporal orientation in patients with brain disease. *Appl. Neurophysiol.* 38: 56.

Levin H. S., Handel S. F., Goldman A. M., Eisenberg H. M., and Quinto F. C. (1985a). Magnetic resonance imaging after "diffuse" nonmissile head injury. *Arch. Neurol.* 42: 963.

Levin H. S., Kalisky Z., Handel S. F., Goldman A. M., Eisenberg H. M., Morrison D., and Von Laufen A. (1985b). Magnetic resonance imaging in relation to sequelae and rehabilitation of head injury. *Semin. Neurol.* 5: 221.

Lezak M. D. (1983). *Neuropsychological Assessment*, 2nd ed. New York: Oxford University Press.

Liepmann H. (1905). Kleine Hilfsmittel bei der Untersuchung von Gehirnkrankheiten. *Dtsch. Med. Wochenschr.* 38: 1.

Lipmann O. (1922). *Handbuch psychologischer Hilfsmittel der psychiatrischen Diagnostik*. Leipzig: Barth.

Lissauer H. (1890). Ein Fall von Seelenblindheit nebst einem Beitrag zur Theorie derselben. *Arch. Psychiatrie Nervenkrankh.* 21: 222.

Loeb J. (1884). Die Sehstörungen nach Verletzung der Grosshirnrinde. *Pflüger's Arch. Ges. Physiol.* 34: 67.

Loeb J. (1885). Die elementaren Störungen einfacher Functionen nach oberflächiger umschriebener Verletzung des Grosshirns. *Pflüger's Arch. Ges. Physiol.* 37: 51.

MacCallum A. G. (1973). Capgras symptoms with an organic basis. *Br. J. Psychiatry* 123: 639.

Marshall J. C. (1986). The description and interpretation of aphasic language disorder. *Neuropsychologia* 24: 5.

Matarazzo J. D. (1972). *Wechsler's Measurement and Appraisal of Adult Intelligence.* New York: Oxford University Press.

Milner B. Taylor L. and Sperry R. W. (1968). Literalized suppression of dichotically presented digits after commissural section in man. *Science* 161: 184.

Munk H. (1878). Weitere Mittheilungen zur Physiologie der Grosshirnrinde. *Arch. Anat. Physiol.* 2: 162.

Nasrallah H. A. (1982). Literality and hemispheric dysfunction in schizophrenia. In Henn F. A. and Nasrallah H. A. (eds.), *Schizophrenia as a Brain Disease,* Chap. 13, New York: Oxford University Press, pp. 273–294.

Natelson B. H., Haupt E. J., Fleischer E. J., Grey L. (1979). Temporal orientation and education. *Arch. Neurol.* 36: 444.

Neary D. and Snowden J. S. (1985). Psychological correlates in presenile dementia. *Interdisc. Topics in Gerontol.* 20: 24.

Oppenheimer H. (1885). Über eine durch eine klinisch bisher nicht verwerthete Untersuchungsmethode ermittelte Form der Sensibilitätsstörung bei einseitigen Erkrankungen des Grosshirns. *Neurol. Zentralbl.* 4: 529.

Perry E. K., Tomlinson B. E., Blessed G., Bergmann K., Gibson P. H., and Perry R. H. (1978). Correlation of cholinergic abnormalities with senile plaques and mental test scores in senile dementia. *Br. Med. J.* 2: 1457.

Pizzamiglio L., DePascalis C., and Vignati A. (1974). Stability of dichotic listening test. *Cortex,* 10: 203.

Poitrenaud J. and Barrere H. (1973). Valeur de l'examen psychométrique dans le pronostic de l'afflaiblissement intellectuel chez le sujet agé. *Rev. Psychol. Appl.* 41: 185.

Poppelreuter W. (1917). *Die psychischen Schädigungen durch Kopfschuss im Kriege 1914–1916.* Leipzig: Voss.

Reitan R. M. (1958). Validity of the Trail Making Test as an indication of organic brain damage. *Percept. Motor Skills* 8: 271.

Rieger C. (1888). *Beschreibung der Intelligenzstörungen in Folge einer Hirnverletzung.* Würzburg: Verlag der Stahelschen Buchhandlung.

Rossolimo G. (1911). Die psychologischen Profil. *Klin. Psych. Nerv. Krankh.* 6: 295.

Roth M., Tomlinson B. E., and Blessed G. (1966). Correlation between scores for dementia and counts of "senile plaques" in cerebral grey matter of elderly subjects. *Nature* 209: 109.

Sapas E. (1918). Zeichnerische Reproduktionen einfacher Figuren durch Geisteskranke. *Schweiz. Arch. Neurol. Psychiatrie* 4: 140.

Schwartzman A. E. Douglas V. I. (1962) Intellectual loss in schizophrenia. *Can. J. Psychol.* 16: 1.

Shipley W. C. (1940). A self-administering scale for measuring intellectual impairment and deterioration. *J. Psychol.* 9: 371.

Sparks R. and Geschwind N. (1968). Dichotic listening in man after section of neocortical commissures. *Cortex* 4: 3.

Sparks R., Goodglass H., and Nickel B. (1970). Ipsilateral versus contralateral extinction in dichotic listening resulting from hemisphere lesions. *Cortex* 6: 249.

Spreen O. and Benton A. L. (1965). Comparative studies of some psychological tests for cerebral damage. *J. Nerv. Ment. Dis.* 140: 323.

Springer S. P. (1986). Dichotic listening. In Hannay H. J. (ed.). *Experimental Techniques in Human Neuropsychology,* Chap. 5, New York: Oxford University Press, pp. 138–166.

Springer S. P. and Gazzaniga M. S. (1975). Dichotic listening in partial and complete split brain patients. *Neuropsychologia* 13: 341.

Springer S., Sidtis J., Wilson D., and Gazzaniga M. (1978). Left ear performance in dichotic listening following commissurotomy. *Neuropsychologia* 16: 305.

Squire L. R., Butters N. (1984). *Neuropsychology of Memory*. New York: Guilford Press.

Todd J. (1954). The syndrome of Capgras. *Psychiatr. Q.* 31: 250.

Tomlinson B. E., Blessed G., and Roth M. (1968). Observations on the brains of non-demented old people. *J. Neurol. Sci.* 7: 331.

Tomlinson B. E., Blessed G., and Roth M. (1970). Observations on the brains of demented old people. *J. Neurol. Sci.* 11: 205.

Wechsler D. (1981). *WAIS-R Manual*. New York: Psychological Corporation.

Weinstein S. and Teuber H-L. (1957). Effects of penetrating brain injury on intelligence test scores. *Science* 125: 1036.

Weinberger D. R. and Wyatt R. J. (1982) Brain morphology in schizophrenia. In Henn F A, Nasrallah H. A. (eds.), *Schizophrenia as a Brain Disease,* Chap. 8. New York: Oxford University Press, pp. 148–175.

Wells F. L., and Reusch J. (1942). *Mental Examiner's Handbook*. New York: Psychological Corporation.

Wilbrand H. (1887). *Die Seelenblindheit als Herderscheinung und ihre Beziehungen zur homonymen Hemianopsie*. Wiesbaden: JF Bergmann.

Wilcock G. K. and Esiri M. M. (1982). Plaques, tangles and dementia. *J. Neurol. Sci.* 56: 343.

Wilcock G. K., Esiri M. M., Bowen D. M., and Smith C. C. T. (1982). Alzheimer's disease. Correlation of cortical choline acetyltransferase activity with the severity of dementia and histological abnormalities. *J. Neurol. Sci.* 57: 407.

Wilcox J. and Waziri R. (1983). The Capgras symptom and non-dominant hemisphere dysfunction. *J. Clin. Psychiatry* 44: 70.

Wu S., Schenkenberg T., Wing S. D., and Osborn A. G. (1981). Cognitive correlates of diffuse cerebral atrophy determined by computed tomography. *Neurology* 31: 1180.

15

The Amusias

"Amusia" is a collective term denoting the loss or impairment of musical capacity that may occur as a consequence of brain disease. The impairment may take a variety of forms. It may be manifested in motor or expressive performances, for example, in loss of the ability to sing, whistle, or hum a tune (oral-expressive amusia); loss of the ability to play an instrument (instrumental amusia or musical apraxia); or loss of the ability to write music (musical agraphia). By definition, the latter two disabilities can be sustained only by trained musicians. On the receptive side, the impairment may be manifested in noteworthy loss of the ability to discriminate between heard melodies (receptive or sensory amusia); loss of the ability to identify familiar melodies (amnesic amusia); or loss of the ability to read musical notation in a person who possessed this skill (musical alexia). Alteration of emotional response to music is still another form. Any of these disabilities may occur singly or in combination. They are encountered frequently in association with aphasic disorders but, as will be seen, this association is not at all obligatory.

Historical Sketch

Disorders in musical appreciation and execution first engaged medical attention when systematic examination of aphasic patients disclosed that many of them had lost one or another musical skill along with their impairment in language.* An early case report by Proust (1866) described loss of the ability to read music

Reprinted with permission from M. Critchley and R. A. Henson (eds.), *Music and the Brain: Studies in the Neurology of Music*. London: William Heinemann Medical Books. © 1977 Butterworth Heinemann Publishers.

* Detailed accounts of the historical development of our knowledge of amusic disorders may be found in Edgren (1895), Henschen (1920), Ustvedt (1937), and Dorgeuille (1966).

in an aphasic musician; however his capacity to recognize music remained intact and he could still sing, play, and even write music. Some years later, Proust (1872) described a different pattern of loss of musical ability in two aphasic patients. One could still read notes, play scales and recognize melodies but could no longer hum a tune. The other, an accomplished musician, could recognize melodies and not only read but also compose music; however, he was no longer capable of humming a tune. An early case report by Fischer (1867) described yet another type of impairment. His patient, who was a music teacher and a composer and who showed both motor and receptive aphasic defects, could discriminate between rhythmic patterns and recognize a melody which he himself had composed. He also handled a violin skilfully and could reproduce an appropriate tune if a scale were played to him. However, he could neither play nor sing a tune that had been sung to him and he had lost his ability to read and write music. In 1870, Finkelnburg described a most unusual case of a left-handed patient who presented with an amnesic aphasia in association with disease of the right hemisphere. This skilled musician could reproduce heard melodies on the violin with fair facility but was unable to do so on the piano.

The *sparing* of musical abilities in patients with congenital or acquired language defects was noted even earlier. Dalin (1745) described a 33-year-old man who suffered a right hemiplegia and complete loss of expressive speech after a stroke but who nevertheless was able to sing the melody and words of hymns that were familiar to him. Bouillaud (1865) reported the case of an aphasic composer who could still play, compose, and hum music, and even accompany singers on the piano. The retention of the ability to sing in an almost speechless aphasic patient of Gowers (1875) was disclosed only when he spontaneously joined another patient who was singing and then continued to sing the words and melody of the second verse by himself.

Conversely, instances of loss of musical skills in patients who were not aphasic were also described. Mann's (1898) patient was a good singer who lost the capacity to sing as well as to whistle after an injury to the right frontal lobe. However, recognition of melodies was well-preserved. At no time did he show any signs of aphasic disorder. Jossmann (1926, 1927) described a patient who presented a very similar picture. This patient showed a transient left hemiparesis without aphasia following ligation of the right common carotid artery and removal of an aneurysm at its bifurcation. However, when he was examined some months later, this trained musician could neither sing nor whistle tunes to command and he could no longer read a score. Recognition of pitch and intensity remained intact and he was quite aware of his errors in expression.

Thus, once attention was directed to the question, a variety of distinctive types of impairment in musical capacity was observed and reported. By the close of the nineteenth century, every form of amusia that is currently recognized had been described and a number of systematic studies (Knoblauch, 1888; Oppenheim, 1888; Brazier, 1892; Edgren, 1895; Probst, 1899) had been devoted to the topic. The most comprehensive of these early studies was that of J. G. Edgren, Professor of Medicine in Stockholm, who presented a critical analysis of the literature with particular reference to those cases on whom autopsy findings were available. From this review and an analysis of his own exhaustively studied case, it seemed clear to Edgren that discrete forms of amusia did occur, that they were closely allied to comparably discrete aphasic disorders and that they had distinctive anatomical bases.

The first full scale monographic treatment of amusia was that of Henschen (1920) who made a detailed analysis of the published literature on the subject as well as of his own extensive case material. Although his primary interest was in questions of localization, Henschen did not neglect the theoretical and clinical aspects of the topic and he devoted considerable attention to the nature of the relationship between aphasic disorders and impairment in musical functions. His classification followed traditional lines in providing for two broad categories of impairment, motor and sensory, within which specific disabilities could be placed. However, he also recognized that a number of auditory capacities, such as pitch discrimination and tonal discrimination, underlay these musical skills and he viewed the central problem as the determination, on the basis of the available anatomo–clinical data, of the degree to which these more elementary capacities can be localized in the brain.

A second monograph on the subject, that of Feuchtwanger (1930), was quite different in character. Covering an extremely broad range of topics, he concluded that impairment in both integrative capacity and in differentiation constituted the fundamental deficits in "amusia." He emphasized the necessity for a thorough knowledge of the premorbid personality of the patient, a requirement that cannot often be satisfied in actual practice. Loosely organized and replete with speculation about the expressive, semantic, and symbolic functions of music, the monograph covered all aspects of musical function in considerable detail; but Feuchtwanger's treatment was generally rather unclear, indeed at times mystifying, and his monumental treatise had no great impact on thinking in the field.

The comprehensive study of Ustvedt (1937) provided a more critical analysis of the problems associated with "amusia" than any work up to its time. Proceeding from a careful review of the literature, Ustvedt pointed out how little is actually known about disturbances in musical functions. He attributed this deficiency to a variety of factors, the primary ones being grossly inadequate techniques of examination, neglect of the premorbid musicality of the patient, and preoccupation with problems of localization without taking account of the complex clinical pictures shown by different patients. With respect to the last point, he emphasized the Jacksonian dictum that localizing the lesions producing amusic disabilities is not equivalent to identifying the neural mechanisms underlying musical functions. In addition, he sharply criticized the proclivity for erecting elaborate theoretical schemata (as reflected, for example, in the writing of Feuchtwanger) that were the product of pure speculation and without empirical foundation.

Ustvedt's own extremely detailed study of a group of patients, all of whom had had musical training and most of whom were also aphasic, led him to conclude that "amusia" is simply a shorthand term for "a heterogenous collection of rather complicated symptom-groups" about which very little is known. Specifically, both the neural mechanisms underlying these symptom pictures and the nature of their relationship to cognitive and linguistic function remain obscure. Nevertheless, he felt that it was of practical value to distinguish disorders of receptive functions and those of expressive functions and that, in the latter group, differentiation between productive as contrasted to merely reproductive activity was useful. The importance of both the emotional and structural aspects of music as potential areas of disturbances was emphasized. Problems of classification were discussed at length but left unresolved in view of the superficial nature of our understanding of these disorders. A major conclusion was that in this field "there has been much overemphasis of the intellectual, cortical factors, and in future research it will be necessary to devote much more attention to the subcortical driving forces of musical function." Ustvedt's monograph, over 700 pages in length, remains the most valuable single contribution to the field. Among more recent work, there is none that approaches it in breadth, detail, and critical acumen.

The Varieties of Musical Disturbance

Numerous classifications of types of amusia have been offered (cf. Henschen, 1920; Kleist, 1934; Wertheim, 1963, 1969; Dorgeuille, 1966; Grison, 1972). Many follow the lines of classical aphasia theory and divide musical disturbances into two broad types, motor and sensory. Thus, for example, Henschen (1920) adopted the following classification as a basis for his analysis.

I. Motor impairments
   A. Loss of the ability to sing (with or without words).
   B. Loss of the ability to write musical notation.
   C. Loss of the ability to play an instrument.
II. Sensory Impairments
   A. "Musical deafness," including loss of recognition of familiar melodies.
   B. Loss of the ability to read musical notation.

Kleist (1928, 1934) also accepted the dichotomy of motor and sensory categories of amusia and he identified specific types of disturbance in each category. Within the motor category, he distinguished between the inability to produce (i.e., sing or whistle) a single tune (*Tonstummheit*) and the inability to produce a melody (*Melodienstummheit; Motorische Amelodie*). Within the sensory category, he distinguished between the inability to discriminate single tones (*Tontaubheit; Perzeptive Sensorische Amusie*), the inability to discriminate melodies (*Melodientaubheit*) and the inability to identify a specific melody (*Musiksinntaubheit*).

Other classifications have been based on a hierarchical principle and have made a fundamental distinction between lower and higher levels of disturbance, contrasting relatively simple performances such as singing and recognizing familiar tunes with more complex, functions such as the composing of music. A particular form of this classification differentiates impairment in comprehending music as a language or symbol system from impairment on the perceptual or motor levels. Still other classifications follow anatomical principles, distinguishing between disorders associated with disease of the left hemisphere and those that occur as a consequence of right hemisphere disease or identifying those types of disorder that appear to be associated specifically with lesions in different loci.

It can be said of all these classifications that they possess the merit of providing a framework within which empirical observations can be fitted. At the same time, it is clear that they are only of limited usefulness since none has been found to be capable of accommodating all the observed facts. Far more is known about the aphasic disorders than about disturbances in musical appreciation and expression. Yet classification in the field of aphasia is still a controversial question, testifying to a lack of certainty about the basic nature of these disorders. This uncertainty is even more pervasive with respect to the amusias and, as a consequence, attempts to develop rigorous classifications are often little more than logical exercises. Given this circumstance, it seems appropriate to acknowledge our present lack of understanding of the basic dimensions along with musical disturbances vary an to proceed on a purely descriptive basis. The forms of disturbance that have been identified by clinical observation will be sketched and their correlates noted without, however, attempting to fit them into a formal schema based on theoretical principles.

Oral-Expressive or Vocal Amusia

Loss of the capacity to sing, hum, or whistle a tune is one of the more frequently described forms of amusia. The loss may be complete in the sense that the patient finds himself unable to produce either a single tone or a melody on verbal command or by imitation. The loss may be partial insofar as the patient may be able to produce a familiar melody but be incapable of reproducing an isolated sound. The loss in oral-expressive capacity may also be partial in the sense that the patient maybe able to carry a tune but his singing proves to be quite poor in terms of melody, intonation, and rhythm.

Two case reports describing patients who showed oral-expressive amusia as their sole or most prominent disability, those of Mann (1898) and Jossman (1926, 1927), were mentioned earlier in the chapter. Neither patient was aphasic and both showed evidence of anterior right hemisphere disease.

The patient described by Botez and Wertheim (1959) presented a very similar picture. After removal of a calcified oligodendroglioma of the right frontal lobe, this 26-year-old man who was an accomplished accordion player showed moderate articulatory disorder and dysprosody in speaking but no paraphasic speech, word-finding difficulties, or impairment in the understanding of language. Reading, writing, and calculation were intact. The slight motor and sensory impairments noted shortly after operation had disappeared. Receptive musical functions were not disturbed: he could discriminate pitch, recognize familiar melodies, and identify intentionally made errors in the playing of a melody. In contrast, expressive musical performances were disturbed to a serious degree. While notes produced by voice were sung accurately, notes produced by an accordion were not. Reproduction of rhythmic patterns was faulty. He made gross errors in intonation when singing a familiar tune to verbal command. The capacity to whistle a familiar tune was even more severely compromised. Although he showed no evidence of generalized praxic difficulties, his ability to play the accordion was grossly impaired. Thus, in this case, the oral-expressive amusia appeared in combination with expressive speech disorder and instrumental amusia. However, the site of the crucial lesion, i.e. the anterior region of the right hemisphere, was the same as in the earlier reported cases.

In other cases, oral-expressive amusia occurs within the setting of pervasive impairment in sensory functions. The patient who was studied postmortem by Pötzl and Uiberall (1937) perceived musical notes as well as other sounds as unpleasant dissonant noises. Human voices, including his own, seemed to him to be too high in pitch. Aside from a very slight word-finding difficulty, he showed no signs of expressive or receptive aphasia. However, he had lost his previously well-developed capacity to sing and he was unable to reproduce auditory rhythmic patterns correctly. In contrast to the finding of frontal lobe disease in the previously mentioned cases, autopsy study of this patient disclosed bilateral lesions involving auditory cortex and its subjacent white matter.

A distinctive feature of the cases of oral-expressive amusia mentioned thus far is that none were aphasic although they might show articulatory difficulties in speaking, as was true of the patient of Botez and Wertheim. The intensively studied case of Jellinek (1933) provides an example of an aphasic patient who also showed motor amusia. Following removal of a left frontal glioma, this professional singer exhibited a nonfluent expressive speech disorder characterized by hesitations, blocking, and repetition of words and syllables as well as impairment in reading, writing and understanding of oral speech. Calculation and design copying were also disturbed. He showed a partial vocal amusia in the sense that he would sing familiar melodies inaccurately and with uncertain intonation. Nor could he sing the notes of the scale accurately. His reproduction of rhythm patterns was also faulty. His perception of music was impaired and his ability to read music was completely lost.

Thus it is evident that loss of the capacity to sing can occur either in more or less isolated form or as part of a more general loss of musical capacity.

Instrumental Amnesia

Loss of the capacity to play an instrument has been the subject of only a few case reports. Moreover, in some instances it appears that the impairment may have been only a specific expression of a more pervasive motor disability. However, instrumental amnesia, which is not attributable to general motor deficit, has been also been clearly described. An excellent example is provided by the patient of Botez and Wertheim (1959) mentioned above. Besides his vocal disabilities, this young man could no longer play the accordion, an instrument which he had practised continuously since he was nine years old. Motor deficits could not be made to account for the striking failure in performance which Wertheim (1963) designated a "bimanual instrumental apraxia."

Musical Agraphia

Two types of impairment in writing have been described under the rubric of "musical agraphia." The first is inability to write a series of heard notes. This can be elicited, of course, only in a trained musician. It typically occurs in combination with other defects in musical function. However, Dorgeuille (1966) has described in trumpeter who showed no noteworthy defects in either language or musical function after head trauma except for some difficulty and hesitation in writing down rhythmic patterns aurally presented to him. The second type of defect is impairment in copying musical notation. This may be simply an expression of visuoperceptive disability and may have no inherent connection with musicality.

Musical Amnesia

This term generally refers to failure to identify melodies which should be familiar to the patient. The patient may be unable to sing a familiar song when given its name although he can sing it after it has been played to him. Or he may be unable to give the name of a familiar melody when it is played to him. A trained musician may not be able to write the main theme of a piece, having been given its name. Thus, one of Dorgeuille's (1966) patients, an accomplished pianist, experienced no difficulty in copying musicl notation, but wrote inaccurate notation when given the name of a familiar melody. She was a fluent aphasic who showed pronounced impairment in both naming and writing. However, failure to identify melodies by name is by no means necessarily associated with the presence of an aphasic disorder. Grison (1972) has described a number of nonaphasic patients with right hemisphere disease who showed this disability.

Disorders of Rhythm

Some writers (e.g., Jellinek, 1933; Döllken, 1935; Dorgeuille, 1966) have laid stress on impairment in the sense of rhythm as a basic component in disturbances in musical function. This impairment is expressed in failure to reproduce rhythmic patterns or to discriminate between them. The clinical literature suggests that disturbances in the recognition and execution of rhythmic patterns are frequently associated with both oral-expressive amusia and apraxic disorders.

Receptive Amusia

Defective perception of music as reflected in failure to discriminate between melodic patterns, timbre, and pitch and in qualitative alterations of acoustic experience. (e.g., hearing sounds as discordant or unpleasant) is a commonly reported type of amusia. In its most striking form, there is inability to discriminate between sounds of different timbre or pitch. An impairment that is so basic in nature necessarily results in grossly defective appreciation of music. However, its consequences extend beyond the field of music to all aspects of auditory experience. Thus most of the patients described in the literature as suffering from defective tonal discrimination were also "word deaf" to a greater or lesser degree, i.e., they suffered from a concomitant impairment in oral language understanding (cf. Vignolo, 1969). However, cases of "auditory agnosia" without receptive aphasic disorder have been observed. For example, the patient of Spreen et al. (1965) showed grossly defective recognition of nonverbal meaningful environmental sounds and performed on a chance level on an easy test of pitch discrimination. Yet a detailed aphasia examination did not disclose clinically significant defects. He showed no receptive or expressive difficulties in conversational speech, repetition, naming or object description. Nor were paraphasias, word-finding difficulties, or agrammatism observed. His reading was slow but accurate and there were not disturbances in writing. However, verbal associative fluency, as measured by a word association test, was impoverished.

In other cases, there is retention of the capacity for tonal discrimination with impairment in melodic discrimination, i.e., in appreciating tonal sequences. It is natural to think of tonal discrimination as being the more basic capacity and to suppose that impairment in tonal discrimination necessarily implies defective appreciation of melodies which are essentially sequences of tones. However, exceptional cases in which the patient could discriminate between melodies and yet showed poor tonal appreciation have been described (cf. Kleist, 1934). But, as a rule, the two types of disability do occur together and in combination with disturbances in the appreciation of rhythm.

Musical Alexia

Loss of the ability to read music in a trained musician has been frequently described and is a clearly recognized type of amusia. It is seen very often in association with acquired verbal alexia. Thus the famous alexic patient of Déjèrine (1892), who was an accomplished singer, could no longer read a single musical note, although he could still sing well. Other cases of musical alexia have been described in association with receptive aphasia and receptive and expressive amusia (Dupré and Nathan, 1911; Jellinek, 1933; Dorgeuille, 1966). Convincing cases of isolated defect in the reading of music without other linguistic or musical disabilities have not been reported.

Assessment of Musical Capacities

The assessment of disturbances in musical function can pose formidable problems, particularly if the question of mild or subtle impairment is raised. There is an extremely wide variation in "musicality" in the population. Some people can read and write music but the majority are musically illiterate. Many people cannot "carry a tune." Others are essentially non-responsive to music and have difficulty in distinguishing one melody from another as well as in remembering tonal sequences. Thus there are no obvious normal standards against which the performances of a patient can be compared, as is usually the case with linguistic capacities. Consequently, in judging whether or not a change in musical capacities has occurred, it is necessary to consider each patient as his own control and make an evaluation of his premorbid musical capacity on the basis of his testimony or that of his relatives. However, one must be cautious about accepting such statements at face value for, as Ustvedt (1937) pointed out, there is a tendency for patients with brain disease to overestimate their endowment, musical or otherwise, and for relatives and friends to offer generalities such as "fairly musical" or "he liked music," which are not very informative. Thus the evaluation of premorbid musical capacity is valid only to the

TABLE 15–1. Functions Assessed in Test Battery of Dorgeuille (1966)

I. Vocal expression
A. Patient is asked to sing familiar songs named by examiner.
B. Patient is asked to sing melodies by imitation
C. Patient is asked to whistle a melody.
D. Patient is asked to reproduce tones presented by voice, piano, etc.

II. Rhythmic expression
Patient is asked to reproduce rhythmic patterns tapped on a table

III. Writing
A. Patient is asked to copy a simple musical text.
B. If task is appropriate for his musical background, patient is asked to transcribe a dictated melody.

IV. Discrimination of sounds
Patient is asked to indicate which of two tones is higher in pitch.

V. Identification of familiar melodies
Patient is asked to identify familiar melodies played on the flute.

VI. Identification of types of music
Patient is asked to indicate the types of music (e.g. dance, military, church) reflected in the playing of representative samples of each genre on the flute or the piano.

VII. Identification of musical instrumemts
Patient is asked to identify the instrument as characteristic pieces are played on the piano, violin, organ, etc.

VIII. Reading
If task is appropriate for his musical background, patient is asked to sight-read musical texts.

extent that it is based on specific information about how well the patient sang or played an instrument, how often he attended concerts, how critical he was, etc.

The desirability of utilizing a systematic examination schedule to ensure that all aspects of musical capacity are assessed and to make possible a meaningful comparison of the performances of different patients has long been recognized. A number of comprehensive batteries have been developed by specialists in the field such as Jellinek (1933) and Wertheim and Botez (1959). These test batteries, which are quite elaborate, provide for the assessment of virtually every aspect of musicality, including the reading and writing of music and instrumental performance. They are fully applicable only to patients who happen to have been trained musicians and only the more elementary parts assessing tonal discrimination, singing, and the recognition of familiar tunes can be used with the average patient. It must also be noted that none of these batteries has been standardized on the basis of performances of normal subjects, in the sense that mental ability tests are standardized.

The test battery developed by Dorgeuille (1966) for his study of the amusias provides an example of a systematic examination that is quite comprehensive and yet not too long for practical application. It covers diverse aspects of musical function, as outlined in Table 15–1. In addition, Dorgeuille assessed the premorbid musical capacities of each patient by a check list that provided specific information about musical training in school, participation in band, chorus, or orchestra, formal musical education and level of skill in instrumental performance, sight reading, and writing music. Evaluation of whether or not the observed level of performance on a particular test was defective could then be made with reference to the patient's premorbid capacity in this respect. Of course, limitation in musical background precluded giving tests assessing the reading or writing of music to many patients.

The test battery, and a systematic neuropsychological examination of language functions, praxis, perception and calculation, were given to 26 right-handed patients with brain disease. Thus it was possible to determine the associations among the different musical performances as well as to determine their relationship to locus of lesion, linguistic functions, and perceptual capacities. The findings of this comprehensive study are considered in the next section.

A more global approach to the problem of assessing premorbid level was taken by Grison (1972) in her study of disturbance of musical function in patients with hemispheric disease. On the basis of anamnestic data, she placed each patient into one of six categories as shown in Table 15–2. Although less rigorous than the method employed by Dorgeuille, this categorization appears to be a useful and practical procedure.

Clinical and Pathological Correlates

More often than not, disturbances in musical function occur in association with aphasic disorders. A survey of the cases reported in the literature suggests that about seven of every ten patients described as amusic suffered from one or another form of aphasia. Moreover, the type of musical disability manifested tends to conform qualitatively to the type of aphasic disorder shown by the patient. Patients with a Broca type of aphasia are likely to show oral-expressive defects without noteworthy concomitant impairment in musical perception or recognition. The occurrence of receptive musical defects is associated with either word-deafness or a Wernicke type of aphasia. Dorgeuille (1966) found five instances of musical agraphia in his series; four showed a concomitant verbal agraphia. He encountered six cases of musical alexia, three of whom showed a concomitant verbal alexia. A predominantly amnesic type of amusia is likely to

TABLE 15–2. Levels of Musical Culture (adapted from Grison, 1972)

1. Showed no interest in music; did not care to listen to it or to sing.
2. Occasionally sang familiar melodies such as nursery rhymes and regional songs; sometimes listened to music on the wireless.
3. Enjoyed singing and had a "repertory" which he maintained and augmented; was a critical listener of music on the wireless; bought gramophone records and listened to them frequently.
4. Played an instrument but was not trained in theory or sight-reading.
5. Played an instrument; fair sight-reading ability and general musical knowledge.
6. Was an excellent musician on both the practical and theoretical levels.

be associated with corresponding amnesic difficulties in speech. For example, one of the patients in the series of Grison (1972) presented with an amnesic aphasia, characterized by word-finding difficulty and circumlocutions in association with fluent speech and mildly defective oral language comprehension. She showed no impairment in the discrimination of notes, melodies, or rhythms and could hum melodies quite accurately. However, she had obvious difficulty in trying to retrieve the names of familiar tunes which she knew quite well.

Nevertheless, despite this close qualitative and quantitative association between disorders of music and language, there is incontrovertible evidence that the two spheres of activity are mediated by distinctive neurobehavioural systems. The long-standing observation that patients with severe expressive language disorder are able to sing is in itself sufficient proof of this. The same dissociation may be observed in patients with receptive language disorder. The word-deaf patient of Klein and Harper (1956) at first experienced oral speech "as an undifferentiated mass of sounds without structure or rhythm." Later, when his condition stabilized, he was able to perceive some familiar words and phrases correctly but was still unable to carry on a conversation. He even heard his own speech as indistinct and, except for vowels, was unable to repeat speech sounds correctly. Nevertheless, he was able to recognize most of the popular melodies played on a gramophone to him. Moreover, he was able to identify the voices of people familiar to him and even to identify different regional accents. Thus his capacity to apprehend the musical aspects of spoken language, as reflected in voice quality and accent, was retained within a setting of defective perception of individual word sounds.

Similarly, Assal (1973) has reported the case of a pianist with a fluent aphasia and marked impairment in verbal understanding, repetition, reading, and writing. He could play the piano quite as well as before his vascular accident and detailed examination disclosed no changes in musical capacities that did not require verbal communication. He continued to play in a professional band specializing in light music.

Nor is the sparing of musical capacity in aphasic patients necessarily limited to relatively simple expressive and receptive functions. Luria et al. (1965) have described the case of a distinguished Russian composer who was rendered severely aphasic after a stroke sustained when he was 57 years old. Some six years earlier he had had a stroke with transient sensory, motor, and speech disturbances from which he recovered completely. After the second stroke, he showed marked impairment in conversational speech, repetition, and verbal comprehension, which persisted until his death at the age of 61 years. Nevertheless, throughout the three-year period between his second stroke and his final illness, he completed a number of compositions begun before the stroke and wrote a substantial series of new compositions which were performed in public by leading artists and which "other musicians considered to be up to standard, and which did not differ significantly from the compositions of his earlier years." Postmortem examination disclosed a massive softening of the temporal and inferior parietal areas of the left hemisphere.

The fact that disturbances in musical function can occur in patients who are free of any aphasic disorder is equally cogent evidence for the independence of the two "language" systems. Patients with purely or predominantly oral-expressive impairment are about as likely to be nonaphasic as aphasic. However, it must be remarked that most of them do in fact show dysprosodic speech, which might be interpreted as another expression of a general defect in the oral production of sounds, rhythms, and melodic intonations. Impaired perception of sounds, tonal sequences, and rhythms is somewhat less frequently observed in nonaphasic patients as compared to those with receptive language disorder but numerous case reports indicate that it is far from being a rare occurrence.

Clinicopathologic correlations with respect to disturbances in musical function are much less abundant than for the aphasic disorders and only a limited amount of information about the site of lesions associated with the amusias has been amassed. Broadly speaking, predominantly expressive amusias with relative preservation of receptive capacities are associated with anteriorly situated lesions, for the most part compromising the frontal lobes, and defects in the perception and recognition of tones and melodies (with or without concomitant expressive impairment) are associated with the presence of disease of the temporal lobes. The analogy with the aphasic disorders, in which a predominantly expressive aphasia is likely to be associated with an anterior lesion and a predominantly receptive aphasia with a temporo–parietal lesion, is evident. There is, however, one quite fundamental difference. Appropriately situated lesions in either hemisphere can produce both expressive and receptive disorders of musical function in a right-handed patient while aphasia in such a patient is almost invariably an expression of left hemisphere disease.

Analysis of the clinical literature suggests that "pure" expressive amusia (vocal or instrumental) with preservation of receptive functions and without aphasia is most likely to be associated with anterior lesions of the right hemisphere. The case reports of Mann (1898), Jossmann (1926, 1927), and Botez and Wertheim (1959) illustrate this relationship. A predominantly expressive amusia in combination with a predominantly expressive aphasic disorder is associated with anterior lesions of the left hemisphere, as illustrated by the inability of many Broca aphasics to reproduce a heard tone or to sing a tune. Thus, setting aside the question of the presence or absence of an associated aphasic disorder, there appears to be no hemispheric bias in respect to the lesions that may produce a disorder of expressive musical function.

Disturbances in receptive musical capacities in combination with aphasic disorder have been found to be associated with lesions involving the middle and posterior parts of the first and second temporal gyri, the transverse temporal gyri, and the anterior temporal region of the left hemisphere. The three surgically explored cases of Dorgeuille (1966) may be cited to illustrate this point. Case No. 19, a fluent aphasic, was examined three years after evacuation of an intracerebral hematoma located in the anterior part of the left temporal lobe. He made many errors in discriminating tones and could not identify the characteristic sounds of different instruments. He also showed defective reproduction of sounds and rhythmic patterns, but he could identify and sing familiar melodies. Case No. 20, examined two weeks after evacuation of an intracerebral hematoma at the tip of the left temporal lobe, also showed a fluent aphasia with paraphasic speech, word-finding difficulties, and mild impairment in oral speech comprehension. She exhibited impairment in the discrimination of tones as well as expressive musical defects. Case No. 22, an accomplished musician, was examined shortly before surgical exploration disclosed a glioblastoma occupying the middle and posterior parts of the first and second temporal gyri of the left hemisphere. She showed a fluent aphasia with significant impairment in oral speech comprehension. She could reproduce isolated tones accurately but showed evident defects in singing melodies with which she had been quite familiar. She would begin to sing the melody correctly but was not able to continue it to completion. She also showed impairment in the perception of tonal sequences.

Receptive amusia without concomitant aphasic disorder has been found to be associated with temporal lobe disease of either hemisphere or of both hemispheres (Schuster and Taterka, 1926; Pötzl and Uiberall, 1937; Pötzl, 1939, 1943; Spreen et al., 1965). These observations, taken together with the circumstance that so many patients with "temporal lobe" aphasia show intact musical capacity, has led to the supposition that music, unlike language, has bilateral hemispheric representation. This may be the case but the facts in themselves indicate only that the left hemisphere dominance characteristic of the mediation of language functions does not hold for musical functions. An equally plausible interpretation is that some individuals show dissociated dominance, i.e., they are left hemisphere dominant for language but right hemisphere dominant for music.

Henschen (1920) and, later, Kleist (1934, 1962) tried to establish extremely precise localizations of the cerebral areas mediating specific musical functions. Henschen, for example, localized a "center" for singing in the upper part of the third frontal gyrus, a "center" for oral musical comprehension in the left temporal pole and a "center" for reading music in the angular gyrus. On his part, Kleist related different aspects of musical perception to different parts of the temporal lobe, e.g., the discrimination of timbre to the transverse gyri and the apprehension of melodic patterns to the architectonically delimited *subregio magna dorsalis* (Hopf, 1954) on the lateral surface of the temporal lobe. These attempts to establish precise anatomic correlates for specific performances often have been derided as being the product of sheer fantasy. In fact, they emerged from painstaking analysis by serious, well-informed investigators of the data available to them; but it is clear that our current fund of anatomical and clinical information is far too meager to provide substantial support for these essentially speculative inferences. Yet they are not without heuristic value in pointing up the necessity for detailed anatomical study and careful clinical investigation.

The idea that each hemisphere makes a distinctive contribution to receptive and expressive musical performance has been proposed. For example, Barbizet (1972; Barbizet et al., 1969) has advanced the concept that the right hemisphere participates primarily on the perceptual and executive levels of musical activity while the left hemisphere mediates the recognition and memory of musical structures, the symbolic processes in reading and writing music, and the higher level integrative functions involved in musical composition.

Only a few definitive statements can be made about the interrelations among the diverse musical deficits. It is clear that there can be a dissociation between expressive and receptive functions. A patient can show significant impairment in singing and instrumental playing without noteworthy perceptual deficit. Conversely, a patient with perceptual defects can be shown by appropriate methods of examination to have intact executive capacities. The abilities to reproduce isolated sounds and to sing a melody may be differentially impaired; however, they are usually lost together. On the other hand, failure to produce a familiar tune when given its name, which is essentially a form of amnesia, frequently occurs within the setting of intact expressive capacity. Impairment in the reading and writing of music shows a close association. There is frequent dissociation between the ability to discriminate isolated sounds and the capacity to recognize melodies or to identify their type (i.e., church music, folk song, etc.). Observations such as these provide some theoretical justification for attempts, such as that of Kleist, to search for distinctive anatomical bases for different aspects of musical reception.

Concluding Remarks

As this survey indicates, a substantial body of information has been amassed about the disturbances in musical function that may occur as a consequence of brain disease. The characteristic forms which these disturbances take have been well-described and some broad correlations between them and the sites of the causative cerebral lesions have been established. Yet our knowledge of the neurological aspects of the problem is still quite fragmentary and major questions remain unanswered.

The nature of the relationship of the amusias to aphasic deficit is one such question. That the two groups of disorders tend to be closely associated is evident. But why one aphasic patient with a focal lesion will show concomitant disturbances in musical function while another patient with a similar type of disorder and lesion will show no musical disabilities is a complete mystery. Obviously, a major determining factor, the nature of which is unknown to us, is operating to produce such individual differences. It is possible that the contribution which each hemisphere makes to the mediation of musical function varies quantitatively from one individual to another. If this should prove to be the case, it could provide an explanation for the individual differences that are observed clinically. But, of course, whether this is in fact the case is not known. Thus a basic question about the hemispheric distribution of the neural mechanisms underlying musical function is posed and remains to be answered. Reliable knowledge about interhemispheric relations in this respect no doubt would go far toward helping us understand a cognate problem, namely, why some patients are rendered amusic as a consequence of disease of the right hemisphere while the majority of patients in this category are not affected.

A number of questions that are perhaps less basic in nature but still of considerable clinical importance also remain unanswered. The relative frequency and severity of disturbances of musical function in patients with brain disease have never been studied. Whether there are sex differences in this regard is unknown. Nor has any attention been given to the question of the frequency and qualitative nature of musical disabilities in left-handed patients. Investigation of this last issue in the field of the aphasic disorders has generated findings that have given much insight into the relations between handedness and hemispheric cerebral dominance for the language functions (cf. Benton, 1965; Subirana, 1969; Hécaen, 1972). Comparable study of the question in the field of the amusias might be as fruitful.

These investigative possibilities presuppose the application of objective and reliable methods for assessing diverse musical performances in relation to premorbid capacities in large groups of patients. Happily Ustved's (1937) strictures about the gross inadequacy of the techniques typically employed in the examination of patients no longer holds. Although much still needs to be done in the way of standardization of procedures and the gathering of normal values in defined populations, nuclear test batteries that can serve as models for further development are now available, thanks largely to the work of Wertheim and Botez (1959) and Dorgeuille (1966). The prospects that methodologically sound clinical assessment, coupled with employment of some of the experimental approaches described in other chapters of this volume, will significantly advance our understanding of the amusias appear to be quite bright.

References

Assal G. (1973). Aphasie de Wernicke chez un pianiste. *Rev. Neurol.* 29: 251.

Ballet G. (1896). *Le Langage Intérieur et les Diverses Formes de l'Aphasie*. Paris: Alcan.

Barbizet J. (1972). Role de l'hémisphère droit dans les perceptions auditives. In Barbizet J., Ben Hamida M., and Duizabo P., eds.) *Le Monde de l'Hémiplégie Gauche*. Paris: Masson.

Barbizet J., Duizabo P., Enos G., and Fuchs D. (1969). Reconnaissance de messages sonores: bruits familiers et airs musicaux familiers lors des lésions cérébrales unilatérales. *Rev. Neurol.* 121: 624.

Benton A. L. (1965). The problem of cerebral dominance. *Canad. Psychol.* 6: 332.

Botez M. I. and Wertheim N. (1959). Expressive aphasia and amusia. *Brain* 82: 186.

Bouillaud J. B. (1865). Sur la faculté du langage articulé. *Arch. Gén. Méd.* 1: 575.

Brazier M. (1892). Du troubles des facultés musicales dans l'aphasie. *Rev. Phil.* 34: 337.

Dalin O. (1745). Berättelse om en dumbe, som kan siunga. K. Swenska Wetensk. *Acad. Handlingar* 6: 114.

Déjèrine J. (1892). Des différentes variétés de cécité verbale. *Mém. Soc. Biol.* 27: 1.

Döllken A. (1935). Ueber Amusie und Spielzeitstörungen. Z. *Neurol. Psychiat.* 154: 32.

Dorgeuille C. (1966). *Introduction à l'Étude des Amusies*. Thèse, Paris.

Dupre E. and Nathan M. (1911). *Le Langage Musical: Étude Médicopsychologique*. Paris: Alcan.

Edgren J. G. (1895). Amusie (musikalische Aphasie). *Dtsch. Z. Nervenhlk.* 6: 1.

Feuchtwanger E. (1930). *Amusie: Studien zur Pathologischen Psychologie der akustischen Wahrnehmung und Vorstellung und ihre Strukturgebiete besonders in Musik und Sprache*. Berlin: Springer.

Finkelnburg F. C. (1870). Asymbolie. *Berlin klin. Wschr.* 7: 449.

Fischer A. (1867). *Ueber zentrale Sprachstörungen mit besonderer Berücksichtigung der Aphasie*. Dissertation. Berlin.

Gowers W. R. (1875). On a case of simultaneous embolism of central retinal and middle cerebral arteries. *Lancet* 2: 794.

Grison B. (1972). *Une Étude sur les Altérations Musicales au Cours des Lésions hémisphériques*. Thèse, Paris.

Hécaen H. (1972). *Introduction à la Neuropsychologie*. Paris: Larousse.

Henschen S. E. (1920). *Klinische und anatomische Beiträge zur Pathologie des Gehirns*, Teil 5: *Ueber Aphasie, Amusie und Akalkulie*. Stockholm: Nordiska Bokhandeln.

Hopf A. (1954). Die Myeloarchitektonik des Isocortex temporalis beim Menschen. *J. Hirnforsch.* I: 208.

Jellinek A. (1933). Zur Phänomenologie der Amusie. *Jahrb f. Psychiat. u. Neurol.* 50: 115.

Jossmann P. (1926). Motorische Amusie (Demonstration). *Zbl. Neurol. Psychiat.* 44: 260.

Jossmann P. (1927). Die Beziehungen der motorischen Amusie zu den apraktischen Störungen. *Mschr. Psychiat. Neurol.* 63: 239.

Klein R. and Harper J. (1956). The problem of agnosia in the light of a case of pure word deafness. *J. Ment. Sci.* 102: 112.

Kleist K. (1928). Gehirnpathologische und lokalisatorische Ergebnisse über Hörstörungen, Geräuschtaubheiten und Amusien. *Mschr. Psychiat. Neurol.* 68: 853.

Kleist K. (1934). *Gehirnpathologie*. Leipzig; Barth.

Kleist K. (1962) *Sensory Aphasia and Amusia: The Myeloarchitectonic Basis*. Oxford: Pergamon Press.

Knoblauch A. (1888). Ueber Störungen der musikalischer Leistungsfähigkeit infolge von Gehirnläsionen. *Dtsch. Arch. klin. Med.* 43: 331.

Luria A. R., Tsvetkova L. S., and Futer D. S. (1965). Aphasia in a composer. *J. Neurol. Sci.* 2, 288.

Mann L. (1898). Casuistische Beiträge zur Hirnchirurgie und Hirnlokalisation. *Mschr. Psychiat. Neurol.* 4: 369.

Oppenheim H. (1888). Ueber das Verhalten der musikalischen Ausdruckbwegungen und des musikalischen Verständnisses bei Aphasischen. *Charité Ann.* 13: 345.

Pötzl O. (1939). Zur Pathologie der Amusie. *Z. Neurol. Psychiat.* 165: 187.

Pötzl O. (1943). Bemerkungen zum Problem der kortikalen Vorgänge bei der akustischen Wahrnehmung. *Mschr. Ohrenhlk.* 77: 422.

Pötzl O. and Uiberall H. (1937). Zur Pathologie der Amusie. *Wiener Klin. Wschr.* 50: 770.

Probst M. (1899). Ueber die Lokalisation des Tonvermögens. *Arch. Psychiat.* 32: 387.

Proust A. (1866). *Arch. Gen. Méd.* Cited by Ballet (1886) and Henschen (1920).

Proust A. (1872). De l'aphasie. *Arch. Gen. Méd.* I: 147.

Schuster P. and Taterka H. (1926). Beitrag zur Anatomie und Klinik der reinen Worttaubheit. *Z. Neurol. Psychiat.* 105: 494.

Spreen O., Benton A. L., and Fincham R. W. (1965). Auditory agnosia without aphasia. *Arch. Neurol.* 13: 84.

Subirana A. (1969). Handedness and cerebral dominance. In Vinken P. J., Bruyn, G. W., Critchley M. and Frederiks J. A. M. (eds.), *Handbook of Clinical Neurology*, Vol. 4 Amsterdam: North-Holland Publishing Co.

Ustvedt H. J. (1937). Ueber die Untersuchung der musikalischen Funktionen bei Patienten mit Aphasie. *Acta Med. Scand.* Suppl. 86.

Vignolo, L. A. (1969) Auditory agnosia: a review and report of recent evidence. In Benton A. L., ed., *Contributions to Clinical Neuropsychology* Chicago: Aldine Publishing Co.

Wertheim N. (1963). Disturbances of musical functions. In Halpern L. (ed.), *Problems of Dynamic Neurology*. Jerusalem: Hadassah University Hospital.

Wertheim N. (1969). The amusias. In Vinken, P. J., Bruyn G. W., Critchley M. and Fredricks A. M. Fredricks (eds.), *Handbook of Clinical Neurology*, Vol. 4. Amsterdam: North-Holland Publishing Co.

Wertheim N. and Botez M. I. (1959). Plan d'investigation des fonctions musicales. *Encéphale* 48: 246.

Wertheim N. and Botez M. I. (1961). Receptive amusia: a clinical analysis. *Brain* 4: 19.

16

Clinical Neuropsychology: 1960–1990

First, I should like to say a few words about the person after whom this lecture is named. There are no more than a handful of people in this room who knew Herbert Birch. And I have a feeling that the great majority of you have no idea who he was, although you may have read some of his papers. Yet he was a founding member of the International Neuropsychological Society (INS) and in fact the organizational meeting at which INS was launched was held in 1968 in his laboratory at the Albert Einstein College of Medicine in New York. He was an active, dedicated member of INS until his untimely death at the age of 54, directly before the 1973 INS meeting in New Orleans. Those of us who knew him were much affected by sad event and it was under these circumstances that this lectureship in his name was established.

Herbert Birch was a remarkable person. For one thing, his educational background was unusual. He began his training in veterinary medicine. However, discovering that he was more interested in the behavior of animals than in their distempers, he soon left that field to take a Ph.D. in comparative psychology. Then, finding that he was at least equally interested in people as in animals, he studied medicine at New York University, all the while holding a full-time teaching position at the City College of New York. He was a most inspiring teacher. The record shows that a surprisingly large number of psychologists acknowledge that their choice of a profession was due to the fact that they took a course or two with Herbert Birch.

Reprinted with permission from *Journal of Clinical and Experimental Neuropsychology*, Vol. 14, No. 3, pp. 407–417.

Herbert Birch Memorial Lecture, held during the 20th Annual Meeting, San Diego, California, February 7, 1992.

His interest in normal and deviant behavioral development led him into the field of pediatrics, primarily as an investigator rather than as a practitioner. The main thrust of his research and scholarship—reflected in 190 papers and 11 monographs—was a resolute attempt to understand the interactions of biological, psychological, social and economic factors in the production of cognitive disabilities and behavior disorders (cf. Bortner, 1979). His grasp of this complex issue was extraordinarily incisive. Theory and practice in clinical neuropsychology would have been greatly enriched if fate had permitted him to continue his far-reaching investigative work that took him from the clinic and laboratory to city slums and Third World countries.

During the past few years we have had the benefit of reviews and assessments of the present status of neuropsychology by many leaders in the field (Costa, 1988; Matthews, 1990; Meier, 1991; Parsons, 1991; Rourke, 1991). Whether there is anything more to say is a real question.

Still each of us sees the past and views the present somewhat differently and we differ in our judgments of what is or is not of prime importance. I have been criticized for not fully appreciating some figures whose achievements are very highly rated by others. Conversely, some of my friends have been puzzled by what they regard as my excessive enthusiasm for certain figures whose contribution they consider to be quite modest in the total scheme of things. No doubt these differences in opinion are determined by each individual's values, special interests, temperament and style. Thus, although what I have to say will repeat in large part what we have already heard in recent years, still another account may be of some interest.

The time period we cover is the recent past from 1960 to 1990. Instead of recounting developments in linear fashion over this time span of 30 years, I will contrast our situation in 1960 with that in 1990 and then consider one or two implications for 1992 and beyond.

In 1960 neuropsychology had not yet come of age. There were no neuropsychological organizations, or even sections of larger organizations, no neuropsychological journals, no examining boards, no standards of training or practice. Nevertheless, neuropsychology had certainly emerged as a distinctive discipline and a distinctive field of clinical practice, one that was recognized as such by at least some neurologists and neurosurgeons and by some colleagues in other areas of psychology. Academic appointments in university departments of neurology and neurosurgery were held by a few people including Ward Halstead, Manfred Meier, Brenda Milner, Ralph Reitan, Hans-Lukas Teuber, and myself. Teuber had just assumed the chairmanship of the Department of Psychology at MIT and was about to establish a major training program which was experimental-theoretical in nature but which did involve normal and brain-injured persons as the primary subjects of study. In Britain, Oliver Zangwill had established close ties with London's leading neurological hospital where his students (George Ettlinger, John MacFie, Malcolm Piercy, and Elizabeth Warrington among them) were engaged in research that generated influential contributions to the field.

It was an exciting time for those who considered themselves to be neuropsychologists. In passing, I might remark that some, for example, Ward Halstead and Lukas Teuber, came to this realization very early while others, like myself, came to it later. Until about 1955, I did not consider myself to be a "neuropsychologist" but rather a clinical psychologist with a special interest in patients with brain disease and in brain–behavior relationships. I would guess that Harold Goodglass also placed himself in the category of a clinical psychologist with a special interest in the aphasic disorders and brain–behavior relationships. (If you are directing a graduate training program in clinical psychology or functioning as chief of clinical psychology in a VA hospital, perhaps you had better call yourself a "clinical psychologist.")

Why were we so enthusiastic about the prospects for this new area of research and practice? Not many years before, our primary tasks had been simply to identify the presence or absence of brain damage in the patient with an unresolved diagnosis and to generate findings that might be useful as a guide to management in the patient with established brain disease.

The reason was that research, both clinical and experimental, in the late 1940s and the 1950s had demonstrated that the behavioral consequences of focal brain disease could be investigated in greater depth and detail and with greater precision than was thought possible before that time. Some of the more prominent contributions may be mentioned.

By 1960 the proposition that the right hemisphere was not a cognitively silent region but instead possessed its own distinctive functional properties was widely, but still not universally, accepted by knowledgeable neurologists and psychologists. This had come about largely through the studies of Oliver Zangwill and the Paris neurologist, Henry Hécaen, who had shown conclusively that impairment in visuospatial and visuocontructional performance was very closely associated with disease of the right hemisphere. The effect of their research was to transform the long-held doctrine of left-hemisphere dominance into that of asymmetry of hemispheric function, according to which each hemisphere serves different, if not contrasting, cognitive functions.

An advance of at least equal importance was the demonstration by Brenda Milner and the neurosurgeon, William Scoville, of the crucial role of the hippocampus in the mediation of learning and memory processes (Scoville and Milner, 1957). The far-reaching impact of that discovery is obvious to all of us.

The comprehensive research program of Lukas Teuber and his able associates, Lila Ghent, Mortimer Mishkin, Rita Rudel, Josephine Semmes, and Sidney Weinstein, at New York's Bellevue Hospital in the 1950s had produced a wealth of empirical findings on the performances of patients with penetrating brain wounds. Dealing with diverse topics including somatosensory performances, spatial orientation, auditory perception, and intellectual functions, their contributions were not only immensely stimulating to researchers but significantly enlarged the possible scope of clinical neuropsychological evaluation.

Reaction time studies by Karl Smith (1947), as well as by my own team in Iowa (Blackburn and Benton, 1955; Benton and Joynt, 1959), reintroduced the question of speed of information processing in brain disease and of its neural mechanisms. The seminal study of Harold Goodglass and Fred Quadfasel in 1954 on the relationships between hand preference and cerebral dominance for speech had disproved long-standing assumptions and reopened the topic for investigation. Donald Broadbent's (1954) introduction of the technique of dichotic listening had—as we well know—profound consequences for the study of hemispheric differences in auditory perception. Analogously, the even earlier tachistoscopic study by Mishkin and Forgays (1952) of lateral differences in visual perception ushered in that program of research.

These and other contributions to knowledge of the variety of cognitive defects that might be shown by brain-diseased patients and, by inference, of the specificity of brain—behavior relationships, testified to the richness of the field of clinical neuropsychology. However, in 1960, neuropsychologists had yet to apply the novel assessment techniques employed in these studies in their own clinical research and practice. Nor had they taken advantage of the many tests described in the literature of clinical neurology and the literatures of educational, vocational, industrial, and applied psychology that might have been adapted for neuropsychological use. For the most part, clinical practice in the 1950s relied on analysis of performance patterns on the Wechsler-Bellevue, which was hardly the optimal instrument for the purpose, or on the first version of the Halstead-Reitan battery. Thus, although these batteries were generally supplemented by a few other tests in the clinical examination, the diagnostic armamentarium of the neuropsychologist was fairly limited. It was also inflexible, the same battery of tests being given to every patient regardless of his complaints and disabilities. It was as if one hoped that something would emerge in the findings that would answer the referral question.

A more serious limitation was the lack of neurodiagnostic techniques that generated information of specific value to the neuropsychologist. Pneumoencephalography and ventriculography, electroencephalography, skull films, and cerebral arteriography were, of course, tremendously useful for neurological and neurosurgical diagnosis; but they provided only indirect and imprecise indications of the locus and extent of lesions. Apart from surgical reports and plotting the path of penetrating brain wounds, both of which in any case have been found to underestimate the extent of brain damage, there was little opportunity to investigate specific brain–behavior correlations directly in the living patient.

Consequently, reliance was placed on the judgment of neurologists as the criterion measure to determine the presence and locus of brain disease in the nonsurgical patient. This procedure was certainly of great value and much important information was gained from it. But it is obvious that it was in large part a circular process since an important component of the neurological examination evaluates the same phenomena that are assessed in a more precise way by the neuropsychological examination. Thus, the situation of the neuropsychologist was similar to that of the psychologist in a psychiatric facility who "validated" his findings on schizophrenic or what was then called "neurotic" patients against "established" psychiatric diagnoses. Nevertheless, enough knowledge was gained to justify an increasing participation of the neuropsychologist in neurological research and practice.

After 30 years of continuous progress, the situation of the neuropsychologist is vastly different. The scope of inquiry and practice has expanded to an amazing degree—I think far beyond what anyone would have anticipated in 1960. The neuropsychological aspects of psychiatric disorders, of diverse medical conditions and toxic states, of dementia and pseudodementia, and of developmental and eduycational disabilities are flourishing, important areas of activity. Child neuropsychology and the neuropsychological rehabilitation of nonaphasic patients were almost unknown in 1960. Today they are major branches of the discipline. Moreover, now neuropsychological research and practice not only cover a much broader territory but are also more incisive and more highly focused.

Undoubtedly, the most important single factor responsible for this progress has been the advent of those remarkable neurodiagnostic techniques, CT scan and MRI, that disclose the locus and extent of structural brain lesions far more accurately and in greater detail than did the older procedures. Their utilization has led to new knowledge (for example, about the significance of hitherto undisclosed white matter lesions in the production of cognitive disability) and to the revision of long-standing assumptions (for example, about the role of Broca's area in the mediation of speech).

In the 1960s, given the lack of precision in specifying the site and size of brain lesions, most neuropsychologists restricted themselves to a quadrantal localization, so to speak—left anterior and posterior, right anterior and posterior—in the assessment of nonsurgical patients. Other neuropsychologists, mindful of the dubious accuracy of even this gross localization, were still more cautious and analyzed their findings only according to a left-hemisphere/right-hemisphere dichotomy.

Today this is all changed. Given the precision of current neurodiagnostic techniques, the neuroradiologists can specify with considerable (but perhaps not absolute) confidence that a lesion is limited, for example, to the territory of the left supramarginal gyrus, to the orbital region of the frontal lobes or to the undersurface of the right occipital lobe. Now the neuropsychologist can determine the behavioral changes associated with these fairly strictly delimited lesions and thus gain knowledge about specific brain–behavior relationships.

Today one often hears the opinion that from a clinical standpoint the utilization of neuropsychological tests to detect the presence of brain disease and to aid in the localization of focal brain lesions is passé. Since CT and MRI do such an excellent job, there is no need for the faltering imperfect efforts of the neuropsychologist. No doubt the clinical application of neuropsychological evaluation for these purposes has declined markedly in importance. Yet I think that this opinion, which reflects an altogether too narrow view of what is meant by "brain disease," is not valid and I believe that it would be most unfortunate if the "detection and localization of lesion" enterprise were abandoned.

We need to keep in mind that, although these neurodiagnostic procedures represent a tremendous advance in lesional localization, they are not the last word on the topic. As we know, taken singly, CT and MRI pick up structural changes that the other does not. For example, MRI often indicates a larger lesion than what is seen on the CT scan and it also is able to pick up white matter lesion and small multifocal lesions that are not detected by CT. Conversely, there are some types of lesion that are better visualized in the CT scan. Taken together, the two procedures are more effective than either one alone and undoubtedly there will be further developments that will make them even more informative.

But the basic and more important consideration is that they disclose structural changes that may or may not carry clinical or behavioral significance. The literature of clinical neurology includes a number of reports describing a lack of correspondence between brain lesions, as visualized by MRI or CT scan, and the expected clinical findings. In part these studies simply confirm some older observations on normal individuals in whom autopsy disclosed gross brain lesions that were clinically silent during life.

These results should not be too surprising. Visualized lesions do not take account of reciprocal relationships between the hemispheres or of restoration of function (or conversely, of diaschisis effects) or of neuronal networks that propagate information throughout the brain. When we speak of "brain–behavior relationships" we mean the relationships between behaviors and the functional mechanisms in the brain that mediate these behaviors, not merely that the destruction of a piece of brain tissue has disrupted behavior. Thus, it seems to me clear that "localization" (which is, admittedly, a hard concept to define precisely) is still of great concern to the neuropsychologist.

An observation worth recalling in this connection is that there are areas of investigation in which neuropsychological assessment serves as the criterion measure in evaluating the significance of the presence (or absence) of pathological findings rather than the other way around. CT, MRI, and autopsy studies of elderly and demented patients are an obvious example. As we know, comparisons of CT and MRI estimates of the amount of loss of brain tissue, as reflected in ventricular enlargement, depth of sulci and the like, with estimates of the degree of mental deterioration have yielded correlation coefficients of fairly modest size, ranging from 0.30 to 0.50. Autopsy studies, involving estimates of the amount of plaques, neurofibrillary tangles and dendritic loss, have produced higher coefficients ranging from 0.40 to an astounding 0.96.

A more important example is provided by the utilization of neuropsychological tests to detect cerebral dysfunction in conditions where there is no evidence of structural cerebral abnormality. Almost everyone would agree that neuropsychological assessment plays an indispensable role in evaluating the sequelae of cardiac surgery, the effects of environmental and occupational toxins, and the cognitive changes associated with metabolic disorders, all of which are conditions in which current neurodiagnostic procedures generally fail to disclose structural abnormality. The utilization of neuropsychological procedures to detect brain abnormality is *not* passé.

Neuropschological test methods (which may be regarded as being in a superficial sense the behavioral counterparts of CT, MRI, and the other neurodiagnostic techniques) showed an explosive growth in the decades after 1960. Tests were conceived and developed for a great variety of purposes and sometimes, it would seem, for no purpose other than the fun of making up a clever test. There was much duplication and hence much redundancy so that, for example, now we have more brief screening tests for early dementia than there are remedies for headache.

But this is the way progress is achieved in most fields. Out of the welter of tests that have been produced, some have proved to be very useful for one or another facet of neuropsychological assessment and they have enjoyed wide use. The Token Test of De Renzi and Vignolo and its many modifications, Rey's Auditory Verbal Learning test and its derivatives, controlled word association and facial recognition tests and the Wisconsin Card Sorting Test are a few examples that come to mind.

These tests were developed or, in some cases, adopted for neuropsychological assessment because they met a specific clinical or research need. Thus, Brenda Milner utilized the Wisconsin Card Sorting Test, which had been devised as an experimental technique, to investigate behavioral flexibility in patients with frontal and nonfrontal lesions. Similarly, she turned the Seashore tests of musical talents into an instrument for determining the consequences of left and right temporal lobe excisions. Broadbent's dichotic listening procedure was elaborated and used to explore the differential hemispheric contribution to auditory perception. Dorothy Gronwall devised the PASAT procedure specifically as an instrument that might disclose slowed information processing in patients with mild head injuries whose complaints could not be validated by either clinical evaluation or conventional neuropsychological assessment. The De Renzi-Vignolo Token Test was deliberately designed to measure oral verbal understanding in the uneducated and sometimes illiterate patient with a limited vocabulary.

As a consequence, today we have a rich armamentarium of test methods at our disposal for assessment purposes. Muriel Lezak's (1983) magisterial treatise on neuropsychological assessment and the new compendium of Otfried Spreen and Esther Strauss (1991) provide more than sufficient evidence on this point.* But on the whole neuropsychologists have yet to take full advantage of the resources that are available to them. There are a number of reasons for this. One is that most neuropsychologists are wedded to a "fixed battery" approach to assessment, in which the same set of tests is given regardless of what the referral question is; for example, whether it is one of dementia, of specific memory impairment, of visuospatial disability, of frontal lobe dysfunction, or of defective interhemispheric integration.

The "fixed battery" approach has a solid justification. It ensures effective communication between specialists. It permits the isolation of distinctive patterns of performance associated with different diagnostic categories and, as experience with it is gained, it affords the opportunity to observe clinically important qualitative characteristics of performance. A standardized approach is a great asset. Yet it has serious limitations. It is doubtful that any fixed neuropsychological test battery, however comprehensive and time-consuming it may be, can be regarded as fully adequate since it cannot possibly answer all the questions that arise in practice or clinical research. The neuropsychologist today is much better off than the neuropsychologist in 1960 in that his assessment battery is more comprehensive and more relevant to clinical problems. Yet in one respect his situation is the same. He gives a battery of tests and *hopes* that some component in it will answer the referral question.

Opposed to the "fixed battery" approach to assessment is the "flexible" approach where both the selection and the sequence of tests given to a patient is determined first by the nature of the referral question and then by observation of performance during the course of examination. Recognizing assessment as a logical, sequential decision-making process, the flexible approach has much to recommend it (not least because it forces the examiner to think about what he is doing). But it, too, has serious weakness. Apart from its idiosyncratic character which surely impedes communication and mutual understanding, there is the risk that this selective procedure may miss an unexpected performance characteristic that might be picked up by a more comprehensive battery.

* Author's Note: Lezak's *Neuropsychological Assessment* is now in a 3rd edition (1995), and an expanded version of *A Compendium of Neuropsychological Tests* by Otfried Spreen and Esther Strauss has also been published (1998). Both events testify to the continued rapid development of the field of clinical neuropsychology.

There must be a way to combine the advantages of the two approaches. Those in the fixed-battery school may maintain that special tests can always be added to the assessment, if they are indicated. But the typical comprehensive battery is already too time-consuming and less cost-effective than it should be. In this regard I have to express two opinions which may not evoke an enthusiastic response. The first is that, like all specialists, neuropsychologists sometimes exaggerate the importance of the contribution that they actually make to diagnosis, management, and rehabilitation. If this is true, then perhaps it behooves us to keep our perceived requirements in terms of time and expense within reasonable bounds. Secondly, possibly because of a narrow clinical experience, too many neuropsychologists are not sufficiently sensitive to the physical condition and affective status of their patients. They are seemingly unaware that the performances which they are eliciting are also determined by a variety of non-neurological factors of a physical, emotional, and motivational nature (particularly fatigue and sagging motivation but also distrust and hostility) that interact with the condition of the brain. I cannot believe that adding special tests to a 3-, 4-, or 6-hour fixed battery is helpful in this respect.

A reasonable response to the problem might be to formulate a relatively brief fixed battery, certainly not more than 1 hour in administration time and preferably somewhat shorter, which is arrived at by consensus but definitely subject to revision from time to time. Care should be taken in the selection of the tests to insure that those measures that are judged to be *generally* most informative are its components. (I doubt that there are many tests in the standard batteries that will satisfy this criterion). It would be expected that this battery will serve as the initial core battery of most neuropsychological examinations. Beyond this the neuropsychologist should be able to call upon a variety of special-purpose tests to evaluate in the greater detail the referral or research questions as well as any that may rise from analysis of the patient's performance on the core battery. While a great many of these tests can be readily applied for clinical or research purpose, there are others which need to be standardized if they are to be used optimally; still others are in embryonic form and will require development.

I do not propose this plan as the solution to the problem. It happens to be the strategy that I finally adopted and some other neuropsychologists have followed the same path. The important point is that the problem has to be faced. Given our present knowledge of brain–behavior relationships, of cognitive processes, and of the influence of cultural, affective, and nonneurological physical factors on test performance, are we doing as well as we can? Are Similarities, Comprehension, Digit Span, and Categories (all of which are of value to answer certain questions) really as broadly informative as other tests that could take their place in a core battery? Are our examinations so long and demanding that they sap the strength of patients whose energies are already depleted by disease, depression, or old age? If so, we are compromising our ability to get at the cognitive functions that we want to assess. These and other questions need to be raised and considered. In short, we should take a hard look at the neuropsychological examination. It deserves its own critical examination.

I have devoted a good deal of time (probably too much time) to neuropsychological assessment. Apart from my special interest in the topic, I have done so because assessment is based on one's understanding of brain functioning and brain–behavior relationships; advances in assessment will come about only to the degree that it is linked to evolving concepts in this domain. By now it is clear that, although it is of great value to neurologists and neurosurgeons in their diagnostic practice, the traditional concept of discrete areal localization, i.e., linking specific functions and cognitive abilities to specific regions of the brain, is dying (if it is not already dead). Neuroscientists now think in terms of extensive, highly complex neural networks, within which there is multiple simultaneous transmission of information, as the mediators of behavioral capacities. Far from being located in a discrete neural aggregate, these networks course through large parts of the brain and their functional properties are defined by dynamic relationships between neural aggregates. It is hard to specify what "localization" means in this context. It means the nature of the interrelations between these aggregates. If a function has to be "localized" somewhere, I suppose it would be in the several synapses of a network. (Now the really hard work begins, namely, to identify these synapses and to describe what happens at these sites.)

This is why MRI and CT, useful as they are for structural lesional localization, can have only limited significance for the theme of the neurological bases of behavior. Instead the newer neurodiagnostic procedures, PET scan, cerebral blood flow determination, and evoked potential recording, that provide measures of *functional* activity in the brain during the course of performances, offer so much greater promise. Neuropsychologists are playing a prominent role in research focused on the behavioral significance of the information generated by these procedures. The results to date, a mélange of positive, negative, and simply puzzling findings, are perhaps best described as "tantalizing." However, both technological advances (as has happened with successive generations of CT and MR equipment), and increased competence in analysis and interpretation on the part of researchers can be expected. Eventually this work will pay substantial dividends for a deeper understanding of brain function and for more effective clinical practice.

In 1960, given the time and inclination, the neuropsychologist could fairly readily learn what was then received knowledge about the structure and function of the brain and what was then received knowledge about cognitive processes. He or she could accomplish this by taking two or three courses or even by independent study.

The revolutions in both basic neuroscience and cognitive psychology between

1960 and 1990 have changed all that. Both fields are now incomparably deeper, more complex, more difficult to master. Today the neuropsychologist requires a much greater breadth and depth of training if he or she is to participate fully in these fast-moving disciplines that form the basis of scientific and clinical service activity. That training is not as easily acquired or as readily available as was its simpler counterpart 30 years ago. It is our collective responsibility to ensure that it is in fact made more available, at least to the young neuropsychologist and to our trainees. (Older neuropsychologists are probably beyond resuscitation.)

We are in fact beginning to meet this responsibility. There are graduate and postgraduate training programs that have made provision for this basic training, more often than not on an optional basis. The excellent series of workshops offered at the meetings of our Society is another example.

But these are only first steps. A much more powerful systematic program needs to be developed. A program such as this will be difficult to implement—it is expensive and we have only a very limited control of resources. However, we should be able to make some progress and achieve at least partial success. If we do, a speaker describing the state of the field at some future INS meeting will have the same satisfaction that I have enjoyed in recounting our progress since 1960.

Summary

Clinical neuropsychology has made significant progress during the past 30 years. Practice and research have expanded remarkably in scope and are more incisive and more highly focused. There has been an explosive development of test methods but clinical neuropsychologists have yet to take full advantage of them. An effort should be made to combine the strengths of the "fixed battery" and "flexible" approaches to assessment. Further advances in neuropsychologist assessment will come about only to the degree that they are linked to evolving concepts of brain behavior relationships. Neuropsychologists now require a deeper understanding of basic neuroscience and cognitive psychology than was true in the past. Steps should be taken to ensure that training to achieve that understanding is provided to the upcoming generation of neuropsychologists.

References

Benton A. L. and Joynt R. J. (1959). Reaction time in unilateral cerebral disease. *Confinia Neurologica* 19: 247–256.

Blackburn H. L. and Benton A. L. (1955). Simple and choice reaction time in cerebral disease. *Confinia Nueurologica* 15: 327–338.

Bortner M. (1979). *Cognitive Growth and Development*. New York: Brunner/Mazel.

Broadbent D. E. (1954). The role of auditory localization in attention and memory span. *J. Exp. Psychol.* 47: 191–196.

Costa L. (1988). Clinical neuropsychology: Prospects and problems. *The Clinical Neuropsychologist* 2: 3–11.

Goodglass H. and Quadfasel F. A. (1954). Language laterality in left-handed aphasics. *Brain* 77: 521–548.

Lezak M. D. (1983). *Neuropsychological Assessment* 2nd ed. New York: Oxford University Press. [3rd ed. New York: Oxford University Press, 1995.]

Matthews C. G. (1991). They asked for a speech. *The Clinical Neuropsychologist* 4: 327–336.

Meier M. J. (1991). Modern clinical neuropsychology in historical perspective. Distinguished Contributions Award Address, 99th Annual Convention, American Psychological Association, San Francisco, CA.

Mishkin M. and Forgays D. G. (1952). Word recognition as a function of retinal locus. *J. Exp. Psychol.* 43: 43–48.

Parsons O. A. (1991). Clinical neuropsychology 1970–1990: A personal view. *Arch. Clin. Neuropsychol.* 6: 105–112.

Rourke B. P. (1991). Human neuropsychology in the 1990s. *Arch. Clin. Neuropsychol.* 6: 1–14.

Scoville W. B. and Milner B. (1957). Loss of recent memory after bilateral hippocampal lesions. *J. Neurol. Neurosurg. Psychiatry* 20: 11–21.

Smith K. U. (1947). Bilateral integrative action of the cerebral cortex in man in verbal association and sensori-motor coordination. *J. Exp. Psychol.* 37: 367–376.

Spreen O. and Strauss E. (1991). *A Compendium of Neuropsychological Tests*. New York: Oxford University Press. [2nd ed. New York: Oxford University Press, 1998.]

Part IV

HEMISPHERIC CEREBRAL DOMINANCE

17

The "Minor" Hemisphere

The purpose of this paper is to sketch the early development of the idea that the "minor" hemisphere in man (i.e., the right hemisphere in right-handed persons) possesses distinctive functional properties with respect to the mediation of behavior in analogy to the predominant role of the left hemisphere with respect to language. The idea of a minor hemisphere derives, of course, from the broader concept of "cerebral dominance" which arose as a consequence of the discovery by Broca of a specific association between motor aphasia and disease of the left frontal lobe (Broca, 1861; Broca, 1863). Soon after the validity of Broca's correlation was confirmed, it became evident that other forms of aphasic disorder, such as impairment in language understanding, disturbances in naming, and loss of reading ability, were related to disease of the left temporal and parietal areas. Inferring the positive from the negative, students of human cerebral function readily concluded that, at least in right-handed persons, language behavior was mediated primarily (if not necessarily exclusively) by neural mechanisms located in the left hemisphere.

The concept of left hemisphere dominance was applied at first only to language functions. However, as continuing clinical study indicated that the left hemisphere apparently subserved a number of other aspects of mentation and cognition, the concept was broadened considerably. To begin with, there was the observation that many aphasic patients showed impairment in intellect which clearly extended beyond their language disabilities. This was a point made by Trousseau as early as 1864 (Trousseau, 1864), and its confirmation fostered the conception (held by many authorities in the field) that "true" aphasia always involved a particular impairment in mentation, an impairment principally involving abstract reasoning and the use of symbols in thought. Thus Hughlings Jackson spoke of the aphasic patient as being "lame in his thinking" (Jackson,

Reprinted with permission from *Journal of the History of Medicine and Allied Sciences,* 27: 5–14, 1972.

1874), Pierre Marie of a defect in higher-level intellectual skills (Marie, 1906), and Kurt Goldstein of a loss of the capacity for "categorical behavior" (Goldstein, 1927). Acceptance of this generalization led inevitably to the conclusion that the left hemisphere must be "dominant" with respect to these distinctively human capacities for reasoning and symbolic thinking as well as for language functions in the strict sense.

A further extension of the concept of left hemisphere dominance took place at the beginning of the twentieth century when the Berlin neurologist Hugo Liepmann established apraxia as a distinctive category of behavioral deficit that might be shown by patients with cerebral disease. Liepmann, 1900). In addition to his analysis of these disturbances in the execution of purposeful movement-sequences, Liepmann was able to show that at least one major type which he had described, ideomotor apraxia, resulted from lesions of the left hemisphere. Some 20 years later, Karl Kleist described the form of visuoconstructive disability which he called "constructional apraxia" (Kleist, 1923; Strauss, 1924); he localized the responsible lesion in the posterior parietal area of the left hemisphere, a region in which visual and proprioceptive information was presumably integrated so that visual guidance of action was made possible.

In the 1920s, Josef Gerstmann described "finger agnosia," i.e., inability to recognize or name the fingers of either hand (Gerstmann, 1924; Gerstmann, 1927). Combining this rather peculiar deficit with three ohter types of behavioral impairment (right-left disorientation, agraphia, and acalculia) into a syndrome, he maintained that his syndrome could occur as a consequence of focal cerebral disease, its locus being in the region of the angular gyrus of the left hemisphere. His explanation was that certain aspects of the bilateral body image find their cerebral representation in the parieto-occipital area of the dominant hemisphere.

These diverse observations coalesced to emphasize the specific importance of the left hemisphere in providing the neural substrate not only for language behavior but also for conceptual thinking, higher-level praxis and orientation to one's body. At the same time, they fostered the idea that the left hemisphere was the 'major' hemisphere insofar as the mediation of higher-level cognitive behavior was concerned.

The designation of the left hemisphere as "major" implied, of course, that the right hemisphere was the minor hemisphere. In this context, the term "minor" evidently had a number of interrelated meanings. First, it indicated that, in accord with the doctrine of contralateral innervation, the right hemisphere mediated motion and sensation on the opposite side of the body; in this respect, it was functionally equivalent to the left hemisphere. Secondly, it meant that the right hemisphere was subordinate to the left in subserving language performances. This was not to say that the right hemisphere did not participate at all in language but rather that under normal conditions, the left hemisphere was the "leading" hemisphere with the right hemisphere playing the role of a minor (and for the most part silent) partner.

The latter conclusion was derived primarily from observation of the language behavior of aphasic patients. It had been noted that, although these patients were incapable of truly propositional language, they did produce automatic, interjectional, and emotional speech; these positive features of an aphasic's language behavior were interpreted as reflecting the operation of mechanisms in his unaffected minor hemisphere. The observation was also made that under special conditions (e.g., in a stressful situation) an aphasic patient might produce perfectly intelligible propositional speech which he could not utter under ordinary circumstances. It was presumed that this speech was produced by the minor hemisphere. This meant that, in the course of language learning, verbal engrams were laid down in the right hemisphere as well as in the left. These minor hemisphere engrams remained inactive because of the specialization of the major hemisphere for language.

The same explanation was applied to account for recovery from aphasic disorder, the assumption being that the right hemisphere had taken over the function of mediating language performances. Since recovery often took place over the course of a few weeks or months, it seemed clear that the minor hemisphere must have participated in the original learning of language. In short, the study of aphasic patients brought forth facts which appeared to be consonant with the idea that the dominance of the left hemisphere for language was of a relative rather than absolute nature. Thus the designation of the right hemisphere as "minor" seemed quite appropriate.

Finally, the term "minor," as applied to the right hemisphere, implied that it had no distinctive functions. It shared certain functional properties with the left hemisphere but, at least with respect to higher-level performances, whatever it could do, the left hemisphere could do better.

However, almost from the very birth of the concept of hemispheric cerebral dominance, there were clinicians who opposed the prevailing opinion that the right hemisphere was merely a weaker version of the left and who insisted that it also possessed distinctive functional properties. The evolution of this trend of thought, as reflected in the publications of the relatively few neurologists, ophthalmologists, and psychologists who advanced the idea over a period of about seventy years (from 1874 to 1941), will be sketched.

The pioneer figure in this movement to give the right hemisphere its due was the British neurologist Hughlings Jackson. In 1874 he published a paper in which he surmised that, while the left hemisphere was specialized with respect to expressive speech functions, the posterior area of the right hemisphere played a crucial role in visual recognition and visual memory (Jackson, 1874). He conceded that the evidence for his generalization was not strong. However, two years later, he was more sure of his ground when he published a case report describing a patient with a tumor in the temporo-occipital region of the right hemisphere (Jackson, 1876). "I diagnosed tumour, and tumour of the right posterior lobe, I may here remark, from the following facts—the kind of mental defect and from its preceding the hemiplegia, from the hemiplegia being left-sided, and because the arm suffered less than the leg" (p. 434).

The "kind of mental defect" shown by Jackson's patient consisted in visual disorientation, failure to recognize persons and dyspraxia for dressing. He designated this constellation of disabilities as "imperception" and argued that it was as specifically characteristic of disease of the posterior right hemisphere as impairment in expressive speech was of disease of the anterior left hemisphere.

Some thirty years later, the German neurologist Conrad Rieger, in all probability unaware of Jackson's thinking, advanced roughly the same idea. In a monograph which appeared in 1909 he postulated the existence of two distinct and interacting "apparatuses" (as he called them) in the brain, one subserving verbal-conceptual functions and the other subserving spatial-practical functions (Rieger, 1909). Pursuing this idea, his student Martin Reichardt concluded from clinico-pathological observations that the spatial "apparatus" was located primarily in the posterior right hemisphere while the verbal "apparatus" was, of course, located in the left hemisphere (Reichardt, 1923).

During the same period there were observations in the field of ophthalmology which pointed to the possibility that the right hemisphere played a particularly important role in subserving certain aspects of visual perception. In the 1880s and 1890s, disturbances in spatial orientation, as reflected in loss of geographic memory, difficulty in locating objects in space, and inability to find one's way from one place to another, were topics of considerable interest to ophthalmologists (Benton, 1969; Critchley, 1953; Faust, 1955; Ajuriagerra and Hécaen, 1960; Gloning, 1965). The fact that this disability might be shown by patients suffering from focal cerebral disease and with intact central visual acuity indicated that it was a "higher-level" disorder and not simply an expression of sensory defect or significant intellectual impairment. The classic case report of Foerster in 1890, describing a patient who first showed a right homonymous hemianopia without complicating disturbances following a stroke and who, after a second stroke, showed a double hemianopia and spatial disorientation with preservation of central vision and intellect, did much to establish the prevailing trend of thinking about the necessary and sufficient conditions for the appearance of visuospatial disorientation, namely, that it could be caused by a focal occipital lesion, but only one which was bilateral in nature and which therefore entailed a loss of visual memory images (Foerster, 1890).

However, this view was challenged by a few ophthalmologists who were impressed by the frequency with which impairment in topographic memory appeared to be associated with disease of the right hemisphere. The first to do so was Thomas D. Dunn who described a patient with a double hemianopia, intact central vision, and "loss of the sense of location" but without impairment in other aspects of visual memory, such as the recognition of faces (Dunn, 1895). Dunn therefore rejected the hypothesis that a general "loss of recollection of optical images" was the underlying disability. The circumstance that his patient showed defects in topographical orientation only after a second stroke which resulted in a left hemianopia being superimposed on a preexisting right hemianopia led him to postulate "a centre (which may, for convenience, be named the geographic centre) on the right side of the brain for the record of the optical images of locality, analogous to the region of Broca for that of speech on the left side in right handed persons" (p. 54). Dunn's hypothesis did not fare well in the hands of the eminent ophthalmologist De Schweinitz, who discussed his paper when it was presented at a meeting of the College of Physicians of Philadelphia. In fact, De Schweinitz did not even deign to mention it but instead advanced the view.

> that the loss of orientation, which has been a marked feature in fully 50 per cent. of the cases of double hemianopsia thus far reported, may be, and, indeed, has been, explained by the greatly contracted visual field, the patient being unable properly to locate landmarks within the field of vision and thus aid his judgment in forming an opinion as to his relation to his surroundings. (p. 55)

A year later, Peters described two patients with visual disorientation, both of whom had only a left homonymous hemianopia (Peters, 1896). Thus a double hemianopia did not appear to be a necessary precondition for the appearance of an orientation defect. Significantly, Peters remarked that he was at first inclined to ascribe a greater influence to the right hemisphere than to the left in the production of disturbances of orientation. However, he was dissuaded from reaching this conclusion by the circumstances that there were case reports in the literature which were not in accord with it. Some ten years later the problem was taken up again by Lenz in a comprehensive study of hemianopic defects (Lenz, 1905). Emphasizing that visual disorientation was by no means a rare feature of the hemianopias following stroke (12% of his case material), he pointed out that no less than seven of his eight cases of homonymous hemianopia with visual disorientation had a left field defect, i.e., involved a lesion of the right hemisphere. Recalling Peters's earlier observations, Lenz also raised (in a rather diffident way) the question of whether "the right occipital lobe is perhaps more strongly related to orientation than the left."

A rather different line of evidence pointing to the possibility of distinctive functional properties of the minor hemisphere was initiated by Babinski's description in 1914 of anosognosia in the specific form of unawareness (or denial) of left hemiplegia (Babinski, 1914). As he and other clinicians observed additional cases showing an apparently specific association between this peculiar partial defect of awareness and disease of the right hemisphere (Babinski, 1918; Babinski, 1923; Barre et al., 1923; Barkman, 1925; Joltrain, 1924), they were led to raise the question of whether a "center" for the integration of somatosensory information with somesthetic memory images might not exist in that hemisphere.

As has been mentioned, it was in the early 1920s that Kleist described constructional apraxia as a distinctive form of behavioral impairment resulting from disease of the left hemisphere (Kleist, 1923). His conception was a fairly precise one. Separating constructional apraxia from other forms of visuoconstructive disability that occur as an expression of impairment in visual perception, he defined it as a disturbance in constructional activity shown by a patient who at the same time has adequate visual form perception and discrimination and preserved ability to localize objects in visual space. He considered that, in its pure form, the disability was neither perceptual nor motor in nature but rather an impairment in translating intact visual perceptions into appropriate motor action and he conceived of a rupture between visual and proprioceptive processes as providing the basis for its appearance.

The broad descriptive aspects of Kleist's concept were readily accepted by subsequent workers and constructional apraxia became recognized as a type of behavioral deficit which might be shown by a brain-damaged patient. However, his precise formulation of the nature of the disability as being neither perceptual nor motor but instead "connectional" in nature was either denied or ignored and the term "constructional apraxia" was used to designate any visuoconstructive disability, regardless of whether or not it appeared within a setting of impairment of visual perception. A number of clinicians in the late 1920s and early 1930s then made the observation that constructional apraxia in this broad sense was shown by patients with lesions of the right hemisphere and indeed with at least as high a frequency as by those with disease of the dominant hemisphere (Potzl, 1928; Schlesinger, 1928; Lange, 1930; Kroll and Stolbun, 1933). They also noted that related visuospatial disabilities occurred with impressively high frequency in patients with right hemisphere disease (Lange, 1936).

Many of these observations were utilized by the French neurologist Dide in a paper which emphasized the importance of the right hemisphere in the mediation of perceptual and motor performances (Dide, 1938). Dide outlined what he called the "syndrome of the right parietal area," the cardinal features of which were certain types of sensory and motor impairment, the anosognosia of Babinski, constructional apraxia, and spatial disorientation. He also discussed the question of the cerebral representation of musical abilities as reflected in singing, musical performance, and the recognition of melodies. The prevailing opinion was that, together with language, musical capacities were mediated by mechanisms in the left hemisphere. Nevertheless, over the decades a few clinicians had raised the question of the importance of the right hemisphere for musical functions. Dide allied himself with this group and advanced the view that musical functions depended upon the integrity of the superior temporal gyrus of the right hemisphere, in analogy to the dependence of language functions on Wernicke's area in the left hemisphere (Milner, 1958; Milner, 1962). He also insisted that a distinctive type of bilateral somesthetic impairment could result from disease of the right hemisphere.

There were two contributions of a psychometric nature during this early period. The monumental study of aphasia by Weisenburg and McBride included consideration of the performances of a group of nonaphasic patients with right hemisphere disease as well as normal control subjects and the target group of aphasic patients (Weisenburg and McBride, 1935). They found that the right hemisphere patients showed a distinctive pattern of performance with significant impairment in some nonverbal performances while verbal abilities were close to the normal level. They made no explicit inferences but did feel impelled to call attention to the qualitative differences between these patients and both the normal and aphasic groups. In 1939 Hebb described the pattern of test performance of a patient who, after having undergone a large excision in the right temporal lobe, showed superior verbal intelligence but markedly defective performances on visuoperceptive and visuoconstructive tests as well as on a test of tactile form recognition (Hebb, 1939). Contrasting the results with his previous findings on patients with left frontal lobe excisions, Hebb concluded that impairment in both visual and tactile form perception may well be a specific consequence of right temporal lobe defect.

One last clinical contribution in this early period deserves mention. In 1941 Russell Brain published a detailed description of spatial disorientation in patients with massive lesions of the right parietal lobe and concluded "that certain syndromes, notably anosognosia, are seen exclusively or almost exclusively as a result of lesions in the right hemisphere" (Brain, 1941).

Discussion

Viewed in retrospect and taken in their totality, these clinical contributions would seem to have produced at least suggestive evidence for the view that the right hemisphere should not be considered simply as a minor hemisphere with no distinctive functional properties. Yet it is clear that at the time they had no significant effect on prevailing conceptions of hemispheric cerebral dominance. One can conjecture about the probable reasons for this lack of impact. First, the contributions were scattered over a period of 70 years, sometimes with decades intervening between them; consequently they had little cumulative effect. At the same time, a counteractive influence may have been exerted by the much larger body of literature pointing to the paramount importance of the left hemisphere for thinking and perception, as well as for language. Secondly, some reports were not widely disseminated; for example, Jackson's papers were published in journals that were not widely read outside of England and the contribution of Rieger was buried in a monograph with a rather limited circulation. Moreover, some authors (e.g., Peters, Lenz, Weisenburg, and McBride) were not prepared to draw conclusions from their observations and such a stance was not likely to encourage others to reflect on the implications of their results. Conversely, some papers, consisting of single case reports and advancing broad generalizations that went far beyond the scanty empirical facts, scarcely constituted evidence that was strong enough to challenge well-established doctrine.

However, these early contributions were not without effect on the next generation of workers, for their influence on O. L. Zangwill and Henry Hécaen, whose studies between 1944 and 1951 initiated the modern period of investigation in this field, is fairly evident. Paterson and Zangwill (1944), in their paper in 1944 on visuospatial deficits associated with right hemisphere disease, cited both the contributions of Brain and Hebb as well as the conclusions of the German neurologist Lange that the right parietal area is of particular importance for the spatial aspects of visual perception. Similarly, in their first papers, Hécaen and Ajuriaguerra called attention to the work of Lange, Dide, and Brain in reporting their own studies of apraxic and visuocostructive disabilities resulting from lesions of the right hemisphere (Hécaen and Ajuriagerra, 1945; Hécaen et al., 1951). Thus, although for the most part ignored at the time when they were published, these pioneer efforts to ascribe distinctive functional properties to the "minor" hemisphere did have an impact on the development of thinking about asymmetry of cerebral hemispheric function in man.

References

Ajuriaguerra J. de and Hécaen H. (1960). *Le cortex cérébral* Paris.

Babinski J. (1914). Contribution à l'étude des troubles mentaux dans l'hémiplegie organique cérébrale (anosognosie). *Rev. Neurol.* 22: 845–848.

Babinski J. (1918). Anosognosie. *Rev. Neurol.* 25: 365–367.

Babinski J. (1923). Sur l'anosognosie. *Rev. Neurol.* 30: 731–732.

Barkman A. (1925). De l'anosognosie dans l'hémiplegie cérébrale: contribution clinique à l'étude de ce symptôme. *Acta Med. Scand.* 62: 235–254.

Barré J. A. Morin L., and Kaiser (1923). Etude clinique d'un nouveau cas d'anosognosie de Babinski. *Rev. Neurol.* 30: 500–503.

Benton, A. L. (1969). Disorders of spatial orientation. In Vinken, P. J. and Bruyn G. W. (eds.) *Handbook of Clinical Neurology*, Vol. 3, *Disorders of Higher Nervous Activity*. Amsterdam.

Brain W. R. (1941). Visual disorientation with special reference to lesions of the right cerebral hemisphere. *Brain* 64: 244–272.

Broca, P. (1861). Remarques sur le siège de la faculté du langage articulé, suivies d'une observation d'aphémie. *Bull. Soc. Anat. Paris* 6: 330–357.

Broca, P. (1863). Localisation des fonctions cérébrales: siège du langage articulé. *Bull. Soc. Anthrop. Paris* 4: 200–203.

Critchley M. (1953). *The Parietal Lobes*. London.

Dide M. (1938). Les désorientations temporo-spatiales et la préponderance de l'hémisphére droit dans les agnoso-akinésies proprioceptives. *Encéphale* 33: 276–294.

Dunn T. D. (1895). Double hemiplegia with double hemianopsia and loss of geographic centre. *Trans. Coll. Phycns. Philad.* 17: 45–56.

Faust C. (1955). *Die zerebralen Herdstörungen bei Hinterhauptsverletzungen und ihre Beurteilung*. (Stuttgart).

Foerster, R. (1890). Ueber Rindenblindheit. *Graefes Arch. Ophthal.* 36: 94–108; a report of the autopsy of Foerster's patient was published by Sachs, H. (1895). Das Gehirn des Förster'schen Rindenblinden. *Arb. Psychiat. Klin. Breslau* 2: 55–122.

Gerstmann, J. (1924). Fingeragnosie: eine umschriebene Störung der Orientierung am eigenen Körper. *Wien. klin. Wschr.* 37: 1010–1012.

Gerstmann, J. (1927). Fingeragnosie und isolierte Agraphie—ein neues Syndrom. *Z. Ges. Neurol. Psychiat.* 108: 152–177.

Goldstein, K. (1967). Die Lokalisation in der Grosshirnrinde. In Bethe A., von Bergmann G., G. Embden, and A. Ellinger (eds.), *Handbuch der normalen and pathologischen Physiologie*, Bd. 10, *Spezielle Physiologie des Zentralnervensystems der Wirbeltiere*. Berlin.

Gloning K. (1965). *Die zerebral bedingten Störungen des räumlichen Sehens und des Raumerlebens*. Vienna.

Hebb, D. O. (1939). Intelligence in man after large removals of cerebral tissue: defects following right temporal lobectomy, *J. Gen. Psychol.* 21: 437–446.

Hécaen H. and Ajuriaguerra de J. (1945). L'apraxie de l'habillage: ses rapports avec la planatopo-kinésie et les troubles de la somatognosie. *Encéphale* 35: 113–143.

Hécaen H. de Ajuriaguerra J., and Massonet J. (1951). Les troubles visuoconstructives par lésion pariéto-occipitale droite. *Encéphale* 40: 122–179.

Jackson, J. H. (1874). On the nature of the duality of the brain. *Med. Press Circ.* 17: 19, 41, 63 (reprinted in *Brain 38*, (1915): 80–103).

Jackson, J. H. (1876). Case of large cerebral tumour without optic neuritis and with left hemiplegia and imperception. *Roy. Ophthal. Hosp. Rep.* 8: 434–444.

Joltrain E. (1924). Un nouveau cas d'anosognosie. *Rev. Neurol.* 31: 638–640.

Kleist, K. (1923) Kriegsverletzungen des Gehirns in ihrer Bedeutung für die Hirnlokalisation und Hirnpathologie. In von Schjerning O. (ed.), *Handbuch der ärztlichen Erfahrung im Weltkriege 1914/1918*, Bd. IV, *Geistes-und Nervenkrankheiten*. Leipzig.

Strauss H. (1924). Ueber konstructive Apraxie. *Mschr. Psychiat. Neurol.* 56: 65–124.

Kroll M. and Stolbun D. (1933). Was ist konstruktive Apraxie? *Z. Ges. Neurol. Psychiat.* 148: 142–158.

Lange J. (1930). Fingeragnosie and Agraphie. *Mschr. Psychiat. Neurol.* 76: 129–188.

Lange J. (1936). Agnosien und Apraxien. In Bumke O. and Foerster O. (eds.), *Handbuch der Neurologie*, BD. VI Berlin.

Lenz G. (1905). *Beiträge zur Hemianopsie*. Stuttgart.

Liepmann, H. (1900). Das Krankheitsbild der Apraxie. *Mschr. Psychiat. Neurol.* 8: 15–44, 102–132, 182–197.

Marie, P. (1906). Revision de la question de l'aphasie: la troisième circonvolution frontale gauche ne joue aucun rôle spécial dans la fonction du langage. *Sem. Médicale* 26: 241–247.

Milner B. (1958). Psychological defects produced by temporal, lobe excision. *Res. Publ. Ass. Res. Nerv. Ment. Dis.* 36: 244–257.

Milner B. (1962). Laterality effects in audition. In Mountcastle V. B. (ed.), *Interhemispheric Relations and Cerebral Dominance.* Baltimore.

Paterson A. and Zangwill O. L. (1944). Disorders of visual space perception associated with lesions of the right cerebral hemisphere. *Brain* 67: 331–358.

Peters A. (1896). Ueber die Beziehungen zwischen Orientirungsstörungen und ein-und doppelseitiger Hemianopsie. *Arch. Augenheilk.* 32: 175–187.

Pötzl O. (1928). *Die Aphasielehre vom Standpunkte der klinischen Pyschiatrie,* Bd. I: *Die optisch-agnostischen Störungen.* Leipzig.

Reichardt. M. (1923). *Allgemeine und spezielle Psychiatrie: ein Lehrbuch für Studierende und Aerzte* III Aufl. Jena.

Rieger, C. (1909). Ueber Apparate in dem Hirn. *Arb. psychiat. Klin. Würzburg* 5: 176–197.

Schlesinger B. (1928). Zur Auffassung der optischen und konstruktive Apraxie. *Z. Ges. Neurol. Psychiat.* 117: 649–697.

Trousseau, A. (1864). De l'aphasie, maladie décrite récemment sous le nom impropre d'aphémie. *Gaz Hôp. Paris* 37: 13–14, 25–26, 37–39, 48–50.

Weisenburg T. and McBride K. (1935). *Aphasia.* New York.

18

Hemispheric Cerebral Dominance Before Broca

A persisting question in the history of neuropsychology is why so many astute clinician-pathologists before 1860 failed to grasp the connection between aphasia and disease of the left hemisphere or, indeed, between aphasia and the occurrence of right hemiplegia. With the benefit of hindsight, one can see that the ingredients for establishing a correlation were already present in ancient medical writings. There is the statement in the Hippocratic corpus that associates temporary speechlessness following convulsions "either with paralysis of the tongue or of the arm and right side of the body" (Chadwick and Mann, 1950, p. 248). Coupled with this is the well-known Hippocratic observation that "an incised wound in one temple produces a spasm in the opposite side of the body" (Chadwick and Mann, 1950, p. 263). Some 500 years later Aretaeus of Cappadocia sought to explain this observation of contralateral motor impairment following a head wound by postulating a crossing of the nerve tracts from the brain to the spinal cord (Adams, 1856, p. 306). It is not unreasonable to think that an integration of these statements would have suggested a specific association between speech disorder and left hemisphere disease.

A possible reason for the failure to make the correlation is that Aretaeus' remarkable conception was by no means universally accepted. Many physicians interpreted the occurrence of paralysis on the side contralateral to the side of injury as being the result of concussion, diffuse inflammation or a contrecoup effect. However, in the eighteenth century these factors were effectively eliminated as putative causes when Pourfour du Petit demonstrated the crossing of the descend-

Reprinted with permission from *Neuropsychologia*, Vol. 22, No. 6. pp. 807–811. © 1984 Pergamon Press Ltd.

Dedicated to the memory of Henry Hécaen.

ing nerve tracts at the level of the pyramids and Morgagni assembled an impressive mass of clinicopathologic case material to support the association between paralysis of one side of the body and disease of the opposite hemisphere.

No doubt a systematic survey of the early medical literature would disclose a trend for "speechlessness," "aphonia," "alalia" and "speech amnesia" to be associated with paralysis of the right side of the body. But at the same time the unbiased compiler would have noted many cases that did not follow the rule, i.e., speechlessness without paralysis or with left-sided paralysis and left hemisphere disease without speech disorder. Thus he would have to conclude there was no obligatory association between aphasia and right-sided paralysis (or left hemisphere disease). Moreover, he would find that the early literature did not yield as rich a harvest as might have been anticipated. These reports were generally only a few lines in length and lacking in essential details. When speechlessness or disordered speech is mentioned, it is usually impossible to determine whether the impairment in expression was aphasic in nature or a reflection of neuromotor disability, stupor, confusion, dementia, or psychosis.

Descriptions of aphasic patients that are sufficiently detailed to be informative first appeared in the late seventeenth century. At least nine such case reports were published before 1800—Schmidt (1673), Rommel (1683), Linné (1745), Dalin (1745), Gesner (1770), two cases), Spalding (1783), Hertz (1791), and Crichton (1798). (Summaries and, in some instances, the complete texts of these reports can be found in the review by Benton and Joynt [1960].) Of the nine patients, three had right-sided paralysis and a nonfluent aphasia. The other six patients had no paralysis and five of them had a fluent aphasic disorder. A reviewer of this series of cases might have noted that, when paralysis was present, it was always on the right side and never on the left. But evidently no student at that time was fortunate enough to be endowed with such serendipity. A possible distraction was the fact that medical interest in the eighteenth century was largely focused on patients showing the more florid forms of fluent aphasia, as reflected in jargon aphasia and "wild" paraphasic utterances, and these patients generally did not show motor disability.

Three monumental treatise on clinical pathology, each of which dealt at some length with brain–behavior relationships, appeared in the eighteenth and early nineteenth centuries—Morgagni's *De Sedibus et Causis Morborum per Anatomen Indigatis* (1761). Bouillaud's *Traité Physiologique et Clinique de l'Encéphalite* (1825) and Andral's *Clinique Médicale* (1829–1840). The present paper attempts an analysis of the basic data in each of these treatises with the aim of evaluating the strength of the latent evidence supporting a specific association between aphasic disorder and disease of the left hemisphere and discusses possible reasons for the failure to perceive the association. The singular story of the one man who did grasp the relationship but who elected at the time to withhold his discovery from the public will then be reviewed.

Morgagni

The first volume of Morgagni's great compilation includes numerous brief descriptions of speechlessness associated with apoplexy, head injury and fever, together with the findings at autopsy. He repeatedly emphasizes the connection between paralysis of one side of the body and the presence of disease in the opposite cerebral hemisphere. Many patients are described as speechless but more often than not the disability is noted within a context of stupor or a rapidly worsening condition resulting in death within hours. Consequently there are relatively few cases that are suitable for our analysis.

From an inspection of the 1769 English translation by Benjamin Holland of *De Sedibus*. I identified 10 cases of unilateral paralysis in patients who were not comatose, stuporous or dying in whom autopsy disclosed a purely or predominantly unilateral hemispheric lesion and in whom it was possible to ascertain whether or not speech was disordered. Five patients had a right-sided paralysis and four of them were impaired in speech. Five patients had a left-sided paralysis and one was impaired in speech.

Bouillaud

Beginning in 1825 and for a half-century thereafter, Jean-Baptiste Bouillaud was the great champion of Gall's localization of the centers of speech and language in the frontal lobes and he argued repeatedly, vigorously and, at times, rancorously that aphasic disorder resulted only from lesions in this territory. In his *Traité . . . de l'Encéphalite* (1825), he presented 29 cases with and without aphasia and with and without lesions in the anterior, middle, and posterior lobes. All of the aphasic patients had lesions that were in or close to the anterior lobes. Neither then nor subsequently could he find a valid example of aphasic disorder that was not a consequence of disease of the anterior lobes.

Inspection of Bouillaud's 29 cases shows that 25 had lesions confined to a single hemisphere, 11 in the left hemisphere and 14 in the right. Eight (73%) of the 11 left hemisphere cases were aphasic. Four (29%) of the right hemisphere cases were aphasic.

Perhaps one reason why Bouillaud did not perceive this trend toward a higher frequency of aphasic disorder in his left hemisphere patients is that not only was he obsessed with the frontal lobe localization of aphasic disorder but he also accepted Gall's dual localization of the centers of speech and language in both hemispheres. Thus whether a lesion was found to be in the left or right hemisphere was a matter of indifference to him.

Andral

Gabriel Andral was one of the luminaries of French clinical pathology in the 1830s and 1840s. His *Clinique Médicale* and *Précis D'Anatomie pathologique* were widely used in France and known throughout the world in English, German, and Italian translations. In Vol. 5 (*Maladies de L'Encéphale*) of the *Clinique Médicale* he addressed the question of the localization of speech disorder with special reference to the Gall–Bouillaud doctrine and presented his conclusions in the following succinct statement:

> M. le professeur Bouillaud a publié, il y a déjâ plusieurs annés, un mémoire rempli de faits curieux desquels il a cru pouvoir déduire la conséquence que la formation de la parole a pour instrument l'extrémité antérieure de chaque hémisphère, attendu qu'il a trouvé cette partie lésée, toutes les fois que pendant la vie la parole elle-même avait été perdue. Voici, à cet égard, ce que nous ont appris nos recherches.
>
> Sur trente-sept cas observés par nous ou par d'autres, relatifs à des hémorrhagies ou à d'autres lésions, dans lesquels l'altération résidait dans un des lobules anterieur ou dans tous les deux, la parole a été abolie vingt-et-une fois, et conservé seize fois.
>
> D'un autre côté, nous avons rassemblé quatorze cas où il y avait abolition de la parole, sans aucune altération dans les lobules antérieurs. De ces quatorze cas, sept étaient relatifs à des maladies des lobules moyens, et sept autres à des maladies des lobules postérieurs.
>
> La perte de la parole n'est donc pas le résultat nécessaire de la lésion des lobules antérieurs, et, en outre, elle peut avoir lieu dans des cas où l'anatomie ne montre dans ces lobules aucune altération [Andral, 1840, p. 368].

It is quite evident from inspection of the *Clinique Médicale* (4th Edition, 1840) that not all 37 cases mentioned by Andral are described in the book. I was able to identify 11 cases of unilateral disease, five with lesions in the left hemisphere and six with lesions in the right hemisphere, where the status of the patient's speech during his illness is described. Of the five left hemisphere cases, three were aphasic. Of the six right hemisphere cases, none was aphasic.

A collaborator and admirer of P. C. A. Louis, who introduced the statistical approach into medical observation, Andral applied the latter's *méthode numérique* to his case material in evaluating Bouillaud's claims. Evidently it did not occur to him to extend its application to the question of a right–left hemisphere difference. The few lines he wrote on aphasia suggests that the topic was not of great interest to him and probably he was content with disproving the Gall–Bouillaud thesis. Bouillaud and Andral were polar opposites in temperament and in their approach to problems. Bouillaud was passionate, polemical and dogmatic: Andral was sober, analytic and wary of speculation. Moreover, the two men were opponents in other respects as well. Andral campaigned vigorously against the practice of bloodletting while Bouillaud was, as Garrison (1929) describes him, "a furious bloodletter" who "favored pitilessly rapid bleeding, *coup sur coup*."

In summary, the observations reported in each of the three treatises show a trend toward a specific association between speech disorder and left-hemisphere disease. However, in no single instance is the trend statistically significant, as assessed by the Fisher Exact Probability Test (two-tailed), although it approaches significance ($P = 0.10$) in Bouillaud's sample. If it is permissible to combine the cases in the three samples and apply a chi-square test to the data, the resulting chi-square (10.3) indicates a between-hemispheres difference which is significant at the 0.002 level.

Some of the possible reasons for the failure to perceive this difference have already been noted, such as the occurrence of exceptional cases, the presence of left-hemisphere disease without speech disorder and the desperate conditions of so many patients. But perhaps the most important single reason is to be found in the circumstance that these men were very busy practitioners who at the same time actively pursued numerous and varied investigative interests. None of them was a specialist in the modern sense of the term, either in their medical practice or in their research. So far as can be seen, Morgagni had no interest in aphasia beyond noting on occasion that a patient was speechless and Andral had only a passing interest which quite clearly had been aroused by Bouillaud's claims.

Aphasia was a topic of major concern only to Bouillaud. Yet, when one considers his subsequent activity, it is understandable that, having embraced Gall's hypothesis of centers of speech in both frontal lobes, he proceeded to defend it vigorously without exploring the matter further. After 1825 he turned his attention to the fields of cardiology and rheumatology, to which he made a number of notable contributions, the most important of which was his demonstration of the association between rheumatic fever and endocarditis. Indeed, it was Bouillaud who introduced the terms "endocardium" and "endocarditis" into medicine (Major, 1954).

Thus it is not unlikely that the major reason why the aphasia–left hemisphere association escaped the attention of Morgagni, Bouillaud, and Andral is that their busy schedule and competing interests did not allow them the time to consider the data bearing on the association. It was left to a thoughtful country doctor with scholarly interests and the time to reflect on the meaning of his own observations and those of others to discover the correlation.

Marc Dax

In about 1836 this physician, who practiced in Sommiéres (about 25 k from Montpellier), wrote a paper purporting to show that aphasic disorder is exclusively associated with lesions of the left hemisphere. Marc Dax was born in 1770 and died in 1837. He was thus about 66 years old when he wrote his famous *mémoire*.

It is a remarkable document. Dax describes the successive observations that led him gradually to the conviction that aphasia was the by product of left hemisphere disease. An aphasic patient with whom he had first become acquainted in 1800 had sustained a left parietal wound. At the time this meant to Dax only that Gall's frontal lobe doctrine could not be altogether correct. In 1809 he had an aphasic patient with an extensive tumor on the left side of the face who died some months later. He attached no special significance to the circumstance that the lesion was left-sided. However, when in 1811 he read that the naturalist Broussonet had become aphasic after a left hemisphere stroke, he reflected on the fact that the three cases with which he was familiar had left hemisphere lesions. From this time onward, Dax had a "prepared mind" and, when he encountered three additional cases of aphasia with presumptive left hemisphere disease over the period of 1812–1814, he formulated his hypothesis. He continued to collect cases over the ensuing 20 years, so that at the time of writing his paper he reported having a series of over 40 cases in whom the diagnosis of left hemisphere disease had been made, primarily on clinical grounds without pathological confirmation. It was on this empirical basis that he wrote:

> De tout ce qui précède, je crois pouvoir conclure, non que toutes les maladies de l'hémisphère gauche doivent altérer la mémoire verbale, mais que, lorsque cette mémoire est altérée par une maladie du cerveau, il faut chercher la cause du désordre dans l'hémisphére gauche, et l'y chercher encore si les deux hémisphères sont malades ensemble.

Marc Dax's paper (M. Dax, 1865) was published in 1865 by his son, Gustav Dax (G. Dax, 1865), who stated that it had been read at a regional medical meeting in Montpellier in 1836. In fact, there is no evidence that he did present the paper on that occasion (Joynt and Benton, 1964). It is not mentioned in accounts of the meeting, nor could anyone be found who remembered having heard it. It seems almost certain that, if the paper had been presented, it would not have been totally neglected and would have had some repercussions.

The tone of Dax's paper is personally modest but firm in conviction. Its style indicates that it was meant to be a communication to his peers. He was quite aware of the importance of his discovery and he made one or two copies which he sent to professional friends. Why he did not make his discovery known at the time through publication or oral presentation is not clear. Perhaps he planned to publish after the collection of further data but death intervened. In any case, whether by intention or not, his manuscript became in effect a *paquet cacheté* that was brought to light only after Broca's discovery.

References

Adams F. (1856). *The Extant Works of Aretaeus, the Cappadocian*. London: The Sydenham Society.

Andral G. (1840). *Clinique Médicale*, 4th ed. Paris: Fortin, Masson.

Benton A. L. and Joynt R. J. (1960). Early descriptions of aphasia. *Arch. Neurol.* 3: 205–222.

Bouillaud J. B. (1825). *Traité Clinique et Physiologique de l'Encéphalite*. Paris: J. B. Baillière.

Chadwick J. and Mann W. N. (1950). *The Medical Works of Hippocrates*. London: Blackwell Scientific Publications.

Dax G. (1865). Notes sur le même sujet. *Gaz. Hebd. Méd. Chir.* 2: 262.

Dax M. (1865). Lésions de la moitié gauche de l'encéphale coincidant avec l'oubli des signes de la pensée. *Gaz. Hebd. Méd. Chir.* 2: 259–262.

Garrison F. H. (1929). *An Introduction to the History of Medicine*. 4th ed. Philadelphia, PA: W. B. Saunders.

Joynt R. J., and Benton A. L. (1964). The memoir of Marc Dax on aphasia. *Neurology* 14: 851–854.

Major R. H. (1954). *A History of Medicine*. Springfield, IL: C. C. Thomas.

Morgani G. (1769). *The Seats and Causes of Diseases Investigated by Anatomy* (trans. by B. A. Alexander). London: A Millar and T. Cadell.

19

The Hécaen–Zangwill Legacy: Hemispheric Dominance Examined

The origin of the concept of hemispheric cerebral dominance is familiar to neuropsychologists. It arose in the 1860s with Broca's (1861, 1863, 1865) demonstration of the association between nonfluent speech disorder (aphemia, motor aphasia) and disease of the anterior left hemisphere. Some 10 years later Wernicke (1874) correlated fluent speech disorder (sensory aphasia) with lesions in the posterior left hemisphere. Together their landmark contributions established the doctrine of left hemisphere dominance for speech and language.

Both Broca and Wernicke had firm ideas about the nature of aphasic disorders, and about the relationship of these disorders to thinking and intellect. Both held the common sense view that speech consisted of the conventional signs of ideas, and that aphasia represented a defect in this system of signs and was *not* an impairment in thinking as such. The patient with motor aphasia knew what he wanted to say—he had the appropriate words in mind—but he could not get them out properly. The patient with sensory aphasia also knew what he wanted to say—his ideas were intact—but he had lost his memory of the conventional relationships between ideas and spoken words; consequently, he had lost his appreciation of the meaning of words (cf. Broca, 1869). Although many aphasic patients did show some degree of cognitive impairment, neither form of aphasic disorder necessarily involved a disturbance of thinking per se. Wernicke was

Reprinted with permission from *Neuropsychology Review,* Vol. 2, No. 4, 1991.

Adapted from an invited address, Division 40, 1991 APA Convention, San Francisco.

particularly insistent on this point, warning that "nothing could be worse for the study of aphasia than to consider the intellectual disturbance associated with aphasia as an essential part of the disease picture" (Wernicke, 1874, p. 35).

However, at the same time a radically different conception of the nature of aphasic disorder that defined it, not as a loss of a system of signs, but as a basic impairment of symbolic thinking itself was also put forward. This conception had its origins in nineteenth century philosophy and linguistics, which equated at least distinctively human thought with language. The conception was succinctly expressed by the linguist Max Müller (1866) when he wrote, "To think is to speak low. To speak is to think out loud." Those who have read John B. Watson, the founder of the American school of behaviorism, will appreciate that he was almost echoing Müller when he defined thinking as subvocal speech or, as he once put it, "talking to ourselves" (Watson, 1924).

This fundamental idea was adopted by some clinicians and applied to the problem of the nature of aphasic disorders. Finkelnburg (1870) introduced the concept of "asymbolia," i.e., a basic impairment in symbolic thinking, and contended that aphasia was a specific manifestation of asymbolia and not a mere instrumental disturbance of speech. To support his position, Finkelnburg cited instances in which aphasic patients no longer understood the value of coins, the import of pantomimed actions, or the meaning of signs of rank. Possibly it was this line of thought that provoked Wernicke's admonition that aphasic disorder should not be confused with intellectual impairment.

In any case, Hughlings Jackson's ideas were eventually far more influential. Jackson (1874) emphasized that aphasia was not a mere loss of speech or a forgetting of words, but an impairment in speech as an integral element of thought. Of necessity the aphasic patient is "lamed in his thinking" since is "speech is a *part* of thought." Jackson's disciple, Henry Head (1926), incorporated this position in his definition of aphasia as a general defect in symbolic formulation and expression that was reflected in a patient's nonverbal as well as his verbal behavior. Consistent with this stance, Head's aphasia examination included nonverbal tasks that presumably made demands on the capacity for symbolic thinking. Pierre Marie (1906) also maintained that "true" aphasia represented a loss of intelligence and not merely a defect in speech communication. The impact of these contributions was to establish the dominance of the left hemisphere for *symbolic thought* as well as for the communication of speech.

Other dimensions were added to the doctrine of left hemisphere dominance by the pathbreaking studies of Liepmann (1900) on apraxia, Kleist (1923) on visuoconstructional defects, and Gerstmann (1930) on impairment of the body schema. All these defects were attributed either to lesions of the left hemisphere or to commissural damage resulting in the isolation of that hemisphere from other parts of the brain. Thus the dominance of the left hemisphere was amplified to encompass some important forms of *nonverbal* mental activity. Truly the left hemisphere was, as the French neurologists characterized it, "the intellectual hemisphere," dominant for thought as well as for speech (cf. Lhermitte, 1929).

Yet almost from the very beginning of this development, a minority view that the right hemisphere might possess its own distinctive functional properties was also voiced. Hughlings Jackson in the 1870s attributed "imperception," i.e., defective visual recognition and orientation, to disease of the posterior right hemisphere and his basic observations were confirmed by a number of clinicians who were unfamiliar with his views. For example, Kleist's correlation between constructional apraxia and left hemisphere disease was challenged by some clinicians who concluded that the disability was in fact more likely to be shown by patients with lesions of the right hemisphere than by those with left hemisphere disease.

Still other authors added further dimensions to the concept of a possible dominance of the right hemisphere. Having described anosognosia in the form of unawareness or denial of left hemiplegia, Babinski (1914) noted an apparently specific association between the defect and right hemisphere disease, and he raised the question of whether the right hemisphere was the locus of a center for the integration of somatosensory information and somesthetic memory images. Dide (1938) postulated the existence of what he called the "syndrome of the right parietal lobe," which included somesthetic disabilities and anosognosia as well as visual disorientation and constructional apraxia. Russell Brain (1941) concluded from his study of some patients with lesions of the right parietal lobe that "certain syndromes, notably anosognosia, are seen exclusively or almost excessively as a result of lesions in the right hemisphere."

Yet for a number of reasons, these contributions had no appreciable effect on the concept of exclusive left hemisphere dominance that prevailed in mainstream neurology. One reason was that there were, in fact, only 10 papers over a time span of six decades that raised the question of the participation of the right hemisphere in cognitive operations. A second reason is that some contributions, such as those of Jackson, were not widely known. Finally, some of the reports were pretty weak. For example, two papers described patients with double hemianopia whose vision was so markedly constricted that their visual capacities were bound to be seriously impaired.

In any case, these scattered communications were not strong enough to counteract the negative findings reported by the neurosurgeon, Walter Dandy (1933). With the intent of prolonging the lives of patients with malignant tumors of the right cerebral hemisphere, Dandy removed the entire hemisphere in a number of cases. Two patients who were studied intensively after this radical surgery showed the anticipated left hemiplegia, left hemianopia, and left hemisensory impairment. Surprisingly, however, they show no apparent defects in cognitive function or changes in personality, as judged from the reports of relatives and friends and from the observations of Dandy himself, a neurologist (Frank R. Ford, later a prominent pediatric neurologist) and a psychologist (Curt P. Richter). Dandy concluded that, from a scientific standpoint, the results were "disappointing" but that he was "still not willing to say that the mentality of the patients was normal; but rather that abnormalities have not been disclosed." Nevertheless, these sweepingly negative findings by an eminent neurosurgeon, who was *not* biased toward regarding the right hemisphere as a cognitively silent area, could only have reinforced the prevailing doctrine of left hemisphere dominance.

In the 1930s, there were two psychologists who were concerned with the behavioral consequences of unilateral brain disease. Katherine McBride, who was largely responsible for a pathbreaking study of aphasia that initiated the modern approach to assessment of the disorder (Weisenburg and McBride, 1935), noted that her nonaphasic patients with right hemisphere lesions performed quite badly on some of the nonverbal performance tests in her battery. Donald Hebb (1939) described the pattern of test performance in a patient who had undergone a right temporal lobe excision and who showed superior verbal abilities, but markedly defective performances on visuoperceptive and visuoconstructional tests as well as on a tactile form perception task. He suggested that impairment in form perception, both visual and tactile, might well be a specific consequence of right temporal lobe defect.

However, neither McBride nor Hebb was prepared to generalize their findings and to mount a challenge to the doctrine of the dominance of the left hemisphere as *the* "major" hemisphere. During and directly after World War II, that challenge arose from the investigative work of the French neurologist Henry Hécaen and the British psychologist Oliver Zangwill, both of whom took the scattered early contributions very seriously. Beginning in 1945, Hécaen and his coworkers undertook a series of studies showing the very high frequency of visuospatial, visuoperceptual, and visuoconstructional deficits associated with lesions of the right hemisphere and by inference of the preminent role of that hemisphere in the mediation of performances of this nature (Hécaen and Ajuriaguerra, 1945; Hécaen et al., 1951; Hécaen et al., 1956). Beginning in 1944, Zangwill and his collegues similarly demonstrated the close association between visuospatial impairment and lesions of the posterior right hemisphere (Paterson and Zangwill, 1944; McFie et al., 1950).

Together Hécaen and Zangwill assembled a mass of empirical evidence about the characteristic deficits resulting from right hemisphere disease that was sufficiently impressive that it shook the belief that distinctive cognitive functions were mediated exclusively by the left hemisphere. The ultimate effect of their efforts was to transform the doctrine of left hemisphere dominance into the more democratic idea of asymmetry of hemisphere function. Another effect was to open the way for scores of psychologists, neurologists, and psychiatrists to investigate the role of the right hemisphere in the mediation of behavior. The field of inquiry extended beyond visuoperceptual and visuoconstructional performances to encompass audition, somesthesis, motor performances, attentional processes, emotional reactions, and psychiatric disorders.

The performances that have been reported as being related to right hemisphere function are so numerous and so diverse as to be almost bewildering. Table 19–1 presents a sampling of the types of performance that have been ascribed to right hemisphere operations. For the most part, the list comes from clinical studies that have found impairment in these performances to be preferentially associated with right hemisphere disease. Studies of the differential hemisphere participation in the performances of normal subjects (made possible through employment of dichotic and lateralized tachistoscopic stimulation) have been generally congruent with these clinical findings. Thus the inference of the positive from the negative, i.e., the assumption that failing performance by a patient with a damaged right hemisphere means that intact performance is mediated by the right hemisphere, appears to be justified.

The very large number of performances listed in Table 19–1 that have been related to right hemisphere operations cannot help but be unsatisfactory from a scientific standpoint. Surely they can be reduced to a smaller number of more basic cognitive dimensions that are differentially related to each hemisphere.

Table 19–2 shows some of the dichotomies that have been proposed for the left and right hemisphere, respectively. As will be seen, a fair number of "basic cognitive dimensions" have been postulated. Nevertheless, some of the contrasts, if they do not represent identical operations, are very closely related to each other, e.g. "logical–pictorial" and "rational–intuitive." Thus it seems evident that in some instances the dichotomies are only different labels for the same cognitive operations.

Tradition and common sense favor the verbal (left hemisphere) vs. nonverbal (right hemisphere) dichotomy. Why have some theorists seen this dichotomy as unsatisfactory? A number of facts have been brought forth to support their position. There is the centuries-old observation that some aphasic patients, if primed, can recite familiar prayers faultlessly (cf. Benton and Joynt, 1960). Some aphasic patients can sing a song (with its words) while some nonaphasic right hemisphere–damaged patients cannot (cf. Benton, 1977; Burkland and Smith, 1977). An aphasic patient who does not understand the propositional content of an utterance may appreciate the import of its prosodic component, i.e. he will know whether the examiner is making a statement, asking a question, or issuing a command. Conversely, the verbal functions of many right hemisphere–damaged patients are not fully intact, with examination disclosing an at least modest decline in performance level as measured by controlled word association and token tests. Another point that is brought up is the sizable number of subjects who show a left ear (i.e., right hemisphere) superiority when proc-

TABLE 19–1. Defective Performances Associated with Right Hemisphere Disease

Vision	
	Discrimination of configurations (e.g., complex shapes)
	Spatial orientation (e.g., route finding, directions, geography)
	Recognition on basis of incomplete information (e.g., fragmented figures)
	Recognition of familiar faces, unfamiliar faces, facial expression
	Stereopsis
	Mental rotation
Audition	
	Sound localization
	Discrimination of pitch, loudness, timbre
	Perception of emotional oral speech
	Identification of persons by voice
	Understanding of metaphoric speech
Somesthesis	
	Object and form perception
	Perception of spatial stimuli (e.g., direction of lines drawn on skin)
Motor	
	Simple reaction time
	Music: instrumental performance
	Singing
	Prosody in speech
	Motor persistence
General	
	Arousal and attention
	Preparatory set
	Awareness of hemispace
	Mood (euphoria/dysphoria)

essing verbal information in dichotic listening studies. These subjects form a minority but they are too numerous to be considered "exceptional."

Observations such as these have impelled some theorists to look for a more basic dichotomy. The leading candidates are the "serial–parallel" and "analytic–holistic" pairs. Speech expression and comprehension, as well as reading text and writing, take place serially in a fixed temporal order. In contrast, the appreciation of a spatial display, whether it be a form, an object, or a face, permits parallel information processing and hence an almost instantaneous grasp of the complex stimulus.

As with the left hemisphere and language, a mass of empirical findings are congruent with this classification of serial-analytic vs. parallel–holistic categories, while some observations are not. One example is the matching of unfamiliar

TABLE 19–2. Left Hemisphere–Right Hemisphere Dichotomies*

Verbal vs. nonverbal	Logical vs. pictorial
Serial vs. parallel	Propositional vs. appositional
Analytic vs. holistic	Rational vs. intuitive
Controlled vs. creative	Social vs. physical

*Drawn from Bradshaw and Nettleton (1981), Trevarthen (1984), and Benton (1988).

faces, which is regarded as a configurational task par excellence. In accord with expectations, one finds a high frequency of failure in patients with right hemisphere disease, particularly those with posterior temporo-occipital lesions where the frequency of failure is about 50%. However, there is a subgroup of patients with posterior *left* hemisphere lesions *and* impaired understanding of speech who also show a notable frequency of failure, in this instance, 35% to 40% (Hamsher et al., 1979). Similarly, tachistoscopic visual field studies of facial recognition in normal subjects find a highly significant left field advantage, indicating a major participation of the right hemisphere in the performance. But again, there is a substantial minority of normal right-handed subjects who exhibit a left field advantage, the proportion being 20–25% (cf. Hilliard, 1973; St. John, 1981).

Thus it appears that each dichotomy accounts for many empirical findings but not all. The verbal–nonverbal dichotomy has considerable, if not perfect, validity; in its defense, it should be pointed out that aphasiologists such as Jackson and Head did not regard singing and recitation as truly linguistic or symbolic processes, but merely as serial performances with no propositional content. The serial–parallel dichotomy is applicable in some instances, as is the analytic–holistic distinction. Given the controversial status of the issue, a pluralistic approach that invokes a number of interrelated principles may be the most reasonable one to adopt at the present time.

Instability in Performance

As has been mentioned, studies of the differential hemispheric participation in the performances of normal right-handed subjects on both verbal and nonverbal tasks have generated a substantial number of deviant cases that do not conform to expectations, i.e., subjects who show a left ear or visual field advantage in processing verbal material, and those who show a right ear or visual field advantage in processing nonverbal material such as faces, the slope of lines, or the location of dots in a display. This is a stumbling block to acceptance of any principle of hemispheric classification.

A set of data that may be helpful in accounting for this state of affairs and in trying to understand the nature of hemispheric cerebral dominance concerns the role of *instability* of performance on these tasks, either from one experimental session to another or within the same session. Dichotic listening studies may serve as an example.

It is no secret that the conventional dichotic listening setup, in which pairs of words, digits, or CVCs are fed into the two ears, generate results of limited reliability. In a study by Pizzamiglio et al. (1974), the usual right ear superiority for digits was found in a sample of 91 college students in both of two testing sessions one month apart. However, no less than 27 subjects (30%) changed their "ear advantage" from the first to the second session: 20% changed from right or left ear superiority to ambilaterality (or vice versa) and 10% changed from right to left ear superiority (or vice versa). A second study by Blumstein et al. (1975) reported almost identical findings for the reception of CVCs. In this instance when subjects were tested two weeks apart, 29% of the subjects shifted with respect to ear difference in one direction or another from the first to the second session. Almost certainly, it is this instability in performance that is responsible for the fact that left-hemisphere dominance for speech is less frequently disclosed by dichotic listening procedures (ca. 80% in normal right-handed patients) than in right-hand patients with unilateral brain disease (95 + percent) or by the Wada test (90 + percent).

The question may be raised as to whether the observed instability is a product of the unreliability of the tests. Are there too few test items and would increasing test length (in accord with time-honored statistical formulas) result in fewer shifts in lateral advantage? This seems quite doubtful. There were 90 trials in the Pizzamiglio study and 120 trials in the Blumstein study. In fact, it is likely that increasing the number of trials would decrease reliability. Participating as a subject in dichotic listening or tachistoscopic visual field study is at best a mildly boring experience. To undergraduate students who are required to participate (on the ground that the experience will give them precious insights into the methods of experimental psychology), the engagement may be more than only mildly boring. Lengthening the test can only intensity the tedium.

Instead, a case can be made that the observed instability is primarily in the subject, not the test. Support for this idea comes from a study by Turkewitz and Ross (1983) of visual field differences in the recognition of tachistoscopically presented faces. Plotting the course of performance over blocks of trials, they observed shifts in field advantage from one block to another. This they interpreted as shifts in the strategy of information processing from a holistic (i.e., right hemisphere) approach to a serial feature detection (i.e., left hemisphere) approach, and vice versa. Moreover, they found that the frequency of these shifts was *positively* related to overall efficiency in the tachistoscopic recognition of faces, i.e., shifts in strategy were characteristic of the better performers.

Additionally, some studies have shown that experimental manipulations of various kinds can influence the direction of half-field advantage in facial recognition. For example, Galper and Costa (1980) found that comments about the social attributes or the physical attributes of a face before it was presented had a differential effect, the social comments favoring *right* field accuracy in identification and the physical comments favoring *left* field accuracy in identification.

The subjects of Turkewitz and Ross showed successive shifts in field advantage spontaneously, i.e., in the absence of experimental manipulation. It is as if they were free to choose (consciously or unconsciously) to attend to either the physical features or the social connotations of faces and to shift their choice over trials. Or they were free to choose one information processing strategy (say a holistic strategy) and then shift to a feature detection strategy. No doubt their choices and shifts in choice were determined by a variety of factors, such as mood, physical condition, previous experience, and associations engendered by items in the task. But they did have the *capacity* to choose.

And why should they not have this capacity? They had healthy brains with unimpeded between-hemispheric transfer of information. Why should they not use one neural network (perhaps one with a strong representation in the right hemisphere) and then use another network (or a modified version of the original network) with a more prominent representation in the left hemisphere—particularly if the original network becomes satiated ("satiation" here being perhaps the neural equivalent of the state of being bored).

Interhemispheric Relationships

We know that by now the concept of areal localization, i.e., endowing specific parts of the brain with specific functional properties, has largely given way to the idea of networks or systems that mediate defined behavioral capacities. The thrust of modern neurophysiological and neuro-psychological thought is that these networks course through large parts of the brain rather than being located in a single discrete neural aggregate (cf. Damasio and Damasio, 1989). They are defined by dynamic sets of interrelationships *between* neural aggregates. The adjective "dynamic" needs to be emphasized. It implies that the networks are fluid or flexible in that their components can change in relative potency as a consequence of the operation of diverse factors. For example, task demands represent such a factor in the case of facial perception where very short exposure times primarily activate the operation of right hemisphere mechanisms while longer exposure times have a bilateral effect. (It will also be appreciated that spontaneous recovery of function would not be possible and neuropsychological rehabilitation efforts would be fruitless *if* the underlying neural networks were *not* flexible.)

At the moment the implications of modern neuropsychological thought for the problem of hemispheric cerebral dominance are both clear and obscure. Clearly, the idea that one hemisphere possesses certain unique neurobehavioral capacities to the *exclusion* of the other is untenable. Yet it is equally clear that each hemisphere *is* particularly adapted to mediate some types of performance and not others; in this respect they differ in important ways. What is not clear is *how* the two hemispheres work together in the healthy brain and what mechanisms are responsible for the differences between them, with the right hemisphere *usually* supporting some cognitive functions and the left hemisphere *usually* supporting others.

One way in which the two hemispheres work together is reflected in the apparent effect of a damaged hemisphere on the functioning of its undamaged counterpart. Studies of tactile sensitivity and perception in unilateral hemispheric lesions may serve as an example. As is well-known, a focal lesion involving the parietal somatosensory region typically produces impairment in tactile sensitivity on the side of the body contralateral to the side of lesion. Although some early case reports indicated otherwise (see Benton, 1972), it was generally believed sensitivity on the ipsilateral side of the body was unaffected in these patients with unilateral lesions. However, the seminal study of Semmes et al. (1960) invalidated that belief. Comparing sensitivity on both sides of the body with normative values, Semmes and her co-workers found that, in addition to the expected contralateral defects in pressure sensitivity, point localization, and two-point discrimination, many patients showed the same defects (generally of lesser severity) on the ipsilateral side as well. Subsequent studies confirmed the basic finding (cf. Vaughn and Costa, 1972; Corkin et al., 1964; Carmon, 1971). In all probability the procedure employed in the conventional neurological examination in which sensitivity on the two sides of the body is compared (i.e., using the patient as his own control) without recourse to normative values was responsible for the delay in recognizing the bilateral effects of a unilateral lesion. Moderate defects on the ipsilateral side might well be missed with this procedure. Carmon's (1971) analysis showed that this was actually the case for the data of Head's (1920) classic study of somesthesis.

It should be emphasized that only a minority of patients with unilateral hemispheric lesions show ipsilateral impairments on these tactile tasks. For example, in the study of Carmon (1971), 17 of 54 patients (31%) showed defective two-point discrimination and 9 (17%) showed a raised threshold of pressure sensitivity on the ipsilateral side of the body. Evidently, this interhemispheric effect is variable, depending upon factors that are as yet not firmly identified. Extent of lesion, the nature of the task, and individual differences in between-hemisphere communication are among the possibilities. Nevertheless, the fact that bilateral impairment in patients with unilateral lesions is not rare supports the idea that under certain conditions a damaged hemisphere does exert an influence on the functioning of the opposite undamaged hemisphere.

This bilateral effect has been found for a number of other performances, for example, choice reaction time (Benton and Joynt, 1959) and some visuoperceptual functions (Teuber et al., 1960). It can be viewed as one illustration of a familiar neuropyschological principle, namely, that a focal lesion typically has both specific and general effects on behavior (cf. Goldstein, 1939; Teuber, 1950). Its significance in the present context is that such an effect cannot help but attenuate observed between-hemispheric differences in the performances of patients with unilateral lesions. In a complementary way, the smooth interhemispheric communication enjoyed by normal subjects results in a similar attenuation.

Epilogue

The legacy of Henry Hécaen and Oliver Zangwill has proved to be a complex one. Asymmetric hemispheric functions take place within a framework of bihemispheric operations and these functions are inevitably modified by changes in bihemispheric operations. In short, "hemispheric dominance" represents a varying condition, depending upon both within-individual and between-individual factors. This is not to say that "cerebral dominance" does not exist. To deny its existence is surely to throw out the baby with the bathwater. But it is a dynamic state of affairs, far more subtle and complicated than was once thought.

The tasks before us are to probe the nature of asymmetry of hemispheric function in a number of respects: in terms of the basic cognitive processes preferentially mediated by each hemispheric, of the neural networks underlying perception and action, and of the factors that produce changes in performance. It is reasonable to anticipate that continued advances in neuroscience and cognitive psychology will enable us to accomplish these tasks.

References

Babinski J. (1914). Contribution a l'étude des troubles mentaux dans l'hémiplegie organique cérébrale (anosognosie). *Rev. Neurobiologique* 22: 845–848.

Benton A. L. (1972). Hemispheric cerebral dominance and somethesis. In Hammer M., Salzinger K., and Sutton S. (eds)., *Psychopathology: Essays in Honor of Joseph Zubin.* New York. Wiley—Interscience.

Benton A. L. (1977). The amusias. In Critchley M., and Henson R. A. (eds.). *Music and the Brain*. London: William Heinemann.

Benton A. L. (1988). *Neuropsychology*: Past, present, future. In Boller F. and Grafman J. (eds.), *Handbook of Neuropsychology* (Vol. 1). Amsterdam: Elsevier.

Benton A. L., and Joynt, R. J. (1959). Reaction time in unilateral cerebral disease. *Confinia Neurologica* 19:247–256.

Benton A. L., and Joynt R. J. (1960). Early descriptions of aphasia. *Arch. Neurol.* 3: 205–222.

Blumstein S., Goodglass H., and Tartter V. (1975). The reliability of ear advantage. *Brain Lang.* 2: 226–236.

Bradshaw J. L. and Nettleton N. C. (1981). The nature of hemispheric specialization in man. *Brain Behav. Sci.* 4: 51–91.

Brain W. R. (1941). Visual disorientation with special reference to lesions of the right cerebral hemisphere. *Brain* 64: 244–272.

Broca P. (1861). Perte de la parole: Ramolissement chronique et destruction partielle du lobe antérieur gauche du cerbeau. *Bull. Soc. Anthropol.* 2: 235–238.

Broca P. (1863). Localisations des fonctions cérébrales: Siége du langage articule. *Bull. Soc. Anthropol.* 4: 200–204.

Broca P. (1865). Sur la faculté du langage articulé. *Bull. Soc. Anthropol.* 6: 337–393.

Broca P. (1869). Sur le siège de la faculté de langage articulé. *Tribune Médicale* 3: 254–256, 265–269.

Burkland C. W. and Smith A. (1977). Language and the cerebral hemispheres. *Neurology* 27: 627–633.

Carmon A. (1971). Disturbances of tactile sensitivity in patients with unilateral cerebral lesions. *Cortex* 7: 83–97.

Corkin S., Milner B., and Rasmussen, T. (1964). Effects of different cortical excisions on sensory thresholds in man. *Trans. Am. Neurol. Assoc.* 89: 112–116.

Damasio H., and Damasio A. R. (1989). *Lesion Analysis Neuropsychology*, New York: Oxford University Press.

Dandy W. E. (1933). Physiological studies following extirpation of the right cerebral hemisphere in man. *Bulletin of the Johns Hopkins Hospital* 53: 31–51.

Dide M. E. (1938). Les désorientations temporo-spatiales et la préponderance de l'hemisphére droit dans les agnoso-akinésies proprioceptives. *Encéphale* 33: 276–294.

Finkelnburg F. C. (1870). Niederrheinsche Gesellschaft: Sitzung von 21 März 1870 in Bonn. *Berlin Klinische Wochenschrift* 7: 449–450. (English translation by Duffy R. J. and Liles B. Z. (1979), *J. Speech Hear. Dis.* 44: 156–168.

Galper R. E., and Costa L. (1980). Hemispheric superiority for recognizing faces depends upon how they are learned. *Cortex* 16: 21–38.

Gerstmann J. (1930). Zur symptomatologie der Hirnläsionen im Uebergangsgebiet der Unterparietal-und mitteleren Occipitalwindung. *Nerenarzt* 3: 691–695.

Goldstein K. (1939). *The Organism.* New York : American Book Company.

Hamsher K., Levin H. S., and Benton A. L. (1979). Facial recognition in patients with focal brain lesions. *Arch. Neurol.* 36: 873–879.

Head H. (1920). *Studies in Neurology*. London: Oxford University Press.

Head H. (1926). *Aphasia and Kindred Disorders of Speech.* London: Cambridge University Press.

Hebb D. O. (1939). Intelligence in man after large removal of cerebral tissue: Defects following right temporal lobectomy. *J. Gen. Psychol.* 21: 437–446.

Hécaen H., and Ajuriaguerra J. de (1945). L'apraxie de l'habillage. *Encéphale* 35: 113–143.

Hécaen H., Ajuriaguerra J. de, and Massonet J. (1951). Les troubles visuoconstructives par lésion pariéto-occipitale droite. *Encéphale* 40: 122–179.

Hécaen H., Penfield W., Bertrand C., and Malmo R. (1956). The syndrome of apractognosia due to lesions of the minor hemisphere. *Arch. Neurol. Psychiatry* 75: 400–434.

Hilliard R. D. (1973). Hemispheric laterality effects on a facial recognition task in normal subjects. *Cortex* 9: 246–258.

Jackson J. H. (1874). On the nature of the duality of the brain. *Medical Press and Circular* 1: 19, 41, 63 (Reprinted in *Brain* 38 (1915): 28–190.)

Kleist K. (1923). Kriegsverletzungen des Gehirns in ihre Bedeutung für die Hirnlokalisation und Hirnpathologie. In von Schjerning O. (ed.), *Handbuch der Aerztlichen Erfahrung im Weltkriege*, 1914/1918 (Vol. 4), Leipzig: Barth.

Lhermitte J. (1929). Le lobe frontal. *L'Encéphale* 24: 87–118.

Liepmann O. (1900). Das Krankheitsbild der Apraxie. *Monatsschrift für Psychiatrie und Neurologie* 8: 15–44; 102–132, 182–197.

Marie P. (1906). Revision de la question de l'aphasie. *Semaine Médicale* 26: 241–247, 493–500, 565–571.

McFie J., Piercy M. F., and Zangwill O. L. (1950). Visual-spatial agnosia associated with lesions of the right cerebral hemisphere. *Brain* 73: 167–190.

Müller M. (1866). *Lectures on the Science of Language*. New York: Charles Scribner's Sons,

Paterson A. and Zangwill O. L. (1944). Disorders of visual space perception associated with lesions of the right cerebral hemisphere. *Brain* 67: 331–358.

Pizzamiglio L., De Pascalis C., and Vignati A. (1974). Stability of dichotic listening test. *Cortex* 10: 203–205.

Semmes J., Weinstein S., Ghent L., and Teuber, H.-L. (1960). *Somatosensory Changes after Penetrating Brain Wounds in Man*. Cambridge: Harvard University Press.

St. John R. C. (1981). Lateral asymmetry in face perception. *Can. J. Psychol.* 35: 213–223.

Teuber H.-L. (1950). Neuropsychology. In Harrower M. R. (ed.), *Recent Advances in Diagnostic Psychological Testing*. Springfield, IL: Charles C. Thomas.

Teuber H.-L., Battersby W. S., and Bender M. B. (1960). *Visual Field Defects after Penetrating Missile Wounds of the Brain*. Cambridge, MA: Harvard University Press.

Trevarthen C. (1984). Hemispheric specialization. *Handbook of Physiology, Section 1: The Nervous System* (Vol. 3), Bethesda, MD, American Physiological Society.

Turkewitz G. and Ross P. (1983). Changes in visual field advantage for facial recognition. *Cortex* 19: 179–185.

Vaughn H. G. and Costa, L. D. (1962). Performances of patients with lateralized cerebral lesions. *J. Nerv. Ment. Dis.* 1973: 1248–1250.

Watson J. B. (1924). *Psychology from the Standpoint of a Behaviorist*, 2nd ed., Philadelphia: Lippincott.

Weisenburg T. and McBride K. E. (1935). *Aphasia*. New York: Commonwealth Fund.

Wernicke C. (1874). *Der Aphasische Symptomencomplex*. Breslau: Cohn und Weigert.

Part V

PEDIATRIC NEUROPSYCHOLOGY

20

Dyslexia: Evolution of a Concept

It was recognized at a relatively early stage of medical history that injury or disease of the brain in adult patients could cause a loss of a specific cognitive skill such as the ability to name objects or the ability to read. Indeed observations of this type were often employed as an argument in favor of localization of function in the brain. Thus specific anomia or "loss of memory for words" was clearly described in the sixteenth century and the syndrome of alexia without agraphia was identified in the seventeenth century.

But neither physicians nor educators were as quick to recognize that children might also suffer from specific cognitive disabilities as a consequence of congenital or early acquired disease. It was only in 1853 that the Dublin otologist William Wilde published his observations on children who were "dumb, but not deaf," i.e., suffering from specific language disability. As we know, developmental dyslexia went unrecognized until the end of the nineteenth century when Morgan published his famous case report. As so often happens, once the attention of physicians was called to the condition, they immediately observed it in their practice and a steady stream of papers on dyslexia appeared in the English and German medical literature between 1900 and 1910. Somewhat later, clinical psychologists recognized dyslexia as a distinctive condition and attempted to relate its occurrence to more basic defects in visualization, auditory perception and associational processes. On the other hand, educators were less ready to accept the real existence of "congenital wordblindness" as a clinical entity.

Reprinted with permission from *Bulletin of The Orton Society*, Vol. 30, 1980.

Presented at the 30th Annual Conference of the Orton Society, Indianapolis, November 1979.

The Early History

Morgan (1896) described a classic case of dyslexia. His patient was an intelligent 14-year-old boy who was severely disabled in reading and writing despite individual tutoring as well as years of conventional school instruction. The boy knew the phonetic value of most letters and could read short, high-frequency words but he could not blend letter sounds and had gained no appreciation of the characteristic spelling patterns of English. Yet he could read three-digit numbers fluently and could solve written problems in algebra. Morgan considered the boy to be "word-blind" but not "letter-blind." Since alexia in adults was known to be related to disease in the territory of the left angular gyrus, he supposed that defective development of this area was responsible for the boy's disability. A very similar case was reported by Bastian (1898), who also ascribed the disability to congenital weakness or early damage of the "visual word centre" in the angular gyrus.

In 1900 James Hinshelwood published the first in what was to be a long series of papers on developmental dyslexia. The two additional cases which he reported added little to what Morgan and Bastian had described. However, Hinshelwood did express the opinion that the condition was "by no means so rare as the absence of recorded cases would lead us to infer. Their rarity is, I think, accounted for by the fact that when they do occur they are not recognized."

There followed a paper by Nettleship (1901) in which he described five cases that he had seen in his practice, two of them dating back to 1882. In addition to confirming the observations of Hinshelwood, Bastian and Pringle Morgan (whom he inexplicably called "Campbell Brown"), Nettleship made a number of new points. He was the first to describe developmental dyslexia in young adults, one of his patients being 23 years old and another 21 years old. He was the first to describe dyslexia in a woman and at the same time also the first to call attention to the preponderance of males with the condition, pointing out that eight of the nine cases reported up to that time were boys or men. Finally, he made a perceptive sociological observation about reading disability. "The detection of congenital word-blindness is easy in the children of well-educated parents whose young children receive much individual attention. It must be much more difficult, both to recognize and deal with, in the children who crowd our Infant Elementary Schools."

Hinshelwood's second paper in 1902 reported two further cases and addressed the problem of teaching dyslexic children to read. He insisted that they should not be taught in the regular classes along with normal readers but by special methods in a separate setting. Since defective development of the "visual word centre" in the angular and supramarginal gyri of the left hemisphere has impaired their visual memory for words and letters, these children need to be taught by methods that utilize the sense of touch to strengthen sight-sound associations.

For this he recommended the employment of block letters which the child could learn to identify by touch as well as vision and which he could use in reading and spelling words.

Over the course of the next few years, case reports from Holland, Argentina, France, Germany and the United States appeared in the medical literature, for the most part in ophthalmologic journals (Lechner, 1903; Wernicke, 1903; Foerster, 1905; Brunner, 1905; Variot and Lecomte, 1906; Claiborne, 1906; Jackson, 1906; Peters, 1908). Although some of these added little to what was already known, they at least demonstrated that dyslexia was not confined to England and Scotland. Claiborne (1906) was the first to raise the question of whether linguistic factors might play a role in the genesis of specific reading disability. Having pointed out the characteristically inconsistent grapheme-phoneme relationships of English, he wrote:

> Those who learn to read English always have this difficulty before them, and it would be interesting to know what difference there is in the relative facility with which children learn English, which is filled with such arbitrary pronunciation, and some other language in which each vowel and consonant has a definite value and the same value always under the same circumstances, such as Italian, Spanish, and German. Compare the English words "tough," "though" and "slough," for example. No such difficulties, I believe, exist in the three other languages mentioned. I believe, and it is reasonable to assume, that word-amblyopia exists more frequently in English-speaking children than in those speaking other languages that have not the difficulties of the English.

The tendency for dyslexia to run in families was noted as early as 1905 by Fisher and by Thomas. Further evidence for a basic hereditary determinant in at least some cases of dyslexia was furnished by the case reports of Stephenson (1907), Hinshelwood (1909) and Plate (1909). Jackson (1906) was the first to suggest that "development alexia" would be a more appropriate designation for the condition than "congenital word-blindness."

The 28 papers on dyslexia published between 1896 and 1910 (15 of them by British authors) provided a substantial amount of information about the disability. They established the real existence of the condition and defined its characteristic features. Many more boys than girls were subject to the disability. An hereditary determinant seemed evident in a proportion of the cases. Cerebral damage resulting from birth trauma probably was causative in other cases and perhaps explained the predominance of dyslexic boys. Linguistic factors may affect the relative frequency of the condition in different countries. A striking dissociation between the ability to read numbers as contrasted to letters and words may be shown. Estimates of the frequency of word-blindness in school children ranged from 1 in 2000 (Fisher, 1905) to 1 in 100 (Warburg, 1911).

However, the growth of empirical knowledge during this period was not accompanied by any basic change in conceptions about the etiology of dyslexia or its underlying mechanisms. The early aphasiologists thought of the territory of the angular gyrus in the dominant hemisphere as being a center in which visual memory images of letters and words were deposited. Injury or faulty development of that center entailed a partial or complete loss of these memory images with consequent impairment in the ability to read. Hinshelwood, the leading theorist of the time, adopted this simplistic conception to "explain" specific dyslexia. The dyslexic child suffered from maldevelopment of the left angular gyrus area with consequent inability to retain the visual memories of letters and words. Hence, he had to use the homologous area in the right hemisphere to learn to read and, since this area was not well adapted for the purpose, his progress was defective. The fact that many dyslexic children could read numbers with greater facility than words was interpreted as meaning that there were separate centers for the visual memories of numbers and words. Hinshelwood contended that the auditory memory of dyslexic children was invariably good, a notion which fit in with his concept of localized pathology and defective visual-verbal imagery.

It was agreed that a child could overcome his disability, at least in part, but special educational arrangements and methods were required to accomplish this. Among other procedures, Fisher (1905) recommended that the "look and say" method calling for global word recognition be employed with these children who experienced so much difficulty with phonemic analysis. Another recommendation was that, since the right hemisphere was subserving the learning of reading by these children with defective left hemispheres, it would be logical to teach them to write with the left hand.

The Psychological Period (1912–1926)

As psycho-educational clinics and child guidance centers were established in the second decade of the twentieth century, educational and clinical psychologists became concerned with dyslexia. Their approach to the problem posed by nonreading children was quite different from that of the ophthalmologists and school doctors who had first described the condition. They were primarily interested in a functional analysis of the dyslexic child with the aim of identifying those basic disabilities that might underlie his failure to learn to read. The psychologists appreciated that reading was more than a matter of simple sight-sound associations, as had been assumed by most of the early workers in the field, and that it involved "perception, interpretation of symbols, memory, comprehension, motor processes, emotions and complex associations" (Bronner, 1917, p. 77). They were, therefore, prepared to investigate all aspects of mentation and cognition in their effort to understand the determinants of reading failure. An early example is the application of the free association test to a dyslexic boy by Voss

(1914) who found that his responses deviated markedly from normative values and who therefore suggested that the basic defect in dyslexia extended beyond visuoverbal processes to encompass oral language as well.

The major studies of this period presented detailed analyses of the performances of disabled readers on diverse perceptual, associational and learning tasks with the aim of identifying the basic disabilities underlying their failure to learn to read. Bronner (1917), for example, found different performance patterns in individual dyslexics. One might be poor in auditory memory and motor speech expression, another might fail nonverbal visual memory tests. From her observation of successful approaches to the remediation of reading disability, Schmitt (1918) concluded that dyslexics were deficient in developing the complex of meanings connected with both oral and written symbols and hence their recognition of these symbols was uncertain and unstable. In essence, she conceived of the basic disability in reading failure as being one of the association rather than of perception and memory. Bronner had expressed the same idea in a rather vague way when she wondered "whether in reading there is not involved some subtle synthetic process which, at the present time, we have no means of studying but defects of which, nevertheless, are of extreme significance." Similarly, Wallin (1920) wrote:

> Although the source of the difficulty has been considered to be a defect in visual word imagery, it is possible that the seat of the trouble may be in the connections between the centers for the images of spoken words and for the images of written words. We suggest this as an important topic for investigation.

In consonance with this conclusion, Wallin reported that his dyslexic children did not show defects in visual imagery or memory, as measured by their performances on the ball-and-field and memory for designs subtests of the Binet. Nor did they show impairment in auditory memory, as measured by auditory-vocal digit span.

Further studies in the 1920s reinforced the concept that dyslexia could not be construed as a purely visuoverbal disability. Fildes (1922) found that many disabled readers showed defects either in visual form discrimination and memory or in auditory memory for numbers and sentences. She therefore concluded that reading disability is partly an expression of a more general impairment involving vision, hearing and their interrelations. Similarly, Hincks (1926) reported that her dyslexic subjects showed a variety of perceptual defects, most notably in visual form perception and pitch discrimination. On the other hand, a dissenting note was sounded by Gates (1922) who found no evidence of defective visual or auditory perception and memory in children who were relatively poor readers (but not necessarily dyslexics). He severely criticized such concepts as faulty "visualization" or "ability to associate auditory and visual symbols" as too poorly defined and too global to be meaningful. Instead, he ascribed poor reading achievement to environmental factors such as inadequate instruction and poor habit training.

Another line of thought that emerged during this period deserves to be mentioned. An association between hand preference, and particularly forced change in preference, with stammering had been noted as early as 1912 by Ballard. Dearborn (1925) extended the association to reading disability, noting that at least one third of the nonreaders whom he had seen were lefthanded. His student, Hincks (1926), who made the same observation, commented:

> Many non-readers are left-handed, and many who are not actually so, show traits that we might call "left-minded." They often begin to read a word at the right instead of the left end. The words "saw" and "was" are apt to be bugbears for all non-readers. Their confusion of letters, numbers and forms alike except for orientation is another characteristic of "left-mindedness." One is inclined to wonder whether some early transfer of handedness may not have caused a disturbance similar to that of stammering, but resulting in reading difficulty. Statistics on a large number of non-readers might prove very enlightening.

Clearly the state of knowledge about dyslexia in the mid-1920s was far more differentiated than it had been in 1910. Attention had shifted from the description of surface characteristics to the analysis of underlying mechanisms. Two schools of thought had emerged. One school postulated diverse perceptual and cognitive disabilities as the basis for the observed failure in learning to read. The other school emphasized environmental and characterological variables, such as faulty instruction, inadequate nurture and poor habits. There was no great interest in identifying a neurological basis for the disorder. However, the theory put forth by Morgan and Hinshelwood that dyslexia arises from focal maldevelopment of the posterior parietal territory of the dominant hemisphere was generally regarded as inadequate.

The Work and Influence of S. T. Orton

A new and highly original neurological theory of dyslexia was advanced by Orton in a series of papers published between 1925 and 1929 (see Orton, 1966). Starting from the observation that dyslexic children tended to show reversals in right-left orientation in the reading of letters and words, he related this disturbance in directionality to a defective interhemispheric organization of cerebral function. Proposing the term "strephosymbolia" (twisted symbols) as a designation for developmental dyslexia, he identified two types of reversals in reading; the reversed reading of letters was designated as static reversals, the reversed reading of words as kinetic reversals.

At the same time, Orton was equally strongly impressed by the high frequency of left-handedness, lack of established hand preference and mixed hand and eye preference in disabled readers as well as in children with speech defects.

Calling attention to the well-known association between mirror writing and left-handedness, he reported that many of his dyslexics read mirror image text as well as they read conventional text. He saw these perceptual and motor deviations as reflecting a specific fault in cerebral development, namely, a failure to establish hemispheric specialization for the visual perception of symbolic stimuli. He pointed out that, while the occipito-parietal areas of the two hemispheres are functionally equivalent at the levels of simple visual perception and object recognition, the occipito-parietal cortex of the dominant hemisphere alone mediates reading, i.e., the recognition of visual symbolic material. This concentration of function in a single hemisphere is necessary for fluent reading in order to effect the suppression of antidromic or mirror image information in the subordinate hemisphere that would compete with correctly orientated information in the dominant hemisphere. Specific reading disability results from a failure to establish this specialization of function in a single hemisphere.

> This suggests that the process of learning to read entails the elision from the focus of attention of the confusing memory images of the nondominant hemisphere which are in reversed form and order, and the selection of those which are correctly oriented and in correct sequence. . . .
>
> The frequency in these cases of reading disability, of reversals of letter pairs, of whole syllables . . . or of the major parts of words strongly suggests that there has been an incomplete elision of the memory patterns in the nondominant hemisphere, and that therefore either right or left sequence may be followed in attempting to compare presented stimuli with memory images, and that this leads to confusion or delay in selection. . . .
>
> The term "congenital word-blindness" because of its association with the acquired condition and the implications therefrom, does not seem to be properly descriptive of this disability and I would therefore like to offer the term "strephosymbolia" . . . as a descriptive name for the whole group of children who show unusual difficulty in learning to read (Orton, 1925, pp. 607–609).

Orton's theoretical formulation decisively influenced the direction of subsequent research on dyslexia. Over the past 50 years no topic in the field has been so thoroughly investigated as has the question of whether specific reading disability is systematically related to incomplete or anomalous hemispheric dominance. As everyone knows, the outcome of this vast amount of research has not led to any firm conclusions. Again and again evidence for an association between reading disability and deviant laterality (e.g., left-handedness, ambidexterity, inconsistent hand-eye preference) has been obtained. On the other hand, many studies have reported negative results. Even discounting this inconsistency, the positive findings do not permit a simple interpretation. For example, a paper may report that indications of left-handedness or ambidexterity were found in 35% of a sample of dyslexic children as compared to a 15% frequency in an age-matched sample of normal readers. The between-groups difference is real enough. But, before inferring any casual relationship, one has to account for the

65% of dyslexics who are purely right-handed and the 15% of adequate readers who show deviant laterality.

The development of techniques such as dichotic listening and tachistoscopic stimulation of the left and right visual fields has made it possible to investigate the auditory and visual information processing capacities of each cerebral hemisphere and thus has provided measures of hemispheric dominance that are more directly related to the Orton theory. As is well known, a right ear (i.e., left hemisphere) superiority in the recognition and recall of verbal stimuli (digits, words) is shown by a majority of normal right-handed adults and older children in the dichotic listening situation. Similarly a right visual field superiority in the recognition and recall of verbal stimuli (words, nonsense syllables) is shown by a majority of normal right-handed adults and older children under the condition of tachistoscopic stimulation of either or both visual fields.

That these measures have serious limitations as indicators of hemispheric specialization for language function must be acknowledged. It is generally accepted that left hemisphere dominance for language is true of almost all right-handed persons. Right hemisphere dominance for language, as reflected in the occurrence of aphasia from a right hemisphere lesion in a right-handed patient is a very uncommon event, occurring in not more than six percent of cases (Conrad, 1949; Russell and Espir, 1961). Similarly, application of Wada's intracarotid sodium amytal test indicates that at least 92% of right-handed subjects are left hemisphere dominant for language (Milner, 1973).

But the experimental auditory and visual tasks have not generated comparable results, for one finds the proportion of normal subjects making performances indicative of left hemisphere dominance for language to be almost always less than 90% and often and often less than 80% (Kimura 1964, 1967; Bryden, 1965; Fontenot and Benton, 1972; Hilliard, 1973; McGlone and Davidson, 1973). Thus, if the clinical findings in aphasic patients with unilateral brain disease and the Wada test results are taken as criterion measures, it is evident that ear advantage and visual field differences are quite imperfect indicators of hemispheric dominance for language.

In any case, studies comparing these measures in normal and dyslexic children have produced the same blend of negative and mildly positive findings as have the studies on handedness (cf. Bryden, 1970; Zurif and Carson, 1970; Witelson and Rabinovitch, 1972; McKeever and Van Deventer, 1975; Yeni-Komshian et al., 1975; Leong, 1976; Thomson, 1976). Nevertheless, while some workers in the field have dismissed laterality as a significant factor in reading failure, others still believe that anomalous or incomplete hemispheric cerebral dominance is characteristic of a specific subgroup of developmental dyslexics (e.g., Zangwill, 1960, 1962). It is possible that the dyslexic cases identified by means of computerized tomography as having a pattern of structural asymmetry opposite of that seen in normal right-handers belong to this subgroup. In a sample of 24 dyslexics, Hier and his co-workers (1978) found 10 who showed a wider parieto-occipital region in the right hemisphere than in the left while the usual finding is a wider region in the left hemisphere (Geschwind and Levitsky, 1968; LeMay, 1976). These dyslexics differed from the other subjects in the sample in their lower WAIS or WISC Verbal Scale IQ and in their more frequent histories of delayed development of oral speech, two characteristics which Zangwill postulated as being part of a specific dyslexic syndrome.

The next development in thought about dyslexia took a rather different direction. In the 1930's, some clinicians and educational psychologists became impressed with the high frequency of behavioral maladjustment and personality disorder in dyslexic children. The impression was perhaps inevitable given the fact that very often these children were brought to clinical attention because of conduct problems and not specific reading failure. Systematic study of the question indicated that an excessively high proportion of cases did in fact show evidence of emotional disturbance (Monroe, 1932; Robinson, 1946). A reasonable interpretation was that the learning disability created stresses and failure experiences which led to the child's emotional disturbances. This was acknowledged but some clinicians viewed the personality disorder as primary and the reading disability as only one expression of it. The practical implication of this view was that psychotherapy was a necessary element in treatment and one which had to precede tutoring or be carried out in conjunction with it (Blanchard, 1935).

Dyslexia Since World War II

After World War II, there was an enormous growth of interest in dyslexia or at least in the failure of children to acquire fully adequate reading skills. Estimates of the prevalence of reading disability ranged from 10% to a hardly credible 30% (Benton, 1975). One reason for this wide variation was that educators and researchers often failed to distinguish between dyslexia, or specific reading disability, and what has come to be called "reading backwardness," i.e., reading failure due to low intelligence, sensory defects or lack of educational opportunity (Benton, 1975; Rutter, 1978). A tremendous expansion of investigative work paralleled this increased interest in reading failure.

Investigation proceeded along various lines. Early themes such as the relationship of deficiencies in visual and auditory perception to dyslexia were taken up again (Benton, 1962; Nielsen and Ringe, 1969; Vellutino et al., 1972; Vellutino, 1978). As already mentioned, Orton's theory continued to be evaluated through the application of newer experimental methods. There were also fresh approaches to the question of the neurological basis of dyslexia. Electroencephalography provided a measure of brain function which could be utilized to assess the presence of diverse types of functional abnormality (Hughes, 1978). Possible structural anomalies have been investigated, as in the CT study of Hier et al. (1978) and the autopsy report of Galaburda and Kemper (1979). Methods of clinical evaluation developed for the assessment of brain injury and anomalous development in children were applied to dyslexics (Denckla, 1977). The confusing results from studies of perceptual functions in dyslexic children led researchers to probe other cognitive processes such as intersensory integration, sequential perception and defects of language function (Birch and Belmont, 1964; Bakker, 1972; Shankweiler and Liberman, 1972, 1976; Vellutino, 1978). Finally, proceeding from the assumption that dyslexia is not the single disorder which it was once thought to be but instead consists of a number of syndromes, each with its own distinctive cognitive characteristics and antecedent conditions, attempts have been made to establish valid and clinically useful classifications of the disorder (Mattis et al., 1975; Doehring and Hoshko, 1977).

The impressive magnitude of this research effort is indicated by the fact that a recent book summarizing the current state of knowledge about dyslexia lists more than 900 monographs, papers and reports published between 1960 and 1977 (Benton and Pearl, 1978). The studies described in these publications investigate dyslexic children from every standpoint—genetic, neurologic, psychologic, educational, and social. As a consequence, we now possess a large body of information about every aspect of dyslexia. But somehow this mass of information has not proved to be as useful as one would have anticipated.

This is not to say that advances in knowledge and practice have not been achieved. Thanks to recent work on the prediction of reading disability, the preschool child at risk for later reading failure can be identified with fair accuracy (Benton, 1976; Jansky, 1978; Satz et al., 1978). This means that remediation can be instituted before the child begins the learning of reading and it offers the possibility that the experience of reading failure at least can be mitigated, if not avoided. This is a first step toward prevention but is not equivalent to prevention which depends upon an understanding of the causes and basic nature of dyslexia. As yet we do not possess this understanding.

Similarly, the dedicated efforts of reading specialists have made a variety of remediation methods available to the teacher who can select those which appear to be most appropriate for an individual child (Johnson, 1978). Yet there is considerable doubt about the effectiveness of many remedial instruction programs since all too often a specific therapeutic effect cannot be demonstrated. The reasons for this are obscure. It may be that the remedial techniques have not been applied skillfully or that their duration and intensity have been inadequate. Whatever the reason, the fact remains that remediation proceeds without knowledge of causation and often seems to be without proven value.

Clinical and experimental observations during the past 20 years have taught us a great deal about the disorder in terms of its genetic, neurologic, behavioral, and social correlates. Yet it is very difficult to integrate these observations into a coherent body of knowledge, particularly since there are so many instances of contradictory empirical findings in the literature. As a consequence, the concept of dyslexia has become quite complex and seems to mean different things to different people. Indeed, the very definition of the disorder is considered to be a serious problem (Eisenberg, 1978; Benton, 1978).

We have yet to find our way out of this impasse. The point is often made that one reason for our failure to find stable correlates of reading failure is that we are dealing with not one but a number of different conditions. Hence the identification of more homogeneous dyslexic syndromes would seem to be a necessary task. Different approaches to the problem of classification have been employed and systems based on the characteristics of reading performance (Boder, 1973; Doehring and Hoshko, 1977), on associated cognitive disabilities (Mattis et al., 1975), on the presence or absence of cerebral electrophysiologic abnormality (Hughes, 1978) or of clinical signs of neurologic abnormality (Rutter et al., 1970; Denckla, 1977) have been investigated. However, for the most part, these classifications have been developed in isolation from each other and their interrelations have not been determined. For example, it has not been established whether or not dyslexic children who show different profiles of reading performance also show different associated cognitive disabilities, although it would seem likely that this is the case. Similarly, neurologic and cerebral electrophysiologic studies of dyslexic children generally have treated them as a homogeneous group without regard to characteristics of their reading performances or the associated cognitive disabilities which they may show. Consequently, it is not known whether neurologic or electrophysiologic abnormality is characteristic of certain types of dyslexic children and not of others. The discordant results of studies on the frequency of neurologic and EEG abnormality in dyslexic children suggest that this may well be the case.

In the 1930s the idea that dyslexia was an expression of a more pervasive personality disorder was advanced. More recent study has shown that, whether the idea is valid or not, emotional disturbance and conduct disorders are indeed frequent correlates of dyslexia (Rutter et al., 1970; Rutter et al., 1970; Wender 1971). However, the meaning of this association and, specifically, the possible role it plays in the genesis of developmental dyslexia remain obscure.

There is another approach to dyslexia that deserves to be considered. At the beginning of this paper I mentioned that, while physicians quickly recognized congenital word-blindness as a distinctive condition once it had been described, teachers were less ready to accept it as a defined entity. Certainly this was not because they did not see children who had failed to learn to read. It was a question of a difference in attitude. Where the physicians saw disease the teachers saw a challenge. As Zigmond (1978) phrased it . . . "failure of the 'dyslexic' to learn is the result of failure of teachers to teach." She has pointed out that learning by its very nature is an interactive process.

> Learning is an interactive process. Whatever learning occurs is a complex product of what the learner brings to the situation and what the situation brings to the learner . . . In this context, failure to learn to read can be seen as the result of something being wrong with the person, *or* the result of something being wrong with the environment (teaching) *or* an interaction of both. While the preponderance of literature on reading disabilities attributes the problem to the person, we must not use the concept of dyslexia as an excuse to condone poor teaching. Teaching which disregards the significant differences among students in motivation, developmental levels, and rate and style of learning in planning instruction is poor teaching. We believe that it produces disabled learners. If "dyslexic" children are placed in educational environments which acknowledge individual differences and which provide for alternative teaching strategies related to these differences, then a significant number of "disabled" learners will begin to learn effectively. These learners could then no longer be viewed as having some "intrinsic specific disorders," leaving only a small minority who continue to have problems to be labelled "dyslexic," i.e., unable to profit from reading instruction as we currently know how to deliver it (Zigmond, 1978, pp. 437–438).

Similarly, Adelman (1970) speaks of "the not so specific learning disability population" and points out how extremely heterogeneous it is with regard to etiology and appropriate remedial strategies.

A number of comments may be made about this point of view. First to the extent that it encourages more vigorous and imaginative teaching, it is of heuristic value. Secondly, support for this interactionist position comes from other sources. We know, for example, that the prevalence of specific reading failure is related to a variety of social and cultural factors, such as size of family and neighborhood. A reasonable interpretation is that the observed educational disability is a product of the interaction of some endogenous defect with environmental forces. Finally, in emphasizing the heterogeneous nature of the problems posed by children diagnosed as dyslexic it is in harmony with current thinking.

Thus we see that the evolution of the concept of dyslexia has been in the direction of a progressively greater degree of differentiation. It is a multifaceted concept which includes genetic, neurologic, cognitive, emotional, educational, and social components. But there is little agreement among experts about which components are primarily and which are secondary or, stated in another way, which components define dyslexia and which do not. We hope and expect that in the 1980s investigative work will be sufficiently comprehensive to take account of this complexity and thus generate findings which will advance our understanding of dyslexic children and enable us to help them more effectively.

References

Adelman H. S. (1970). Learning problems: An interactional view of causality. *Academy Therapy* 6: 117–123.

Bakker D. (1972). *Temporal Order in Disturbed Reading*, Rotterdam: University Press.

Ballard P. B. (1912). Sinistrality and speech. *Journal of Experimental Pedagogy* 1: 298–310.

Bastian H. C. (1898). *A Treatise on Aphasia and Other Speech Defects*. London, H. K. Lewis; New York: Appleton and Company.

Benton A. L. (1962). Dyslexia in relation to form perception and directional sense. In Money J. (ed.), *Reading Disability: Progress and Research Needs in Dyslexia*. Baltimore, Johns Hopkins Press.

Benton A. L. (1975). Developmental dyslexia: Neurological aspects. In Friedlander W. J. (ed.), *Advances in Neurology*, Vol. 7). New York: Raven Press.

Benton A. L. (1976). Developmental dyslexia. *J. Ped. Psychol.* 1: 28–31.

Benton A. L. (1978). Some conclusions about dyslexia. In Benton A. L. and Pearl D. (eds.) *Dyslexia: An Appraisal of Current Knowledge*. New York: Oxford University Press.

Benton A. L. and Pearl D. (eds.) (1978). *Dyslexia: An Appraisal of Current Knowledge*. New York: Oxford University Press.

Birch H. G. and Belmont L. (1964). Auditory-visual integration in normal and retarded readers. *Am. J. Orthopsychiatry*. 34: 852–861.

Blanchard P. (1935). Psychogenic factors in some cases of reading disability. *Am. J. Orthopsychiatry* 5: 361–374.

Boder E. (1973). Developmental dyslexia: A diagnostic screening procedure based on three characteristic patterns of reading and spelling. In Bateman B. (ed.), *Learning Disorders*. Seattle: Special Child Publications.

Bronner, A. F. (1917). *The Psychology of Special Abilities and Disabilities*. Boston: Little, Brown.

Brunner W. E. (1905). Congenital word-blindness. *Ophthalmology* 1: 189–195.

Bryden M. P. (1965). Tachistoscopic recognition, handedness, and cerebral dominance. *Neuropsychologia* 3: 1–8.

Bryden M. P. (1970). Laterality effects in dichotic listening: Relationships with handedness and reading ability in children. *Neuropsychologia* 8: 443–450.

Claiborne J. H. (1906). Types of congenital amblyopia. *JAMA* 47: 1813–1816.

Conrad K. (1949). Ueber aphasische Sparchstörungen bei hirnverletzten Linkshändern. *Nervenarzt* 20: 148–154.

Dearborn W. F. (1925). The etiology of congenital word blindness. *Harvard Monogr. Educ.* Ser. 1, Vol. 1, No. 1, 50–76.

Denckla M. B. (1977). Minimal brain dysfunction and dyslexia: Beyond diagnosis by exclusion, In Blaw M. E. Rapin I., and Kinsbourne M. (eds.), *Topics in Child Neurology*. New York: Spectrum Publications.

Doehring D., and Hoshko I. M. (1977). Classification of reading problems by the Q-technique of factor analysis. *Cortex* 13: 281–294.

Eisenberg L. (1978). Definitions of dyslexia: Their consequences for research and policy. In Benton A. L. and Pearl D. (eds.), *Dyslexia: An Appraisal of Current Knowledge*. New York: Oxford University Press.

Fildes L. G. (1922). A psychological inquiry into the nature of the condition known as congenital word-blindness. *Brain* 4: 286–307.

Fisher J. H. (1905). Case of congenital word-blindness (inability to learn to read). *Ophthalmic Rev.* 24: 315–318.

Foerster R. (1905). Beiträge zur Pathologie des Lesens und Schreibens (congenitale Wortblindheit bei einem Schwachsinnigen). *Neurol. Centralbl.* 24: 235–236.

Fontenot D., and Benton A. L. (1972). Perception of direction in the right and left visual fields. *Neuropsychologia* 10: 447–452.

Galaburda A. M., and Kemper T. L. (1979). Cytoarchitectonic abnormalities in developmental dyslexia: A case study. *Ann. Neurol.* 6: 94–100.

Gates A. I. (1922). *The Psychology of Reading and Spelling with Special Reference to Disability.* Teachers College Contr. Educ. No. 129.

Geschwind N. and Levitsky W. (1968). Human brain: Left-right asymmetries in temporal speech region. *Science* 161: 186–187.

Hier D. B., LeMay M., Rosenberger P. B. and Perlo V. P. (1978). Developmental dyslexia: Evidence for a subgroup with a reversal of cerebral asymmetry. *Arch. Neurol.* 35: 90–92.

Hilliard R. D. (1973). Hemispheric laterality effects on a facial recognition task in normal subjects. *Cortex* 9: 246–258.

Hincks E. M. (1926). Congenital word-blindness. *Lancet* 1: 1506–1508.

Hinshelwood, J. (1900). Congenital word-blindness, with reports of two cases. *Ophthalmic Rev.* 21: 91–99.

Hinshelwood, J. (1909). Four cases of congenital word-blindness occurring in the same family. *Br. Med. J.* 2: 1229–1232.

Hughes, J. R. (1978). Electroencephalographic and neurophysiological studies in dyslexia. In Benton A. L. and Pearl D. (eds.), *Dyslexia: An Appraisal of Current Knowledge.* New York: Oxford University Press.

Jackson E. (1906). Developmental alexia (congenital word-blindness). *Am. J. Med. Sci.* 131: 843–849.

Jansky J. J. (1978). A critical review of "some developmental and predictive precursors of reading disabilities." In Benton A. L. and Pearl D. (eds.), *Dyslexia: An Appraisal of Current Knowledge.* New York: Oxford University Press.

Johnson D. J. (1978). Remedial approaches to dyslexia. In Benton A. L. and Pearl D. (eds.), *Dyslexia: An Appraisal of Current Knowledge.* New York: Oxford University Press.

Kimura D. (1964). Left-right differences in the perception of melodies. *Qt. J. Exp. Psychol.* 16: 355–358.

Kimura D. (1967). Functional asymmetry of the brain in dichotic listening. *Cortex* 3: 163–178.

Lechner C. S. (1903). Aangeboren woordblindheid. *Ned Tijdschr. Geneeskunde.* 39: 235–244.

LeMay M. (1976). Morphological cerebral asymmetries of modern man, fossil man, and nonhuman primates. *Ann. N. Y. Acad. Sci.* 280: 349–366.

Leong, C. K. (1976). Lateralization in severely disabled readers in relation to functional cerebral development and synthesis of information. In Knights R. M. and Bakker D. J. (eds.), *The Neuropsychology of Learning Disorders.* Baltimore: University Park Press.

Mattis S., French J. H. and Rapin I. (1975). Dyslexia in children and young adults: Three independent neuropsychological syndromes. *Dev. Med. Child Neurol.* 17: 150–163.

McGlone J. and Davidson W. (1973). The relationship between cerebral speech laterality and spatial ability with special reference to sex hand preference. *Neuropsychologia* 11: 105–113.

McKeever W. F. and Van Deventer A. D. (1975). Dyslexic adolescents: Evidence of impaired visual and auditory language processing associated with normal lateralization responsivity. *Cortex* 11: 361–378.

Milner B. (1973). Hemispheric specialization: Scope and limits. *The Neurosciences: Third Study Program.* Cambridge, Massachusetts: M.I.T. Press.

Monroe M. 1932. *Children Who Cannot Read.* Chicago: University of Chicago Press.

Morgan W. P. (1896). A case of congenital word-blindness. *Br. Med. J.* 2: 1378.

Nettleship E. (1901). Cases of congenital word-blindness (inability to learn to read). *Ophthalmic Rev.* 20: 61–67.

Nielson H. H. and Ringe K. (1969). Visuo-perceptive and visuo-motor performance of children with reading disability. *Scand. J. Psychol.* 10: 225–231.

Orton S. T. (1925). "Word-blindness" in school children. *Arch. Neurol. Psychiat.* 14: 581–615.

Orton S. T. (1966). *"Word-blindness" in School Children and Other Papers on Strephosymbolia (Specific Language Disability-Dyslexia) 1925–1946.* Towson, Maryland: The Orton Society.

Peters A. (1908). Ueber kongenitale Wortblindheit. *Münchener Med. Wschr.* 55: 1116–1119.

Plate E. (1909). 4 Fälle von kongenitale Wortblindheit in einer Familie. *Münchener Med. Wschr.* 56: 1793–1796.

Robinson H. M. (1946). *Why Pupils Fail in Reading.* Chicago: Univ. Chicago Press.

Russell W. R. and Espir M. L. E. (1961). *Traumatic Aphasia.* London: Oxford University Press.

Rutter M. (1978). Prevalence and types of dyslexia. In Benton A. L. and Pearl D. (eds.), *Dyslexia: An Appraisal of Current Knowledge.* New York: Oxford University Press.

Rutter M., Graham P. and Yule W. (1970). *A Neuropsychiatric Study in Childhood.* London: Heinemann.

Rutter M., Tizard J. and Whitmore K. (1970). *Education, Health and Behavior.* London: Longman.

Satz P., Taylor H. G., Friel J. and Fletcher J. (1978). Some developmental and predictive precursors of reading disabilities: A six year follow-up. In Benton A. L. and Pearl D. (eds.), *Dyslexia: An Appraisal of Current Knowledge.* New York: Oxford University Press.

Schmitt C. (1918). Developmental alexia. *Elem. School J.* 18: 680–700, 757–769.

Shankweiler D. and Liberman I. Y. (1972). Misreading: A search for causes. In Kavanaugh J. F. and Mattingly I. G. (eds.). *Language by Ear and by Eye.* Cambridge, Massachusetts: MIT Press.

Shankweiler D. and Liberman I. Y. (1976). Exploring the relations between reading and speech. In Knights R. M. and Bakker D. J. (eds.), *The Neuropsychology of Learning Disorders.* Baltimore: University Park Press.

Stephenson S. (1907). Six cases of congenital word-blindness affecting three generations of one family. *Ophthalmoscope* 5: 482–484.

Thomas C. J. (1905). Congenital "word-blindness" and its treatment. *Ophthalmoscope* 3: 380–385.

Thomson M. E. (1976). A comparison of laterality effects in dyslexics and controls using verbal dichotic listening tasks. *Neuropsychologia* 14: 243–246.

Variot G. and Lecomte (1906). Un cas de typholexie congénitale (cécité congénitale verbale). *Bulletins et Memories de la Société-Medicale des Hôpitaux de Paris* 23: 995–1001.

Vellutino F. F. (1978). Toward an understanding of dyslexia: Psychological factors in specific reading disability. In Benton A. L. and Pearl D. (eds.) *Dyslexia: An Appraisal of Current Knowledge*. New York: Oxford University Press.

Vellutino F. F., Steger J. A. and Kandel G. (1972). Reading disability: An investigation of the perceptual deficit hypothesis. *Cortex* 8: 106–118.

Voss G. 1914. Ueber die Assoziationsprüfung bei Kindern nebst einem Beitrag zur Frage der "Wortblindheit." *Z. Neurol.* 26: 340–351.

Wallin J. E. W. (1920). Congenital word blindness—some analyses. *Training School Bulletin* 17: 76–84; 93–99.

Warburg F. (1911). Ueber die angeborene Wortblindheit und die Bedeatung ihrer Kenntnis für den Unterricht. *Z. Kinderforschung* 16: 97–113.

Wender P. (1971). *Minimal Brain Dysfunction in Children*. New York: Wiley-Interscience.

Wernicke O. (1903). Ceguera verbal congenita. *Rev. Soc. Med. Argentina* 11: 477–485.

Wilde W. (1853). *Practical Observations on Aural Surgery*. London: J. Churchill; Philadelphia: Blanchard and Lea.

Witelson S. F. and Rabinovitch M. S. (1972). Hemispheric speech lateralization in children with auditory-linguistic deficits. *Cortex* 8: 412–426.

Yeni-Komshian G. H., Isenberg D. and Goldberg H. (1975). Cerebral dominance and reading disability: Left visual field deficit in poor readers. *Neuropsychologia* 13: 83–94.

Zangwill O. L. (1960). *Cerebral Dominance and Its Relationship to Psychological Function*. Edinburgh: Oliver and Boyd.

Zangwill O. L. (1962). Dyslexia in relation to cerebral dominance. In Money J. (ed.), *Reading Disability: Progress and Research Needs in Dyslexia*. Baltimore: Johns Hopkins Press.

Zigmond N. (1978). Remediation of dyslexia: A discussion. In Benton A. L. and Pearl D. (eds.), *Dyslexia: An Appraisal of Current Knowledge*. New York: Oxford University Press.

Zurif E. B. and Carson G. (1970). Dyslexia in relation to cerebral dominance and temporal analysis. *Neuropsychologia* 8: 351–361.

21

Developmental Neuropsychology: Its Present Status

The origins of developmental neuropsychology can be traced back to the early nineteenth century when neuropathologic study related severe mental retardation to structural malformation of the brain. In the middle of the century, the otologist William Wilde (1853) published his observations on children who were not mentally retarded but who were, as he phrased it, "dumb but not deaf," i.e., suffering from severe expressive speech disorder. These children were later described under the labels of "audimutitas" and "congenital aphasia."

Yet I think it is fair to say that the field in its modern form really began with the brief description by Morgan (1896) of a case of congenital wordblindness, a contribution that was as far-reaching in its consequences for developmental neuropsychology as were Broca's papers in the early 1860s for the evolution of concepts about the neurological basis of adult aphasia. As is well-known, Morgan's observations were quickly confirmed and his supposition that congenital wordblindness resulted from a congenital or early acquired abnormality in the territory of the angular gyrus of the left hemisphere was generally accepted. No less than 28 papers on the topic were published in the first decade of the twentieth century (cf. Benton, 1980). Thus the disability can be regarded as the first specific topic in the field and indeed one that is as important today as it was 80 years ago.

An event some 20 years later added another dimension. This was the pandemic of encephalitis that swept through Europe and North America from 1916 to 1924 and left in its wake thousands of surviving children presenting conduct disorders, specific cognitive impairments without obvious global mental retardation, hyperactivity, and defective impulse control. Clinical study of these chil-

---

Reprinted with permission from A. Benton, H. Levin, G. Moretti & D. Riva (Eds.), *Neuropsicologia dell'Età Evolutiva/Developmental Neuropsychology.* Milan, FrancoAngeli © 1992.

dren in the 1930s gave rise to the concept of the nondefective brain-injured child (cf. Kahn and Cohen, 1934). After World War II, under the rubric of "minimal brain dysfunction," the concept was broadened (and, one should say, diluted) to include children who showed no evidence or history of brain disease but whose behavior could plausibly (but not always correctly) be ascribed to brain dysfunction (cf. Strauss and Lehtinen, 1947; Bax and Mackeith, 1963; Clements and Peters, 1962; Benton, 1973; Strother, 1973). This development took place in the face of considerable opposition from many psychiatrists and psychologists who adhered to the then prevailing view that the behavioral and cognitive disturbances of these children were determined by psychogenic factors. Even specific reading and arithmetic disabilities were interpreted in this way (cf. Blanchard, 1946; Benton, 1962).

This was more or less the state of affairs as late as 1970. Since that time there has been an enormous expansion of interest and activity in the field. This expansion has been characterized by: the introduction of new techniques of study—anatomic, physiologic, and psychologic; new modes of treatment (chiefly pharmacologic); investigation of the neuropsychologic manifestations of diverse organic and psychiatric conditions; more carefully formulated theoretical conceptions; and, the circumstance that many highly competent young clinical researchers entered the field.

As a consequence, both the experimental and clinical aspects of pediatric neuropsychology are major fields of endeavor today. Neurologically oriented behavioral study of normal children, which was almost unknown 30 years ago, is now a prominent feature of child psychology. On the clinical side, the fact that functional neurologic abnormality is responsible for many of the conduct problems and school failures encountered in children is now generally recognized by doctors, teachers, and parents.

In this presentation, I shall try to assess our present understanding (or lack of understanding) of a number of normative and clinical topics in the field. While some topics will be considered in detail, others can receive only brief mention.

Developmental Dyslexia

Among the specific determinants of school failure and conduct disorder, defective development of language abilities is surely the most important. The linguistic disability that has received the most attention is specific reading failure or developmental dyslexia. Our present understanding of the nature and determinants of this still puzzling disability needs to be assessed.

During the first decade of the century, when it was taken for granted (without any evidential basis) that developmental dyslexia was the childhood analogue of acquired wordblindness in adult patients, only one or two clinicians expressed reservations about this rather naive assumption (cf. Nettleship, 1901; Wernicke, 1903). However, as the disability became more widely recognized, conflicting findings and controversy arose about not only its neurological basis but also its nature and causes and even its existence as an entity.

These conflicting findings and conceptual disagreements are still with us today. In the early years some educators denied that developmental dyslexia was a specific entity and instead ascribed specific failure in reading to such factors as bad work habits, lack of motivation, and poor teaching (cf. Gates, 1922). This position is still held by a few educational specialists who have written about what they call the "nonsense" about dyslexia and the "mystique" of learning disability (cf. Sirch, 1975; Coles, 1987). This nihilistic position, reminiscent in some ways of Ivan Illich's (1976) scathing attack on modern medicine, is untenable but it does find a basis of support in the widespread habit of professional workers in clinics and schools of overdiagnosing "dyslexia" and "learning disability."

A more considered approach is that of Zigmond (1978), who contends that most children who have been classified as dyslexic are, in fact, children who have not benefited from routine methods of teaching reading and that "they read poorly because our instruction has been inadequate—these children will learn to read if instruction were more personalized and individualized." Conceding that there is a small group of children who are truly dyslexic, she discusses instructional programs that are designed to match teaching methods to the characteristics of the individual child.

Both the intemperate attacks on the concept of dyslexia and Zigmond's reservations raise the question of how the disability is defined and what criteria can be utilized to make the diagnosis. No single set of criteria has been universally adopted so that different investigators inevitably deal with different populations of subjects. As it happens, the most popular performance criterion, i.e., that the child's reading achievement is two or more years below his grade level, is grossly inadequate. It does not take account of the child's intelligence (e.g., whether his IQ is 85 or 125), of his grade level (e.g., whether he is in the early or late school years), of his cultural background or of the quality of the school which he is attending. There are much better methods for establishing criteria, for example, the use of regression equations in which a child's reading level is compared with that predicted from correlations with his age, intelligence and educational history (cf. Thorndike, 1963; Yule, 1967; Rutter, 1978).

Some definitions are extremely restrictive and specify that the child must be of at least average intelligence, must come from an adequate cultural background and must have had the benefit of conventional reading instruction (cf. Critchley, 1970). The simple "two or more years below grade level" criterion leads to overdiagnosis, e.g., by classifying a 14-year-old child who is reading at a 12-year-old level as "dyslexic." The very stringent definitions underdiagnose the condition, e.g., by considering a 14-year-old child with an IQ of 80 who cannot read at all as not dyslexic. A good deal of confusion has been engendered by this inconsistency in definition. Yet, in spite of the confusion, a number of advances in our knowledge of dyslexia have been gained in recent years.

We know that even when dyslexia is defined in rather strict terms, dyslexic children differ among themselves in showing a variety of neurological signs, behavioral characteristics, and patterns of test performance. This heterogeneity has led to attempts to develop classifications of types of dyslexia on the basis of one or another criterion. One such classification is a division into "pure dyslexia" (i.e., without "soft" neurological signs) and "dyslexia plus" (i.e., with these signs) proposed by Denckla (1977). This classification has an appeal to neurologists because it at least indicates the setting within which the failure in reading is manifested. While it is not clear that these "soft" signs have a direct connection with the failure in reading, longitudinal study has indicated that they do have predictive significance for the adjustment of learning-disabled children in later life (cf. Spreen, 1988).

Dyslexic children show a variety of errors in their reading. They may confuse letters and words that are similar in shape. In the English language at least they may reverse words, reading "god" for "dog" and "saw" for "was." They may mispronounce the sounds of letters, particularly, vowels and terminal consonants. They may even make semantic errors of the paraphasic type, reading "bad" for "evil" or "girl" for "woman." This diversity has encouraged efforts to develop a classification according to the kinds of errors a child makes in his reading. The most prominent classification is a division into an audiophonic (or phonological) type and a visuospatial (or "eidetic") type (cf. Ingram et al., 1970; Boder, 1970, 1971, 1973). Most dyslexic children fall into the audiophonic category or a "mixed" category. Only a very small proportion (less than 10%) show predominantly visual errors.

A third approach to a typology of dyslexia identifies children in terms of characteristic patterns of cognitive function, as disclosed by their performance on a battery of verbal and nonverbal tests (cf. Mattis et al., 1975; Denckla, 1977; Mattis, 1978; Watson and Goldgar, 1988). The overall result of these studies has been to document the very high frequency of defects in oral language and motor speech in dyslexic children. Visuospatial and visuomotor defects are quite uncommon, accounting for no more than 5% of the cases. We should also note that a substantial proportion of children (about 25%) cannot be placed in any category, either because they do not show an identifiable pattern of defects or because their test performances are normal.

The question of a visual type of developmental dyslexia deserves comment. It was a very popular concept some years ago and there is a school of thought today that ascribes reading disability to unstable binocular control of visual fixation (cf. Dunlop et al., 1973; Dunlop and Dunlop, 1974a, b; Stein and

Fowler, 1984, 1985; Stein et al., 1986). It is true, of course, that some dyslexics do show visuospatial and visuomotor problems. But it is not at all clear that their difficulties are related in any significant way to their reading disability. In fact, the weight of evidence suggests that we are dealing here with concurrence and not causality (cf. Benton, 1984; Dorman, 1987). If visuospatial disability were responsible for the dyslexia, one would expect that these children would show a preponderance of orientational errors in their reading; but, in general, they are indistinguishable from most dyslexics who show a mixture of phonological and orientational errors. Nor, is there evidence that specific remedial procedures designed to correct orientational errors are more effective with these children than is phonological training (Lyon, 1985).

The past decade has seen a renewal of interest in investigating the neurological bases of dyslexia, along both anatomic and physiologic lines. The postmortem studies of Galaburda (1989; Galaburda et al., 1985) indicate that the brains of dyslexic adults show an absence of the bilateral asymmetry of the planum temporale which is typical of the brains of normal right-handed persons and also that architectonic abnormalities are present throughout the brain, particularly in the language-associated perisylvian area. On the physiological side, new techniques of EEG study have reported abnormalities in both the left parietotemporal and the bifrontal areas of dyslexic subjects (cf. Duffy et al., 1980). These fresh observations are provocative and perhaps they will prove to be pathbreaking. What is needed at this time are equally detailed anatomic and physiologic studies of an adequate number of the brains of nondyslexics and replication of the findings by other investigators.

In any case, whatever reservations we may have about the cogency of one or another specific finding, there is no longer any doubt that organic factors are a significant component of specific reading disability in the majority of cases. Recent genetic studies, which confirm the high familial incidence of the disorder and provide indications about its mode of inheritance, support this conviction (cf. Pennington, 1989). Of course, this does not mean that remediation efforts will be any less effective. New approaches to remediation, inspired by recent research, have been adopted and there is an increasing emphasis on early intervention by identifying preschool children at risk for dyslexia through review of their family histories and the administration of "reading readiness" tests (cf. Fox and Routh, 1983; Mann, 1984; Fiedorowicz, 1986; Morais, 1987; Fletcher et al., 1989).

Specific Arithmetic Disability

Other forms of learning disorder include specific arithmetic disability which, I think, is also overdiagnosed. The acquisition of mathematical skills makes substantial demands on sustained attention, perseverance, and the capacity for reflection. These are behavioral traits that are notoriously lacking in many children and it is only to be expected that some of them will experience difficulty in mastering arithmetic operations. Children who have sustained a head injury show a much poorer subsequent development of mathematical skills as compared to reading skills, probably because of disturbances in attention and concentration (cf. Levin and Benton, 1986). However, "pure" (or "inexplicable") specific arithmetic disability does exist and it poses the same problems of interpretation and the same formidable remedial challenge as does developmental dyslexia. The two disabilities are sometimes seen in combination. In turn, both arithmetic and reading disability are generally counted as components of the "developmental Gerstmann syndrome." However, many cases of children with one or more Gerstmann deficits who are adequate readers have been described (cf. Spellacy and Peter, 1978). There is one fundamental difficulty with this area of arithmetic disability. Most of the studies concerned with the topic have not been sufficiently well-designed and executed to allow confident interpretation of their findings. In any case, the neurological basis of specific arithmetic disability remains obscure.

"Right Hemisphere" Learning Disability

Poor arithmetic achievement is also part of an assemblage of deficits, including poor visuospatial and perceptuomotor skills, attentional difficulties, shyness, depression, aprosodic speech, and impaired interpersonal relations, that has been postulated as reflecting developmental dysfunction of the right hemisphere (cf. Rourke, 1982; Weintraub and Mesulam, 1983; Tranel et al., 1987). Diverse partial combinations of these characteristics are observed clinically and only in the broadest sense of the term can these behavioral traits be considered to form a "syndrome." The inference that the clinical pictures are referable to dysfunction of the right hemisphere comes from both behavioral observation and neurologic examination. On the behavioral side, one finds that verbal attainments such as vocabulary level, range of information, reading, and verbal reasoning are better developed than are nonverbal capacities; this is reflected in a generally higher Verbal Scale IQ than Performance Scale IQ on the Wechsler test batteries. Neurologic examination has disclosed evidence of right-hemisphere dysfunction (e.g., hyperreflexia and extensor plantar responses on the left side, deviant posturing of the left arm, slowness in performance on the left in speed tests) in about 30 percent of these patients. The great majority of them are described as clumsy and awkward. No doubt many would be placed in the diagnostic category of "developmental dyspraxia" (cf. Gubbay, 1975). When interpersonal difficulties, depression, and shyness are prominent features of this syndrome, the child or adolescent is often regarded as an odd or difficult personality. However, if it represents a developmental learning disability, the indicated course of action is cognitive remediation and behavior modification.

Developmental Prosopagnosia

A specific disability that is possibly related to the right-hemisphere "syndrome" is developmental prosopagnosia, i.e., an inability to recognize familiar people that can be dated back to the early years of life (cf. McConachie, 1976; Tranel and Damasio, 1989; Young and Ellis, 1989). The impairment is described in case reports as ranging from moderate to quite marked in severity and it can lead to disturbed social interactions and interpersonal difficulties. Like the adult prosopagnosic, these children often show defects in color perception, topographic orientation, and difficulty in identifying animals, coins, and specimens of handwriting. A history of early brain damage with involvement of the right hemisphere is evident in some cases. Beyond this, very little is known about its neurological background. It is difficult to assess the clinical significance of this unusual disability which must pose problems for a child in his/her daily intercourse with other people. The little information we possess suggests that prosopagnosic children may be less disturbed than those with "right-hemisphere" learning disabilities; however, this may be a matter of selective attention to the presenting complaint. On the other hand, it has been proposed that developmental prosopagnosia and, especially, impaired ability to interpret facial expressions, may play a role in the genesis of autism (cf. Fotheringham, 1987).

Minimal Brain Dysfunction

In the 1960s, the term and concept of minimal brain dysfunction was steadily expanded as a diagnosis for almost every behavioral deviation observed in children that could not be covered by more firmly established diagnoses such as epilepsy, mental retardation, or obvious cerebral disease. Hyperactivity and underactivity, impulsivity and inhibition, aggressiveness and passivity, anxiety and depression, as well as all types of learning disability, were interpreted as reflecting minimal brain dysfunction. The adjective "minimal" was intended to indicate that there was no substantial neurological evidence to support the diagnosis. At best, minor signs of equivocal significance, designated as "soft" signs, could be elicited.

Inevitably a reaction set in (cf. Benton, 1973; Ingram, 1973; Rutter, 1982). The concept was said to be hopelessly vague, amorphous, and broad. As one pediatric neurologist phrased it, minimal brain dysfunction was equivalent to "maximal neurologic confusion" (Gomez, 1967). Another clinician stated that "the diagnosis of minimal brain dysfunction, at best, is just an uncertain hypothesis, which is usually not open to testing in the individual child and, at worst, creates a neuromythology, which provides a rather pretentious cloak for ignorance" (Rutter, 1982).

Yet, the term persists. It persists because clinicians are convinced that many children exhibiting hyperactivity, attention deficit disorder, mood disturbances, and specific learning disabilities are suffering from some type of primary or secondary cerebral dysfunction and are not simply reacting to psychosocial stresses even though factors of this type may be part of the total situation.

Both Denckla (1977, 1978) and Rutter (1982) have addressed this problem and have suggested approaches to it that may resolve the conflict between the unsatisfactory nature of the concept of minimal brain dysfunction and the conviction that it does possess an important meaning. "Minimal brain dysfunction" is a suspicion, not a diagnosis. One then proceeds to determine whether or not the suspicion can be confirmed and whether or not more specific signs of cerebral abnormality can be identified from EEG and clinical neurological findings or from nonneurological organic disease. The investigation should indicate the degree to which a diagnosis of cerebral dysfunction is justified. Of equal importance, it may give some indications of the etiology and nature of the cerebral dysfunction. Since minimal brain dysfunction is an umbrella term covering a great variety of behavior disorders, one attempts to identify specific syndromes within the broad category. Denckla (1978) and Rapin (1982) have outlined a number of such syndromes. Thus, although the global concept has proved to be defective, it is serving us well as starting point for the empirical verification of more meaningful limited forms of organically conditioned behavior disorders.

Frontal Lobe Functions

A number of clinicians have suggested that some of the symptoms of minimal brain dysfunction, such as disturbances of attention, defective impulse control, hyperactivity, and distractibility may be related specifically to impairment in frontal lobe functioning. In view of the absence of hard neurological signs in these children (as is so often the case in adults), the idea is an intriguing one.

But it has not been easy to test this hypothesis. Apart from studies of children with acquired aphasia resulting from left frontal lobe disease, there has been very little usable case material for evaluating the behavioral effects of disease of the prefrontal region in children. Until recently, there has been very little opportunity to make direct comparisons of the symptoms of minimal brain dysfunction with those produced by focal disease of the prefrontal region. Now the application of refined neurodiagnostic procedures make this a distinct possibility (see Price et al., 1990).

The question has been approached indirectly by comparing the behavior of human infants and very young children, in whom the structural and functional properties of the frontal lobes are still in process of development, with that of normal and prefrontally injured monkeys (cf. Diamond, 1985; Diamond and Doar, 1989; Welsh and Pennington, 1988). The comparison provides an opportunity to determine whether or not behavioral test performances that have been found to be sensitive to the integrity of the prefrontal region in monkeys can be utilized as measures of prefrontal functioning in children. Delayed response tasks are a prime example. Normal monkeys and very young children perform these tasks successfully. Monkeys with lesions of dorsolateral prefrontal cortex and human infants under the age of one year fail. There are a number of other task performances that have been shown to be vulnerable to dysfunction of the prefrontal region (cf. Levin et al., 1991). Given these results, their application to normal and minimally brain damaged children of school age might well advance our understanding of the possibility that a subgroup of children in the category of "minimal brain damage" in fact do suffer from abnormality of the prefrontal region.

Early Brain Damage

A final topic that merits our attention concerns recent studies of the behavioral consequences of diseases in early life that involved damage to the brain, e.g., hydrocephalus, meningitis, acute lymphocytic leukemia, and closed head injury. Replacing the impressionistic judgments of earlier years, the findings of these studies have provided reliable indications of the wide range of behavioral outcomes that may follow cerebral insult in childhood.

The studies of Taylor (1987; Taylor et al., 1984, 1990) of children surviving an attack of influenzal meningitis in early life provide one example of the useful information that can be gained by systematic objective investigation. The essential findings were that, as compared to their unaffected siblings, the children had somewhat lower WISC Full Scale and Performance Scale IQs. However, their Verbal Scale IQ was not different from the controls and they performed on a normal level on 8 of 11 neuropsychological tests. Their mean academic achievement and overall behavioral adjustment were also comparable to that of their unaffected siblings. As a group, the postmeningitis children were more variable than their siblings, e.g., three had IQs of less than 80. Certain factors (e.g., younger age at admission, longer duration of fever, high protein level in the cerebrospinal fluid) were found to be significant but somewhat limited predictors of behavioral outcome.

A second example is the study of children with congenital or early acquired vascular disease by Riva et al. (1990), who found that the size and locus of the lesions as well as the age of onset were significant predictors of the status of certain aspects of the children's cognitive functioning. Still another example is the study of Donders et al. (1990) on the intellectual sequelae of infantile hydrocephalus.

Carefully designed studies, such as those of Taylor et al. serve to correct global impressions that are derived from a necessarily limited experience and that often lead to erroneous conclusions; for example, with respect to influenzal meningitis, that the prognosis is either very good or very bad. It is neither. It may be relatively good or relatively poor depending upon certain antecedent conditions and the specific abilities that are compromised. More importantly, the findings of these studies can provide valuable indications for the management of children surviving early life-threatening disorders (cf. Fletcher and Copeland, 1988). In the case of prematurely born children, for example, it has been shown that a systematic program of instruction and advice to the parents results in significantly better behavioral competence and health status than is found in an untreated group (cf. Gross and Ramey, 1990).

Epilogue

I think that this review demonstrates that we have made significant advances in understanding the neuropsychological problems of children as well as some progress in their management. It also points to unanswered questions that now need to be addressed. Moreover, it makes it clear that, as always, the issues are much more complicated than they once seemed to be. The intelligent employment of the remarkable neurodiagnostic methods now at our disposal should elucidate the neurological basis of these problems. The intelligent use of relevant behavioral test methods should identify the basic cognitive and affective factors that, in combination with environmental influences, give rise to these problems.

References

Bax M. and MacKeith R. (eds.) (1963). *Minimal Brain Dysfunction.* London: W Heinemann.

Benton A. L. (1962). Some aspects of the concept of psychogenic mental deficiency. Proceedings, *London Conference on the Scientific Study of Mental Deficiency* 1: 243–250.

Benton A. L. (1973). Minimal brain dysfunction from a neuropsychological point of view. *Ann. N. Y. Acad. Sci.* 205: 29–37.

Benton A. L. (1980). Developmental dyslexia: Evolution of a concept. *Bulletin of the Orton Society* 30: 10–26.

Benton A. L. (1984). Dyslexia and spatial thinking. *Ann. Dyslexia* 34: 69–85.

Blanchard P. (1935). Psychogenic factors in some cases of reading disability. *Am. J. Orthopsychiatry* 5: 361–374.

Boder E. (1970). Developmental dyslexia: A new diagnostic approach based on the identification of three subtypes. *J. Sch. Health* 40: 289–290.

Boder E. (1971). Developmental dyslexia: A diagnostic screening procedure based on three characteristic patterns of reading and spelling. In Bateman B. (ed.), *Learning Disorders*. Seattle: Special Child Publications.

Boder E. (1973). Developmental dyslexia: A diagnostic approach based on three atypical reading patterns. *Dev. Med. Child Neurol.* 15: 663–687.

Clements S. D. and Peters J. E. (1962). Minimal brain dysfunctions in the school-age child. *Arch. Gen. Psychiatry* 6: 185–197.

Coles G. (1987). *The Learning Mystique*. New York: Pantheon Books.

Critchley M. (1970). *The Dyslexic Child.* Springfield, Ill.: CC Thomas.

Denckla M. B. (1977). The neurological basis of reading disability. In Roswell F. G. and Natchez G (eds.), *Reading Disability*. New York: Basic Books.

Denckla M. B. (1978). Minimal brain dysfunction. In Chall J. S. and Mirsky A. F. (eds.), *Education and the Brain.* Chicago: University of Chicago Press.

Diamond A. (1985). Development of the ability to use recall to guide action, as indicated by infants' performance on AB. *Child Dev.* 56: 868–883.

Diamond A. and Doar B. (1989). The performance of human infants on a measure of frontal cortex function, the delayed response task. *Dev. Psychobiol.* 22: 271–294.

Donders J., Canady A. I., and Rourke B. P. (1990). Psychometric intelligence after infantile hydrocephalus. *Childs Nerv. Syst.* 6: 148–154.

Dorman C. (1987). Reading disability subtypes in neurologically impaired children. *Ann. Dyslexia* 37: 166–188.

Duffy F. H., Denckla M. B., Bartels P. H., and Sandini G. (1980). Dyslexia: Regional differences in brain electrical activity by topographic mapping. *Ann. Neurol.* 7: 412–420.

Dunlop D. B. and Dunlop P. (1974a). New concepts of visual laterality in relation to dyslexia. *Aust. J. Ophthalmol.* 2: 101–111.

Dunlop D. B. and Dunlop P. (1974b). Orthoptic assessment of children with learning difficulties. *Aust. J. Ophthalmol.* 2: 113–116.

Dunlop D. B., Dunlop P., and Fenelon B. (1973). Vision-laterality analysis in children with reading disability. *Cortex* 9: 227–236.

Fiedorowicz C. A. M. (1986). Training of component reading skills. *Ann. Dyslexia* 36: 318–334.

Fletcher J. M. and Copeland D. R. (1988). Neurobehavioral effects of central nervous system prophylactic treatment of cancer in children. *J. Clin. Exp. Neuropsuychol.* 10: 495–538.

Fletcher J. M., Levin H. S., and Satz P. (1989). Neurological and intellectual assessment of children. In Kaplan H. I. and Sadock B. J. (eds.), *Comprehensive Textbook of Psychiatry.* Baltimore: Williams & Wilkins.

Fotheringham J. B. (1987). Facial recognition cells and autism. *Science* 238: 1496–1497.

Fox B. and Routh D. K. (1983). Reading disability, phonemic analysis and dysphonetic spelling. *J. Clin. Child Psychol.* 12: 28–32.

Galaburda A. M. (1985). Developmental dyslexia: Four consecutive cases with cortical anomalies. *Ann. Neur.* 18: 222–233.

Galaburda A. M. (1989). Ordinary and extraordinary brain development. *Ann. Dyslexia* 39: 67–80.

Gates A. I. (1922). *The Psychology of Reading and Spelling with Special Reference to Disability*. Teachers College Contributions to Education. N. 129.

Gomez M. R. (1967). Minimal cerebral dysfunction (maximal neurologic confusion). *Clin. Pediatr*. 6: 589–591.

Gross R. T. and Ramey C. T. (1990). Enhancing the outcome of low birth-weight, premature infants. *JAMA* 263: 3035–3042.

Gubbay S. S. (1975). *The Clumsy Child*. Philadelphia: WB Saunders.

Illich I. (1976). *Medical Nemesis*. New York: Pantheon Books.

Ingram T. T. S. (1973). Soft signs. *Dev. Med. Child Neurol*. 15: 527–530.

Ingram T. T. S., Mason A. W., and Blackburn I. M. (1970). A retrospective study of 82 children with reading disability. *Dev. Med. Child Neurol*. 12: 271–281.

Kahn E. and Cohn L. H. (1934). Organic drivenness. *N. Engl. J. Med*. 210: 748–756.

Levin H. S. and Benton A. L. (1986). Developmental and acquired dyscalculia in children. In Flehming I. and Stern L. (eds.) *Child Development and Learning Behavior*. New York: Gustav Fisher Verlag.

Levin H. S., Eisenberg H. M, and Benton A. L. (1991). *Frontal Lobe Function and Dysfunction*. New York: Oxford University Press.

Lyon G. R. (1985). Educational validation studies of learning disabilities subtypes. In Rourke B. P. (ed.), *Neuropsychology of Learning Disability Subtypes*. New York: Guilford Press.

Mann V. A. (1984). Longitudinal prediction and prevention of reading disability. *Ann. Dyslexia* 34: 117–135.

Mattis S. (1978). Dyslexia syndromes. In Benton A. L., and Pearl D. (eds.), *Dyslexia*, New York: Oxford University Press.

Mattis S., French J. H., and Rapin I. (1975). Dyslexia in children and young adults. *Dev. Med. Child Neuro*. 17: 150–163.

McConachie H. R. (1976). Developmental prosopagnosia. *Cortex* 12: 76–82.

Morais J. (1987). Segmental analysis of speech and its relation to reading ability. *Ann. Dyslexia* 37: 126–141.

Morgan W. P. (1986). A case of congenital world-blindness. *Br. Med. J*. 2: 1378.

Nettleship E. (1901). Cases of congenital word-blindness (inability to learn to read). *Ophthalmic Rev*. 20: 61–67.

Pennington B. F. (1989). Using genetics to understand dyslexia. *Ann. Dyslexia* 39: 81–93.

Price B. H., Daffner K. R., Stowe R. M., and Mesulam M. M. (1990). The comportmental learning disabilities of early frontal lobe damage. *Brain* 113: 1383–1393.

Rapin I. (1982). *Children with Brain Dysfunction*. New York: Raven Press.

Riva D., Miiani N., and Pantaleoni C. (1990). Neuropsychological functioning in children with vascular lesions. *Neurology* 40 (Suppl. 1): 199.

Rourke B. P. (1982). Central processing deficiencies in children. *J. Clin. Neuropsychol*. 4: 1–18.

Rutter M. (1978). Prevalence and types of dyslexia. In Benton A. L. and Pearl D. (eds.) *Dyslexia*. New York: Oxford University Press.

Rutter M. (1982). Syndromes attributed to "minimal brain dysfunction" in childhood. *Am. J. Psychiatry* 129: 21–33.

Shankweiler D. and Liberman I. Y. (1989). *Phonology and Reading Disability*. Ann Arbor: University of Michigan Press.

Sirch K. (1975). *Der Unfug mit der Legasthenie*. Stuttgart: Klett Verlag.

Spellacy F. and Peter B. (1978). Dysscalculia and elements of the developmental Gerstmann syndrome. *Cortex* 14: 192–206.

Spreen O. (1988). *Learning Disabled Children Growing Up: A Follow-up into Adulthood.* New York: Oxford University Press.

Stein J. F. and Fowler S. (1984). A physiological theory of visual dyslexia. In Rose F. C. (ed.), *Progress in Aphasiology*. New York: Raven Press.

Stein J. F. and Fowler S. (1985). Effect of monocular occlusion on visuomotor perception and reading in dyslexic children. *Lancet* 2: 69–73.

Stein J. F., Riddel P. M., and Fowler S. (1986). The Dunlop test and reading in primary school children. *Br. J. Ophthalmol.* 70: 317–320.

Strauss A. A. and Lehtinen L. (1947). *Psychopathology and Education of the Brain-Injured Child.* New York: Grune & Stratton.

Strother C. R. (1973). Minimal brain dysfunction: A historical overview. *Ann. N.Y. Acad. Sci.* 205: 6–17.

Taylor H. G. (1987). Childhood sequelae of early neurological disorders. *Dev. Neuropsychol.* 3: 153–164.

Taylor H. G., Michaels R. H., Mazur P. M., Bauer R. E., and Liden C. B. (1984). Intellectual, neuropsychological and achievement outcomes in children six to eight years after recovery from *Haemophilus influenzae* meningitis. *Pediatrics* 74: 198–205.

Taylor H. G., Mills E. L., Ciampi A. et al. (1990). The sequelae of *Haemophilus influenzae* meningitis in school-age children. *N. Engl. J. Med.* 323: 1657–1663.

Thorndike R. L. (1963). *The Concepts of Over- and Underachievement.* New York: Teachers College, Columbia University.

Tranel D., and Damasio A. R. (1989). Developmental prosopagnosia. *Soc. Neurosci. Abstr.* 15: 303.

Tranel D., Hall L. E., Olson S., and Tranel N. N. (1987). Evidence for a right hemisphere developmental learning disability. *Dev. Neuropsychol.* 31: 113–127.

Watson B. U. and Goldgar D. E. (1988). Evaluation of a typology of reading disability. *J. Clin. Exp. Neuropsychol.* 10: 432–450.

Weintraub S. and Mesulam M. M. (1983). Developmental learning disabilities of the right hemisphere. *Arch. Neurol.* 40: 463–468.

Welsh M. C. and Pennington B. F. (1988). Assessing frontal lobe functioning in children. *Dev. Neuropsychol.* 4: 199–230.

Wernicke C. (1903). Ceguera verbal congenita. *Revista Sociedad Medica Argentina* 11: 477–485.

Wilde W. (1853). *Practical Observations on Aural Surgery*. London: J. Churchill.

Young A. W. and Ellis H. D. (1989). Childhood prosopagnosia. *Brain Cogn.* 9: 16–47.

Yule W. (1967). Predicting reading ages on Neale's analysis of reading ability. *Br. J. Educ. Psychol.* 37: 252–255.

Zigmond N. (1978). Remediation of dyslexia. In Benton A. L. and Pearl D. (eds.), *Dyslexia.* New York: Oxford University Press.

Index